# REVIEWERS

Lois Angelo, RN, CS
Massachusetts General Hospital
Boston, Massachusetts

Vicki Britt, ARNP
Process Improvement / Staff Development
Fairfax Hospital
Kirkland, Washington

Jacqueline Rosenjack Burchum, DNSc, APRN, BC
Family Nurse Practitioner.
Assistant Professor
The University of Memphis
Memphis, Tennese

Dorothy A. Varchol, MSN, MA, RN, BC
Nursing Instructor
Cincinnati State Technical and Community College
Cincinnati, Ohio

Barbara Jones Warren, PhD, APRN, BC
Associate Clinical Professor
College of Nursing
The Ohio State University
Columbus, Ohio

Judith A. Wilson, MS, RN, CS
Clinical Nurse Specialist
University of Alabama at Birmingham Hospital
Birmingham, Alabama

## STUDENT REVIEWERS

Sonia Alvarado
Evelyn Chin
Patrick Cusack
Joshua Flores
Tyisha Hardy
Gloria Onyekwere
Natasha Parker
Shantinea Tackson
Hostos Community College
Bronx, New York

# PREFACE

It is hoped that this clinical guide will enable students and practitioners alike to plan realistic nursing care individualized to their client's present level of functioning and priority of needs. It is for that reason that **assessment tools** are included for most mental disorders and psychiatric emergencies. Accurate and thorough assessments are crucial for the planning of appropriate, effective, and safe interventions. These assessment tools can readily be found in Appendix D in this edition.

In addition to updates to the content, slight revision of the format for easier access, and addition of more nursing care plans, this edition has added **outcomes, long-term goals**, and **short-term goals,** as requested by some students and faculty.

The chapter on **psychopharmacology** will hopefully help the reader to better understand the uses and workings of the psychotropic agents. When a specific neurotransmitter (e.g. $5\text{-}HT_1$, $D_1$, $D_2$, $H_1$) is either increased or decreased for the purpose of improving symptoms, the effectiveness of a drug may also be accompanied by certain adverse reactions and toxic effects. Through an understanding of transmitter-receptor actions, health care professionals can identify agents that would best serve individual client needs. When a client is able to mitigate the effects of adverse reactions, client medical compliance may be increased. Therefore, **client and family teaching tools** are included at the end of the discussion of each psychotropic agent in this chapter. An overview of specific medications and dosages, as well as drug tables, remain in the relevant clinical chapters.

*Wishing you success,*
*Elizabeth Varcarolis*

# ACKNOWLEDGMENTS

I wish to thank Cherrill Colson for her excellent and thorough chapter on child and adolescent disorders. She identifies useful and concrete interventions that can easily be adapted to any level of nursing practice.

I was truly blessed to have excellent reviewers work beside me on this edition. Their attention to detail and wide breadth of knowledge is responsible for the best parts of this book. This is especially evident in the psychopharmacology chapter, for which the clinical and didactic knowledge of the reviewers was a tremendous guide. I also took some important cues from student reviewers, who gave me perspectives from a "bird's eye view," so to speak. I am grateful to you all.

I want to express my genuine gratitude to three people at Elsevier who were supportive, imaginative, and more than helpful to me during the revision process:

- My Editor, Tom Wilhelm, whose creative ideas, energy, and enthusiasm ignited *my* enthusiasm for this project.
- My Developmental Editor, Jennifer Stoces, for her contribution to this update.
- Project Manager, Kathy Teal, for her tireless reworking of this project.

# PART I

# ASSESSMENT TOOLS AND GUIDELINES FOR PLANNING PSYCHOSOCIAL CARE

# CHAPTER 1

# The Nursing Process and Assessment Tools

The nursing process continues to be the basic framework for nursing practice with clients. A client can be an individual, a family, a group, or a community. The Scope and Standards of Psychiatric-Mental Health Nursing Practice (American Nurses Association [ANA], 2000) are authoritative statements that describe the responsibilities for which nurses are accountable and provide direction for professional nursing practice and a framework for the evaluation of practice. The Psychiatric-Mental Health Clinical Nursing Practice standards define the nursing process within the context of six standards of care (Figure 1-1):

| | |
|---|---|
| **Standard I—Assessment:** | Gathering and organizing data |
| **Standard II—Nursing diagnosis:** | Identifying areas for intervention |
| **Standard III—Outcome identification:** | Setting outcome criteria |
| **Standard IV—Planning:** | Planning actions to meet the outcome criteria |
| **Standard V—Implementation:** | Carrying out those actions |
| **Standard VI—Evaluation:** | Evaluating whether the desired outcomes have been achieved; if not, identifying alternative plans of action |

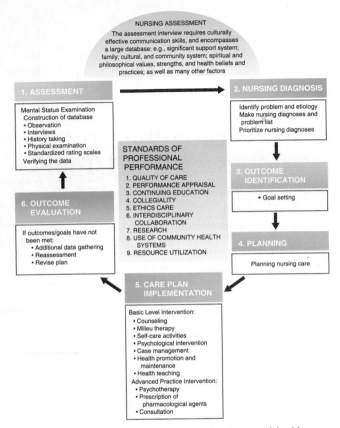

**Figure 1-1** The nursing process in psychiatric mental health nursing. (From Varcarolis, E. [2002]. *Foundations of psychiatric mental health nursing* [4th ed.]. Philadelphia, WB Saunders, p. 199; reprinted by permission.)

## ASSESSMENT

The assessment of a client's *psychosocial status* is a part of any nursing assessment, along with assessment of the client's physical health. Depression, suicidal thoughts, anger, disorientation, delusions, and hallucinations might be encountered in medical-surgical wards, obstetric and intensive care units, outpatient settings, extended-care facilities, emergency departments, community centers, and home settings.

The purpose of the assessment is to identify and clearly articulate specific problems in the individual's life that are causing physical or mental disequilibrium or harm. To help clients and their families, nurses define client problems/processes that warrant intervention in very specific terms called *nursing diagnoses*. The assessment is the first step in identifying key nursing diagnoses.

The purpose of the *psychosocial assessment* is to:

- **Establish a rapport**
- **Obtain an understanding of current illness**
- **Understand how this illness/process has affected the client's life** (self-esteem, loss of intimacy, role change, change in family dynamics, lifestyle change, employment issues)
- **Identify recent life changes or stressors** (refer to Chapter 5 for a useful tool)
- **Obtain information on previous psychiatric problems or disorder(s)**
- **Gather current lifestyle information** (social patterns, interests and abilities, stress factors, substance use and abuse, relationship issues, social supports)
- **Perform a mental status examination** (to identify dysfunctions in emotional, cognitive, or behavioral spheres) (see Chapter 12)
- **Formulate a plan of care**

A psychiatric nursing assessment contains both *subjective* and *objective* components. The basic components of the *psychosocial/psychiatric nursing assessment* include a client history (predominantly subjective) and a mental and emotional status evaluation (predominantly objective) (e.g., mental status examination). Because it is always preferable to verify the client's data, family members should be a part of the assessment whenever possible. It is helpful for the nurse to know (1) if there is anything going on in the family, (2) how the family defines the problem(s), and (3) how the client's problems affect the family.

Friends and neighbors can also verify or contradict the client's self-perception and actions and might add data. If a police officer is the one who brought the client into the psychiatric emergency department, it is important for the nurse to know as much as possible about what the client was doing that warranted police intervention. Old charts and medical records can also offer background information. This is particularly important if the client is too psychotic, withdrawn, or agitated to provide a history. In many places, this information might be easily available through the use of computer-based client records (CBRs). Laboratory reports also provide important information. Abnormal body chemistry can cause personality changes and violent behavior. For example, abnormal liver enzymes can explain irritability, depression, and lethargy.

The use of a standardized nursing assessment tool facilitates the assessment process. Many assessment forms are easily available; for example, hospitals and clinics often have their own assessment tools. Even if an assessment tool is used, it is best to gather information from the client in an informal fashion, with the nurse clarifying, focusing, and exploring pertinent data with the client. This method allows clients to state their perceptions in their own words and enables the nurse to observe a wide range of nonverbal behaviors. When the order and the questions on the assessment tool are too rigidly applied, spontaneity is reduced. Assessment is a skill that is learned over time. Practice, supervision, and patience enhance the development of this skill. A personal style of interviewing congruent with the nurse's personality develops as comfort and experience increase.

Table 1-1 is an example of an assessment tool for use in the clinical area. Tables 1-2, 1-3, and 1-4 can help the nurse identify and define specific unfamiliar terms.

Another helpful tool that can give nurses and other health care workers important information about the client is the multiaxial assessment system of the American Psychiatric Association (American Psychiatric Association [APA], 2000) (Box 1-1).

| Box 1-1 | DSM-IV-TR Multiaxial Assessment System |
|---|---|
| **Axis I** | Clinical Disorders<br>Other Conditions That Might Be a Focus of Clinical Attention |
| **Axis II** | Personality Disorders<br>Mental Retardation |
| **Axis III** | General Medical Conditions |
| **Axis IV** | Psychosocial and Environmental Problems |
| **Axis V** | Global Assessment of Functioning |

From American Psychiatric Association. (2000). *Diagnostic and statistical manual of mental disorders* (4th ed., text revision). Washington, DC: American Psychiatric Association.

Table 1-1 **Comprehensive Nursing Assessment Tool**

1. **Client History**
I. **GENERAL HISTORY OF CLIENT**
   Name _____ Age _____ Sex _____
   Racial and ethnic data _____
   Marital status _____
   Number and ages of children/siblings _____
   Living arrangements _____
   Occupation _____
   Education _____
   Religious affiliations _____
II. **PRESENTING PROBLEM**
   A. Statement in the client's own words of why he or she is hospitalized or seeking help
   B. **Recent difficulties**/alterations in
      1. Relationships
      2. Usual level of functioning
      3. Behavior
      4. Perceptions or cognitive abilities
   C. **Increased feelings of**
      1. Depression
      2. Anxiety
      3. Hopelessness
      4. Being overwhelmed
      5. Suspiciousness
      6. Confusion
   D. **Somatic changes,** such as
      1. Constipation
      2. Insomnia
      3. Lethargy
      4. Weight loss or gain
      5. Palpitations
III. **RELEVANT HISTORY—PERSONAL**
   A. **Previous hospitalizations and illnesses** _____
   B. **Educational background** _____
   C. **Occupational background** _____
      1. If employed, where? _____
      2. How long at that job? _____
      3. Previous positions and reasons for leaving _____
      4. Special skills _____
   D. **Social patterns**
      1. Describe friends _____
      2. Describe a usual day _____

Adopted from Varcarolis, E. (2002). *Foundations of psychiatric mental health nursing* (4th ed.). Philadelphia, WB Saunders, p. 203–205; reprinted by permission. *Continued*

Table 1-1 **Comprehensive Nursing Assessment Tool—cont'd**

E. **Sexual patterns**
   1. Sexually active? _____
   2. Sexual orientation _____
   3. Sexual difficulties _____
   4. Practice safe sex or birth control? _____
F. **Interests and abilities**
   1. What does the client do in his or her spare time?_____
   2. What is the client good at? _____
   3. What gives the client pleasure? _____
G. **Substance use and abuse**
   1. What medication does the client take? _____
      How often? _____ How much?_____
   2. Any herbal or over-the-counter medications? _____
      How often? _____ How much? _____
   3. What psychotropic drugs does the client take?_____
      How often? _____ How much? _____
   4. How many drinks of alcohol does the client take
      per day? _____Per week? _____
   5. Does the client identify use of drugs as a
      problem? _____
H. **How does the client cope with stress?** _____
   1. What does the client do when he or she gets
      upset? _____
   2. Whom can the client talk to? _____
   3. What usually helps to relieve stress? _____
   4. What did the client try this time? _____
IV. **RELEVANT HISTORY–FAMILY**
   A. **Childhood**
      1. Who was important to the client growing up? _____
      2. Was there physical or sexual abuse? _____
      3. Did the parents drink or use drugs? _____
      4. Who was in the home when the client was growing
         up? _____
   B. **Adolescence**
      1. How would the client describe his or her feelings in
         adolescence? _____
      2. Describe the client's peer group at that time. _____
   C. **Use of drugs**
      1. Was there use or abuse of drugs by any family
         member? _____
         Prescription _____ Street _____ By whom? _____
      2. What was the effect on the family? _____

Table 1-1 **Comprehensive Nursing Assessment Tool—cont'd**

   D. **Family physical or mental problems**
      1. Is there any family history of violence or physical/sexual abuse? _____
      2. Who in the family had physical or mental problems? _____
      3. Describe the problems. _____
      4. How did it affect the family? _____
   E. Was there an unusual or outstanding event the client would like to mention? _____
2. **Mental and Emotional Status**
   A. **Appearance**
      Physical handicaps _____
      Dress appropriate _____ Sloppy _____
      Grooming neat _____ Poor _____
      Eye contact held _____ Describe posture _____
   B. **Behavior**
      Restless _____ Agitated _____ Lethargic _____
      Mannerisms _____ Facial expressions _____
      Other _____
   C. **Speech**
      Clear _____ Mumbled _____ Rapid _____
      Slurred _____
      Constant _____ Mute or silent _____ Barriers to communications _____
      Specify (e.g., client has delusions or is confused, withdrawn, or verbose) _____
   D. **Mood**
      What mood does the client convey? _____
   E. **Affect**
      Is the client's affect bland, apathetic, dramatic, bizarre, or appropriate? Describe _____
   F. **Thought process**
      1. Characteristics
         Describe the characteristics of the person's responses:
         Flights of ideas _____
         Looseness of association _____ Blocking _____
         Concrete _____
         Confabulation _____
         Describe _____
      2. Cognitive ability
         Proverbs: Concrete _____ Abstract _____
         Serial sevens: How far does the client go? _____
         Can the client do simple math? _____
         What seems to be the reason for poor concentration? _____
         Orientation to time (?), place (?), person (?) _____

*Continued*

Table 1-1 **Comprehensive Nursing Assessment Tool—cont'd**

G. **Thought content**
   1. Central theme: What is important to the client? _____
      Describe _____
   2. Self-concept: How does the client view himself or
      herself? _____
      What does the client want to change about himself
      or herself? _____
   3. Insight: Does the client realistically assess his or her
      symptoms? _____
      Realistically appraise his or her situation? _____
      Describe _____
   4. Suicidal or homicidal ideation? _____ What is
      suicide potential? _____ Family history of suicide
      or homicide attempt or successful completion? _____
      Explain _____
      Preoccupations. Does the client have hallucinations?
      _____ Delusions? _____
      Obsessions? _____ Rituals? _____ Phobias? _____
      Grandiosity? _____
      Religiosity _____ Worthlessness _____ Describe ___

ASK CLIENT:

H. **Spiritual assessment**
   What importance does religion or spirituality have in
   your life? _____
   Do your religious or spiritual beliefs influence the way
   you take care of yourself or your illness? How? _____
   Who or what supplies you with hope? _____

I. **Cultural influences**
   With what cultural group do you identify? _____
   Have you tried any cultural remedies or practices for
   your condition? If so, what? _____
   Do you use any alternative or complementary
   medicines/herbs/practices? _____

Axes IV and V can give the nurse and others information
that is important for setting realistic goals and planning
effective care. **Axis IV—Psychosocial and Environmental
Problems** identifies things going on in the client's life that
might greatly impact the client's life and might become the
primary focus of clinical attention. Examples of Axis IV-TR
problems include (APA, 2000):

- **Problems with primary support groups** (death, illness,
  divorce, sexual/physical abuse, neglect of child, discord
  with siblings, birth of a sibling)

Table 1-2 **Abnormal Motor Behaviors**

| Behavior | Definition | Example |
|---|---|---|
| **Echopraxia** | Repeating the movements of another person. | Every time the nurse moved or gestured with her hands, the client copied her gestures. |
| **Echolalia** | Repeating the speech of another person. | The nurse said to the client, "Tell me your name." The client responded, "Tell me your name, tell me your name." |
| **Waxy flexibility** | Having one's arms or legs placed in a certain position and holding that same position for hours. | The nurse lifted the client's arm to check the pulse, and the client left his arm extended in the same position. |
| **Parkinson-like symptoms** | Making mask-like faces, drooling, and having shuffling gait, tremors, and muscular rigidity. Seen in people who are on antipsychotic medication, such as phenothiazines. | The nurse noticed that the client's face held no emotion. He walked very stiffly, leaning forward, almost robot-like. |
| **Akathisia** | Displaying motor restlessness, feeling of muscular quivering; at its worst, patient is unable to sit still or lie quietly. | The client's leg kept jiggling up and down when he talked to the nurse. When his feet were still, his arm constantly jiggled during the interview. |
| **Dyskinesia** | Having distortion of voluntary movements, such as involuntary muscular activity (e.g., tic, spasm, or myoclonus). | The client had a marked facial tic around his mouth, which was distracting to the nurse during the interview. |

From Varcarolis, E. (1998). *Foundations of psychiatric mental health nursing* (3rd ed.). Philadelphia, WB Saunders, p. 999; reprinted with permission.

Table 1-3 **Summary of Abnormal Thought Processes**

| Thought Process | Definition | Example |
| --- | --- | --- |
| **Tangentiality** | Association disturbance in which the speaker goes off the topic. When it happens frequently and the speaker does not return to the topic, interpersonal communication is destroyed. | The nurse asked the client to talk more about his family. The client continuously left the topic and talked about boats, animals, his apartment, and so forth. Each time the nurse tried to help the client to focus, he went off on another topic. |
| **Neologisms** | Words a person makes up that have meaning only for the person himself, often part of a delusional system. | "I am afraid to go to the hospital because the *norks* are looking for me there." |
| **Looseness of association** | Thinking is haphazard, illogical, and confused. Connections in thought are interrupted. Seen mostly in schizophrenic disorders. | "Can't go to the zoo, no money, Oh . . . I have a hat, these members make no sense, man . . . What's the problem?" |
| **Flights of ideas** | Constant flow of speech in which the person jumps from one topic to another in rapid succession. There is a connection between some topics, although it is sometimes hard to identify. Characteristically seen in manic states. | "Say babe, how's it going . . . Going to my sister's to get money . . . money, honey, you got any bread . . . bread and butter, staff of life, ain't life grand?" |

From Varcarolis, E. (1998). *Foundations of psychiatric mental health nursing* (3rd ed.). Philadelphia, WB Saunders, p. 1000; reprinted with permission.

Table 1-3 **Summary of Abnormal Thought Processes—cont'd**

| Thought Process | Definition | Example |
|---|---|---|
| **Blocking** | Sudden cessation of a thought in the middle of a sentence. Person is unable to continue his/her train of thought. Often sudden new thoughts crop up that are unrelated to the topic. Can be disturbing to the individual. | "I was going to get a new dress for the . . . I forgot what I was going to say." |
| **Circumstantiality** | Before getting to the point or answering a question, the person gets caught up in countless details and explanations. | "Where are you going for the weekend, Harry?" "Well, I first thought of going to my mother's, but that was before I remembered that she was going to my sister's. My sister is having a picnic. She always has picnics at the beach. The beach that she goes to is large and gets crowded. That's why I don't like that beach. So I decided to go someplace else. I thought of going to my brother's house. He has a large house on a quiet street . . . I finally decided to stay home." |

*Continued*

Table 1-3 **Summary of Abnormal Thought Processes—cont'd**

| Thought Process | Definition | Example |
|---|---|---|
| **Perseveration** | Involuntary repetition of the same thought, phrase, or motor response to different questions or situations. Associated with brain damage. | N: How are you doing, Harry?<br>H: Fine, nurse, just fine.<br>N: Did you go for a walk?<br>H: Fine, nurse, just fine.<br>N: Are you going out today?<br>H: Fine, nurse, just fine. |
| **Confabulation** | Filling in a memory gap with detailed fantasy believed by the teller. The purpose is to maintain self-esteem; seen in organic conditions, such as Korsakoff's psychosis. | The nurse asked Harry, who spent the weekend at home, what he did for the weekend. "Well, I just came back from California after signing a contract with MGM for a film on the life of Roosevelt. We had the most marvelous tour of the studio . . . went to lunch with the director . . ." |
| **Word salad** | Mixture of words and phrases that have no meaning. | "I am fine . . . apple pie . . . no sale . . . furniture store . . . take it slow . . . cellar door . . ." |

- **Problems related to the social environment** (death or loss of friends, inadequate social support, living alone, difficulty with acculturation, discrimination, adjustment to life-cycle transition [e.g., retirement])

Table 1-4 **Preoccupation in Thought Content**

| Thought Process | Definition | Example |
|---|---|---|
| **Hallucinations** | A sense of perception for which no external stimuli exist. Hallucinations can have an organic or a functional etiology. | |
| | *Visual:* Seeing things that are not there. | During alcohol withdrawal, he kept shouting, "I see snakes on the walls." |
| | *Auditory:* Hearing voices when none are present. | "I keep hearing my mother's voice telling me I am bad. She died a year ago." |
| | *Olfactory:* Smelling smells that do not exist. | "I smell my stomach rotting." |
| | *Tactile:* Feeling touch sensations in the absence of stimuli. (Also referred to as *haptic*.) | A paranoid man feels electrical impulses "from outer space" entering his body and controlling his mind. |
| | *Gustatory:* Experiencing taste in the absence of stimuli. | A paranoid woman tastes poison in her food while eating at her son's wedding. |
| **Delusions** | A false belief held to be true even with evidence to the contrary. Three common delusions follow: | |
| | *Persecution:* The thought that one is being singled out for harm by others. | An intern believes that the chief of staff is plotting to kill him to prevent the intern from becoming too powerful. |

From Varcarolis, E. (1998). *Foundations of psychiatric mental health nursing* (3rd ed.). Philadelphia, WB Saunders, p. 1001; reprinted with permission.

*Continued*

Table 1-4 **Preoccupation in Thought Content—cont'd**

| Thought Process | Definition | Example |
|---|---|---|
| | *Grandeur:* The false belief that one is a very powerful and important person. | A newly admitted patient told the nurse that he was God, and he was here to save the world. |
| | *Jealousy:* The false belief that one's mate is going out with other people. The person might misinterpret every-day occurrences as *"proof."* | Sally "knew" that her husband, Jim, was being unfaithful. Even when Sally's brother swore he and Jim really did play pool Friday nights, Sally declared Jim's not being home then was her "proof." |
| **Obsessions** | An idea, impulse, or emotion that a person cannot put out of his or her consciousness. Can be mild or severe. | A young mother, Jane, told the nurse that she was hounded by constant thoughts that something terrible was going to happen to her baby. She knew that this was crazy, but she could not get the thought to stop. |
| **Rituals** | Repetitive actions that people must do over and over until either they are exhausted or anxiety is decreased. Often done to lessen the anxiety triggered by an obsession. | Jane stated to the nurse that the only way she could temporarily get these obsessions to cease was to say three "Hail Marys" and knock on wood twice to reassure herself that "nothing terrible was happening." |

Table 1-4 **Preoccupation in Thought Content—cont'd**

| Thought Process | Definition | Example |
| --- | --- | --- |
| **Phobias** | An intense irrational fear of an object, situation, or place. The fear persists even though the object of the fear is perfectly harmless, and the person is aware of the irrationality. | Although she was aware that cats would not harm her, Mary was deathly afraid of cats and refused to visit her sister and friends who had cats. |

- **Educational problems** (illiteracy, academic problems, discord with teachers or classmates, inadequate school environment)
- **Occupational problems** (unemployment, threat of job loss, stressful work schedule, difficult work conditions, job dissatisfaction, job change, discord with boss or co-workers)
- **Economic problems** (extreme poverty, inadequate finances, insufficient welfare support)
- **Problems with access to health care services** (inadequate health care services, transportation to health care facilities unavailable, inadequate health insurance)
- **Problems related to interaction with the legal system/crime** (arrest, incarceration, litigation, victim of crime)

**Axis V—Global Assessment of Functioning** is the clinician's judgment of the client's overall level of functioning. This information helps the health care team plan treatment and predict outcomes. See Box 1-2 for the Global Assessment of Functioning Scale.

After the initial assessment, it is useful to summarize pertinent data with the client. This summary provides clients with reassurance that they have been heard, and it allows them the opportunity to clarify any misinformation. They should then be told what will happen next. For example, if the initial assessment takes place in the hospital, the nurse should tell the client whom else the client will be seeing. If a psychiatric nurse in a mental health

| Box 1-2 | DSM-IV-TR Global Assessment of Functioning (GAF) Scale |
| --- | --- |

Consider psychologic, social, and occupational functioning on a hypothetical continuum of mental health-illness. Do not include impairment in functioning caused by physical (or environmental) limitations.

**Code**   (**Note**: Use intermediate codes when appropriate; e.g., 45, 68, 72.)

100 | **Superior functioning in a wide range of activities, life's problems never seem to get out of hand, is sought out by others because of his or her many positive qualities. No symptoms.**

91

90 | **Absent or minimal symptoms** (e.g., mild anxiety before an examination), **good functioning in all areas, interested and involved in a wide range of activities, socially effective, generally satisfied with life, no more than everyday problems or concerns** (e.g., an occasional argument with family members).

81

80 | **If symptoms are present, they are transient and expectable reactions to psychosocial stressors** (e.g., difficulty concentrating after family argument); **no more than slight impairment in social, occupational, or school functioning** (e.g., temporarily falling behind in schoolwork).

71

70 | **Some mild symptoms** (e.g., depressed mood and mild insomnia) **OR some difficulty in social, occupational, or school functioning** (e.g., occasional truancy, or theft within the household), **but generally functioning pretty well, has some meaningful interpersonal relationships.**

61

60 | **Moderate symptoms** (e.g., flat affect and circumstantial speech, occasional panic attacks) **OR moderate difficulty in social, occupational, or school functioning** (e.g., few friends, conflicts with peers or co-workers).

51

| Box 1-2 | DSM-IV-TR Global Assessment of Functioning (GAF) Scale—cont'd |
|---|---|

**50**

**Serious symptoms** (e.g., suicidal ideation, severe obsessional rituals, frequent shoplifting) **OR any serious impairment in social, occupational, or school functioning** (e.g., no friends, unable to keep a job).

**41**

**40**

**Some impairment in reality testing or communication** (e.g., speech is at times illogical, obscure, or irrelevant) **OR major impairment in several areas, such as work or school, family relations, judgment, thinking, or mood** (e.g., depressed man avoids friends, neglects family, and is unable to work; child frequently beats up younger children, is defiant at home, and is failing at school).

**31**

**30**

**Behavior is considerably influenced by delusions or hallucinations OR serious impairment in communication or judgment** (e.g., is sometimes incoherent, acts grossly inappropriately, is preoccupied with suicide) **OR inability to function in almost all areas** (e.g., stays in bed all day; has no job, home, or friends).

**21**

**20**

**Some danger of hurting self or others** (e.g., suicide attempts without clear expectation of death; frequent violence; manic excitement) **OR occasionally fails to maintain minimal personal hygiene** (e.g., smears feces) **OR gross impairment in communication** (e.g., largely incoherent or mute).

**11**

**10**

**Persistent danger of severely hurting self or others** (e.g., recurrent violence) **OR persistent inability to maintain minimal personal hygiene OR serious suicidal act with clear expectation of death.**

**1**

**0**

Inadequate information

From American Psychiatric Association. (2000). *Diagnostic and statistical manual of mental disorders* (4th ed., text revision). Washington, DC: American Psychiatric Association.

clinic conducts the initial assessment, the nurse will let the client know when and how often they will meet to work on the client's problems. If the nurse thinks a referral is necessary (e.g., to a psychiatrist, social worker, or medical physician), he or she will discuss this with the client.

## Assessment of a Non–English-Speaking Client

More and more English-speaking nurses are caring for clients who are non–English speaking. If a nurse does not speak the client's language, data gathering can be extremely difficult. It is to a nurse's benefit, when working primarily with clients who speak a specific language (e.g., Spanish), to learn at the very least relevant words, phrases, and questions in that language. The Americans with Disabilities Act (ADA) has established federal standards that ensure that communication does not interfere with equal access to health care for all people. All health care establishments are to establish systems for identifying available language interpreters, interpreters trained in sign language, telecommunication devices for the deaf (TDDs), closed-caption decoders for televisions, and amplifiers on phones (Gorman et al., 1996).

Therefore, nurses must often rely on interpreters. Interpreters can be family members, friends or neighbors, employees within the health care institution who have other responsibilities, or professional interpreters. Each group can have drawbacks. For example, a family interpreter might want to protect the client and filter out information given to the client. Conversely, the family member might want to filter out information about a problem or crisis in the family, and not clearly relay the information back to the nurse. It is best to avoid a family member acting as an interpreter.

Family members acting as interpreters should be avoided altogether when the client is a child. Employees with other jobs who speak English as a second language might have difficulty understanding the information you wish to convey. Friends and neighbors might find it embarrassing to discuss private and personal matters. The nurse might want to explore the use of the AT&T Interpreter Service.

Gorman and associates (1996) make the following suggestions when working through an interpreter:

- **Address the client directly** rather than speaking to the interpreter. Maintain eye contact with the client to ensure client involvement and to strengthen personal contact.
- **Avoid interrupting the client and interpreter.** At times, their interaction might take longer because of the need to clarify issues. Descriptions might require more time because of dialect differences, or the interpreter's awareness that the client needs more preparation before being asked a particular question.
- **Instruct the interpreter to give you verbatim translations.**
- **Avoid using medical jargon** that the interpreter or the client might not understand.
- **Avoid talking or commenting to the interpreter at length;** the client might feel left out and distrustful.
- **Always ask for permission to discuss intimate or emotionally laden topics** first, and prepare the interpreter for the content of the interview.
- **Be aware that asking intimate or emotionally laden questions might be difficult for the client as well as for the interpreter.** Lead up to these questions slowly.
- **Whenever possible, arrange for the interpreter and the client to meet each other ahead of time** to establish some rapport.
- **Try to use the same interpreter** for subsequent interviews with the client.

When an interpreter is not immediately available, aids such as picture charts or flash cards can help the nurse and the client communicate important basic information about the client's immediate needs (e.g., degree of pain or need for elimination). Because of cultural backgrounds or wanting to be helpful, some clients with limited English might seem agreeable and nod "yes" even though they do not understand. Asking questions that require more than a yes or no answer can provide a better idea of the client's level of understanding.

# NURSING DIAGNOSIS

A nursing diagnosis is a clinical judgment about individual, family, or community responses to actual or potential health problems/life processes (North American Nursing Diagnosis Association [NANDA International], 2005–2006).

This clinical judgment is derived through a deliberate, systematic process of data collection and analysis. A nursing diagnosis provides the basis for selection of nursing interventions chosen to achieve outcomes for which the nurse is accountable (NANDA International, 2005-2006). A nursing diagnosis is expressed concisely and includes the etiology ("Related To's") of the condition and is supported by objective and subjective data ("As Evidenced By's"). (See Appendix B for currently used nursing diagnoses.) Nursing diagnoses are updated every 2 years by NANDA International, in *NANDA Nursing Diagnosis: Definitions & Classification*. Nursing diagnoses are added and updated based on research and clinical evaluation.

Physicians and researchers also have formulated clear and accurate guidelines for identifying and categorizing clinical psychiatric disorders and syndromes. The APA provides specific criteria that must be met before a medical psychiatric diagnosis can be reached. The most current of these criteria are found in the *Diagnostic and Statistical Manual of Mental Disorders*, Fourth Edition, Text Revision (DSM-IV-TR) (APA, 2000). In each clinical chapter in this manual, the DSM-IV-TR criteria is provided as well as the appropriate nursing diagnosis. The classification system used for medical diseases and medical treatments is found in the *International Statistical Classification of Diseases and Related Health Problems*, Tenth Edition (ICD-10) (World Health Organization, 1992).

Therefore, the psychiatric-mental health nurse uses nursing diagnoses and standard classifications of mental disorders (DSM-IV-TR), as well as the standard international classification of diseases (ICD-10), to develop a treatment plan based on assessment data and theoretical premises.

A nursing diagnosis has three structural components: (1) problem/process, (2) etiology (Related To's), and (3) supporting data (As Evidenced By's).

## Problem/Process

The nursing diagnostic title states what should change; for example:
**Risk for injury**

## Etiology (Related To's)

The etiology includes probable cause or factors that contribute to or are *related* to the development or maintenance of a nursing diagnosis title. Stating the etiology or probable cause tells what needs to be done to effect change, and identifies causes that the nurse can treat through interventions. Etiology is linked to the diagnostic title with the words "related to." Therefore, the "related to" component of the nursing diagnosis needs to be defined as clearly as possible, because it discerns what needs to be targeted; for example:

**Risk for injury:** *related to extreme agitation and constant, uncontrollable motor activity*

This activity is a probable nursing diagnosis for a client in the manic phase of bipolar disorder. In this case, the potential for injury is *related to* uncontrollable hyperactivity in a person who is unable to use his or her usual problem-solving skills to avoid harm. Contrast this with the same nursing diagnostic title for a woman who is being constantly battered by her mate:

**Risk for injury:** *related to mate's poor impulse control and rage reaction*

In this case, probable cause for injury is *related to* a woman living with a physically violent partner, in a situation that she believes she cannot leave (fear for her life, no way to support herself financially, fear for her children).

## Supporting Data (As Evidenced By's)

Supporting signs and symptoms (As Evidenced By's) are the defining characteristics that cluster in patterns and support the validity of the diagnosis (NANDA International, {2005-2006}). Therefore, one can assume that, after interventions have been made and are successful, these signs and symptoms would no longer be present or present a problem for the client.

For example, using the situation above, manic clients might have observable signs and symptoms that alert the medical staff that injury or potential for injury is present and requires nursing/medical intervention. The client might have bruises or wounds resulting from falls, might suffer from lack of sleep as a result of constant physical activity, might have dehydration from not drinking or eating (related to hyperactivity or an inability to concentrate on the task of eating/drinking), and might be near exhaustion or even cardiac collapse. A complete nursing diagnostic statement would then read:

**Risk for injury: related to extreme agitation and constant, uncontrollable motor activity** *as evidenced by fewer than 2 hours rest a night, poor skin turgor, and abrasions on hands and arms*

Members of the health team could expect to see the client obtain adequate rest or sleep (e.g., 6 hours per night), good skin turgor, and an ability on the client's part to rest and refrain from agitated physical activity for frequent periods during the day as the final outcome of effective medical and nursing interventions.

## Summary

From data, nurses make clinical judgments about an individual's, family's, or community's response to actual or potential health problems/life processes and formulate nursing diagnoses accordingly. The nurse then plans and provides nursing actions that target the client's health problem or life process.

# OUTCOME IDENTIFICATION

Outcome criteria describe in behavioral or measurable terms the desired results of nursing interventions planned for a client. Outcome criteria also provide the basis for evaluating the effectiveness of care. Outcome criteria are the desired results of care. The nurse sets short- and long-term goals that (once met) will help ensure the outcome criteria are met. The short- and long-term *goals* are stated in behavioral or measurable terms and might have time factors (in 1 week, by discharge, within 2 days) or end results, or hoped-for results. They might also indicate a future steady state; for example:

- Client will function independently in the community with aid of social support.
- Client will refrain from self-harm.

These goals can be evaluated and revised as the client progresses. They are always client centered (not staff centered) and can be short-term or long-term. Goals are only useful if they are reasonable and attainable within a specified period of time. The short-term goals for each nursing diagnosis can include several steps that lead to the final outcome criteria. The amount of time needed to attain some of these goals will vary among clients. For some clients, the final outcome criteria might not be realistic goals, whereas for other clients the goals might be not only realistic but easily attainable. For these reasons, the nurse needs to use good judgment based on the client's database to identify realistic outcome criteria and to select appropriate goals for reaching the outcome criteria.

For example, for the Previously-stated nursing diagnosis:

**Risk for injury: related to extreme agitation and constant, uncontrollable motor activity as evidenced by fewer than 2 hours rest a night, poor skin turgor, and abrasions on hands and arms**

Possible outcome criteria might include:

- By discharge, client will be sleeping 6 to 8 hours per night.
- Client will willingly maintain an adequate diet (1500 to 2000 cal/day) and sufficient daily fluid intake by the time of discharge.
- Client will be free from infections, and abrasions/wounds will be in final healing stages by time of discharge.
- Client will continue attendance at support group within the community.
- Client will adhere to medication regimen.

Possible short-term goals (outcomes) might include:

- Client will sleep 3 to 4 hours per night within 2 days, with the aid of medication.
- Client will drink 8 oz of fluid (juice, milk, milkshake) every hour with the aid of nursing intervention.
- Client's skin turgor will be within normal limits within 24 hours.
- Client will spend 10 minutes in a quiet, nonstimulating area with nurse each hour during the day.

## PLANNING

Each stated goal should include nursing interventions, which are instructions for all people working with the client. These written plans aid in the continuity of care for the client and are points of information for all members of the health team. Increasingly units, in both inpatient and community-based facilities, use standardized care plans or clinical/critical pathways for clients with specific diagnoses. However, even standardized care plans and critical pathways must be tailored to specific clients, and there are often spaces on the standardized forms for client-centered revisions. Nursing interventions planned for meeting a specific goal should be:

*Safe:* They must be safe for the client as well as for other clients, staff, and family.

*Appropriate:* They must be compatible with other therapies and with the client's personal goals and cultural values, as well as with institutional rules.

*Effective:* They should be based on scientific principles.

*Individualized:* They should be realistic: (1) written within the capabilities of the client's age, physical strength, condition, and willingness to change; (2) based on the number of staff available; (3) reflective of actual available community resources; and (4) within the student's or nurse's capabilities.

The Nursing Outcome Classification (NOC) (2004) is a useful guide for identifying appropriate guidelines for intervention. NOC outcomes used in this text are flagged with a ■ preceding them.

## IMPLEMENTATION

Implementation is the action the nursing staff takes to carry out the nursing measures identified in the care plan to achieve the expected outcome criteria. Nursing interventions might be called actions, approaches, nursing orders, or nursing prescriptions. When carrying out the nursing interventions, additional data might be gathered and further refinements of the care plan can be made.

The Scope and Standards of Psychiatric–Mental Health Nursing Practice (ANA, 2000) identifies 10 areas for intervention for psychiatric nurses. Recent graduates and practitioners new to the psychiatric setting will participate in many of these activities. Interventions at the *basic level* include:

• Counseling
• Milieu therapy
• Self-care activities
• Psychobiologic interventions
• Health teaching
• Case management
• Health promotion and health maintenance

The psychiatric-mental health advanced practice registered nurse is prepared at the master's level or beyond. *Advanced practice interventions* include:

- Psychotherapy
- Prescription of pharmacologic agents (in several but not all states)
- Consultations and referrals

## EVALUATION

Evaluation is often the most neglected part of the nursing process. Ideally, evaluation should be part of each phase in the process. Evaluation of short- and long-term goals can have three possible outcomes: The goal is met, not met, or partially met. Using our original example for the nursing diagnosis:

**Risk for injury: related to extreme agitation and constant, uncontrollable motor activity as evidenced by fewer than 2 hours rest a night, poor skin turgor, and abrasions on hands and arms**

For the short-term goal (outcome):

- Client will drink 8 oz of fluid (juice, milk, milkshake) every hour during the day with the aid of nursing intervention.

In evaluation, the nurse might chart:

*Goal met:* **Client takes frequent sips of fluid equaling 8 oz an hour provided in portable containers with lid, during the hours of 9 AM to 4 PM, with reminders from nursing staff.**

For the short-term goal (outcome):

- Client will spend 10 minutes in a quiet, nonstimulating area with nurse each hour during the day.

In evaluation, the nurse might chart:

*Goal partially met:* **After 2 days, client continues restless and purposeless pacing up and down the halls, and is only able to stay quiet with nurse for 4 to 6 minutes an hour.**

For the short-term goal (outcome):

- Client's skin turgor will be within normal limits within 24 hours as evidenced by skin pinched over sternum and released; raised area disappears in 3 seconds or fewer.

In evaluation, the nurse might chart:

*Goal not met:* **At 8:00 AM this morning client's skin turgor still poor. Pinched skin over sternum disappeared 4 seconds postrelease. Evaluate need for increasing daytime fluids from 9 AM to 9 PM.**

The chapters in Parts II and III of this book present specific psychiatric clinical disorders and phenomena that might require nursing interventions. Under each disorder or phenomenon, the most common nursing diagnoses are presented. Suggested outcomes and short-term goals are offered for each nursing diagnosis. Outcome criteria are the final long-term goals that signal that the nursing diagnosis should no longer be a target for intervention.

Keep in mind that all goals are tailored to each client's current level of functioning and realistic potential. Therefore, one person's short-term outcome might be appropriately another's long-term outcome.

For each nursing diagnosis, specific nursing actions are suggested with supporting rationales. This clinical reference guide is intended to help nurses formulate well-stated nursing diagnoses and to set realistic outcome criteria with suggested steps (short-term goals) to reach the final outcome. Realistic and appropriate nursing interventions are provided, and nurses identify those that are appropriate for their clients. Some of the interventions are well within the student's realm; others might be better suited to a more advanced practitioner. They are all included to help give a more thorough overview of what constitutes nursing interventions. This clinical nursing guide is intended for students in planning care, as a guide to staff members who are new to a psychiatric unit, and for clinicians as a quick clinical reference.

## INTERNET SITES

**Nursing Net**
http://www.nursingnet.org
Information and web links for students as well as seasoned nurses

**American Nurses Association**
http://www.nursingworld.org

# CHAPTER 2

# Maximizing Communication Skills

Peplau (1952) identified two main principles that guide the communication process during the nurse-client interview. Those two main principles are (1) clarity and (2) continuity. *Clarity* means that the meaning of the message is accurately understood by both parties. *Continuity* promotes the connection among ideas "and the feelings, events, or themes conveyed in those ideas." This chapter offers a way to use and categorize your communication techniques, and it is hoped it will help you to enhance your ability to follow both of these principles.

Communication and interviewing techniques are acquired skills. Nurses learn to increase their ability to use communication and interviewing skills through practice and supervision. Communication is a complex process that can involve a variety of personal and environmental factors that might distort the sending and receiving of messages. Examples include:

*Personal Factors:* emotions (mood), knowledge level, language use, attitudes, and bias

*Social Factors:* previous experience, culture, language, and health beliefs and practice

*Environmental Factors:* physical factors (background noise, lack of privacy, uncomfortable accommodations) and societal factors (presence of others, expectations of others)

Communication consists of *verbal* and *nonverbal* elements. Communication is approximately 10% verbal and 90% nonverbal (Shea, 1998). Nonverbal communication consists of an amalgam of feelings, feedback, local wisdom, cultural rhythms, ways to avoid confrontation, and unconscious views of how the world works. When we try to communicate in words only, the results range from the humorous to the destructive (Hall, 1983).

## VERBAL COMMUNICATION

Verbal communication comprises all words a person speaks. Talking is our most common activity. Talking links us with others, it is our primary instrument of instruction, and it is one of the most personal aspects of our private life. When we speak, we:

- Communicate our beliefs, values, attitudes, and culture
- Communicate perceptions and meanings
- Convey interests and understanding *or* insult and judgment
- Convey messages clearly *or* convey conflicting or implied messages
- Convey clear, honest feelings *or* disguised, distorted feelings

Verbal communication can become misunderstood and garbled even among people with the same primary language and/or from the same cultural background. In our multiethnic society, keeping communication clear and congruent takes thought and insight. Communication styles, eye contact, and touch all have different meanings and are used and interpreted very differently among cultures. Ensuring that your verbal message is what you mean to convey, and that the message you send is the same message that the other person receives, is a complicated skill.

At times people convey conflicting messages. A person says one thing verbally, but conveys the opposite in nonverbal behavior. This is called a **double message** or **mixed message**. As in the saying, "actions speak louder than words," actions are often interpreted as the true meaning of a person's intent, whether that intent is conscious or unconscious. For example:

A young man goes to counseling because he is not making good grades in school and fears that he will not be able to get into medical school. He appears bright and resourceful, and states he has good study habits. In the course of the session, he tells the nurse that he is a star on the tennis team, is president of his fraternity, and has an active and successful social life, "If you know what I mean." Implied in this exchange appears to be a double message.

The verbal message is "I want good grades to get into medical school." The nonverbal message is that what is important to him is spending a great deal of time excelling at a sport, heading a social club, and engaging in dating activities.

Dee (1991) suggests that one way a nurse can respond to verbal and nonverbal incongruity (double messages) is to reflect and validate the individual's thoughts and feelings. For example:

"You say you are unhappy with your grades and as a consequence might not be able to get into medical school. Yet, from what I hear you say, you seem to be filling up your time excelling in so many other activities that there is very little time left for adequate preparation for excelling in your main goal, that of getting into medical school. I wonder what you think about this apparent contradiction in priorities?"

# NONVERBAL COMMUNICATION

Nonverbal communication consists of the behaviors displayed by an individual. Tone of voice and manner in which a person paces speech are examples of nonverbal communication. Other common examples of nonverbal communication (called *cues*) are facial expressions, body posture, amount of eye contact, eye cast (emotion expressed in the eyes), hand gestures, sighs, fidgeting, and yawning. Table 2-1 identifies some key components of nonverbal communication.

Sometimes gestures and other nonverbal cues can have opposite meanings, depending on culture and context. For example, eye contact can be perceived as comforting and supportive or as invasive and intimidating. Touching a client gently on the arm can be experienced as supportive and caring, or threatening or sexual. Facial expressions such as a smile can appear to convey warmth and interest, or hide feelings of fear or anger.

Many nonverbal cues have cultural meaning. For example, in some Asian cultures, avoiding eye contact shows respect. Conversely, in many people with French, British, and African backgrounds, avoidance of eye contact by another person might be interpreted as disinterest, not telling the truth, avoiding the sharing of important information, or dictated by social order.

Table 2-1 **Nonverbal Behaviors**

| Type | Possible Behaviors | Example |
| --- | --- | --- |
| **Body behavior** | Posture, body movements, gestures, gait | The client is slumped in a chair, puts her face in her hands, and occasionally taps her right foot. |
| **Facial expressions** | Frowns, smiles, grimaces, raised eyebrows, pursed lips, licking lips, tongue movements | The client grimaces when speaking to the nurse; when alone, he smiles and giggles to himself. |
| **Eye cast** | Angry, suspicious, and accusatory looks | The client squints his eyes, the pupils dilated. |
| **Voice-related behaviors** | Tone, pitch, level, intensity, inflection, stuttering, pauses, silences, fluency | The client talks in a loud, sing-song voice. |
| **Observable autonomic physiologic responses** | Increase in respirations, diaphoresis, pupil dilation, blushing, paleness | When the client mentions discharge, she becomes pale, her respirations increase, and her face becomes diaphoretic. |
| **General appearance** | Grooming, dress, hygiene | The client is dressed in a wrinkled shirt and his pants are stained; his socks are dirty and he wears no shoes. |
| **Physical characteristics** | Height, weight, physique, complexion | The client appears grossly overweight for his height, and his muscle tone appears flabby. |

From Varcarolis, E. (2002). *Foundations of psychiatric mental health nursing* (4th ed.). Philadelphia, WB Saunders, p. 250; reprinted with permission.

There are numerous ways to interpret verbal and non-verbal communications for each cultural and subcultural group. Even if a nurse is aware of how a specific cultural group responds to, for example, touch, the nurse could still be in error when dealing with an individual within that cultural group. Sustaining effective and respectful communication is very complex. It is the task of nurses to identify and explore the meaning of clients' nonverbal and verbal behaviors. Listed at the end of the chapter are Internet sites that provide further cultural information for health care professionals.

# EFFECTIVE COUNSELING AND COMMUNICATION TECHNIQUES

## Degree of Openness

Any question or statement can be classified as (1) an open-ended verbalization, (2) a focused question, or (3) a closed-ended verbalization. Furthermore, any question or statement can be classified along the *continuum of openness*. There are three variables that influence where any given verbalization sits on this openness continuum (Shea, 1998):
1. The degree to which the verbalization tends to produce spontaneous and lengthy response
2. The degree to which the verbalization does not limit the client's answer set
3. The degree to which the verbalization opens up a moderately resistant client
   Refer to Table 2-2 during the following discussion.

### Open-Ended Questions

Open-ended questions require more than one-word answers (e.g., a "yes" or "no"). Even with a client who is sullen, resistant, or guarded, open-ended questions can encourage lengthy information on experiences, perceptions of events, or responses to a situation. Examples of an open-ended question are: "What are some of the stresses you are grappling with?" "What do you perceive to be your biggest problem at the moment?" "Will you tell me something about your family?"

Shea (1998) encourages the use of frequent open-ended questions or gentle inquiries (e.g., "Tell me about . . ."Share with me . . ."). This is especially helpful when beginning a

Table 2-2 **Degree of Openness Continuum**

| Verbalization | Example |
| --- | --- |
| **Open-ended** | These questions are to be stated with a gentle tone of voice while expressing a genuine interest. They invite the client to share personal experiences. They cannot be answered with a "yes" or a "no." |
| 1. Open-ended questions (giving broad openings) | 1. What would you like to discuss?<br>2. What are your plans for the future?<br>3. How will you approach your father?<br>4. What are some of your thoughts about the marriage? |
| 2. Gentle commands (encouraging descriptions of perceptions) | 1. Tell me something about your home life?<br>2. Share with me some of your hopes about your future.<br>3. Describe for me the problem with your boss. |
| **Focused** | These questions represent a middle ground with regard to openness. When the relationship is strong, these questions can result in spontaneous lengthy speech. Used with a resistant client, these questions might be answered tersely. |
| 1. Exploring/ focusing | 1. Can you describe your feelings?<br>2. Can you tell me a little about your boss?<br>3. Can you say anything positive about your marriage?<br>4. Can you tell me what the voices are saying? |
| 2. Qualitative questions | 1. How's your appetite?<br>2. How's your job going?<br>3. How's your mood been? |
| 3. Statements of inquiry (restating, reflecting, paraphrasing, clarifying) | 1. You say you were fifth in your class?<br>2. So you left the marriage after 3 years?<br>3. So when she cries you feel guilty?<br>4. You seem to be saying that you're viewed as the bad guy in the family?<br>5. Give me an example of your being "no good." |

Adapted from Shea, S.C. (1998). *Psychiatric interviewing: The art of understanding* (2nd ed.). Philadelphia, WB Saunders, p. 82; reprinted with permission.

Table 2-2 **Degree of Openness Continuum—cont'd**

| Verbalization | Example |
| --- | --- |
| 4. Empathetic statements (making observations, sharing perceptions, seeking clarification) | 1. It sounds like a troubling time for you.<br>2. It's difficult to end a marriage after 10 years.<br>3. It looks like you're feeling sad.<br>4. You seem very disappointed about . . . |
| 5. Facilitatory statements (accepting, offering general leads) | 1. Uh-huh<br>2. Go on.<br>3. I see. |
| **Closed-ended** | **These techniques tend to decrease a client's response length. However, they can be effective in focusing a wandering client. Closed-ended questions help obtain important facts or ask for specific details. Closed-ended statements give information or explanations, or have an educational slant.** |
| 1. Closed-ended questions (seeking information) | 1. How long have you been hearing voices?<br>2. Are you feeling happy, sad, or angry?<br>3. What medications are you taking? |
| 2. Closed-ended statements (giving information) | 1. Anxiety can be helped with behavioural therapies.<br>2. This test will determine . . .<br>3. I read in your chart that you tried suicide once before.<br>4. We will begin by taking a blood sample to check your medication level. |

relationship and in the early interviews. Although the initial responses might be short, with time the responses often become more informative as the client becomes more at ease. This is an especially valuable technique to use with clients who are resistant or guarded, but is a good rule for opening phases of any interview and especially in the early phase of establishing a rapport with an individual.

## Closed-Ended Questions

Closed-ended questions, in contrast, are questions that ask for specific information (dates, names, numbers, yes-or-no information). These are closed-ended questions because they limit the client's freedom of choice. For example:

"Is your mother alive?"

"When were you born?"

"Did you seek therapy after your first suicide attempt?"

"Do you think the medication is helping you?"

Closed-ended questions give specific information when needed, such as during an initial assessment or intake interview, or to ascertain results, as in "Are the medications helping you?" They are usually answered by a "yes," a "no," or a short answer. When closed-ended questions are used frequently during a counseling session, or especially during an initial interview, they can close an interview down rapidly. This is especially true with a guarded or resistant client.

Other useful tools for nurses in communicating with their clients are (1) clarifying/validating techniques, (2) the use of silence, and (3) active listening.

## Clarifying/Validating Techniques

Understanding depends on clear communication, which is aided by verifying with a client the nurse's interpretation of the client's messages. The nurse must request feedback on the accuracy of the message received from verbal and nonverbal cues. The use of clarifying techniques helps both participants to identify major differences in their frames of reference, giving them the opportunity to correct misperceptions before they cause any serious misunderstandings. The client who is asked to elaborate on or clarify vague or ambiguous messages needs to know that the purpose is to promote mutual understanding. For example, "I hear you saying that you are having difficulty trusting your son after what happened. Is that correct?"

## Paraphrasing

For clarity, the nurse might use paraphrasing, which means to restate in different (often fewer) words the basic content of a client's message. Using simple, precise, and culturally relevant terms, the nurse can readily confirm interpretation of the client's previous message before the interview proceeds. By prefacing statements with a phrase such as "I am not sure I understand" or "In other words, you seem to be saying . . .," the nurse helps the client form a clearer perception of what might be a bewildering mass of details. After paraphrasing, the nurse must validate the accuracy of the restatement and its helpfulness to the discussion. The client might confirm or deny the perceptions through nonverbal cues or by directly responding to a question such as "Was I correct in saying . . .?" As a result, the client is made aware that the interviewer is actively involved in the search for understanding.

## Restating

With restating, the nurse mirrors the client's overt and covert messages; therefore, this technique can be used to echo feeling as well as content. Restating differs from paraphrasing in that it involves repetition of the same key words the client has just spoken. If a client remarks "My life has been full of pain," additional information might be gained by restating, "Your life has been full of pain." The purpose of this technique is to explore more thoroughly subjects that might be significant. However, too frequent and indiscriminate use of restating might be interpreted by clients as inattention or disinterest. It is very easy to overuse this tool and become mechanical. Inappropriately parroting or mimicking what another has said might be perceived as ridiculing, making this nondirective approach a definite drawback to communication. To avoid overuse of restating, the nurse can combine restating with use of other clarifying techniques that encourage descriptions. For example:
"Tell me about how your life has been full of pain."
"Give me an example of how your life has been full of pain."

## Exploring

A technique that enables the nurse to examine important ideas, experiences, or relationships more fully is exploring. For example, if a client tells the nurse that he does not get along well with his wife, the nurse should explore this area further. Possible openers might include:

"Tell me more about your relationship with your wife."

"Describe your relationship with your wife."

"Give me an example of you and your wife not getting along."

Asking for an example can greatly clarify a vague or generic statement made by a client:

*Mary:* No one likes me.

*Nurse:* Give me an example of one person who doesn't like you.

*Jim:* Everything I do is wrong.

*Nurse:* Give me an example of one thing you do that you think is wrong.

## Use of Silence

In many cultures in our society, including nursing, there is an emphasis on action. In communication, we tend to expect a high level of verbal activity. Many students and practicing nurses find that, when the flow of words stops, they become uncomfortable. The effective use of silence, however, is a helpful communication technique.

Silence is not the absence of communication. Silence is a specific channel for transmitting and receiving messages. The practitioner needs to understand that silence is a significant means of influencing and being influenced by others.

In the initial interview, the client might be reluctant to speak because of the newness of the situation, the unfamiliarity with the nurse, self-consciousness, embarrassment, shyness, or anger. Talking is highly individualized: some find the telephone a nuisance, whereas others believe they cannot live without it. The nurse must recognize and respect individual differences in styles and tempos of responding.

Although there is no universal rule concerning how much silence is too much, silence has been said to be worthwhile only as long as it is serving some function and not frightening the patient. Knowing when to speak during the interview is largely dependent on the nurse's perception about what is being conveyed through the silence. Icy silence might be an expression of anger and hostility. Being ignored or "given the silent treatment" is recognized as an insult and is a particularly hurtful form of communication. Ingram (1991) points out that silence among some African-American clients might relate to anger, insulted feelings, or acknowledgment of a nurse's lack of cultural sensitivity.

Silence can also convey: a person's acceptance of another person; comfort in being with someone and sharing time together; that a person is pondering an idea or forming a response to what has just been said; or that a person is comfortable when there is nothing more to say at that moment. Successful interviewing might be dependent on the nurse's "will to abstain"—that is, to refrain from talking more than necessary. Silence might provide meaningful moments of reflection for both participants. It gives each an opportunity to contemplate thoughtfully what has been said and felt, to weigh alternatives, to formulate new ideas, and to gain a new perspective of the matter under discussion. If the nurse waits to speak and allows the client to break the silence, the client might share thoughts and feelings that could otherwise have been withheld. Nurses who feel compelled to fill every void with words often do so because of their own anxiety, self-consciousness, and embarrassment. When this occurs, the nurse's need for comfort tends to take priority over the needs of the client.

Conversely, prolonged and frequent silences by the nurse can hinder an interview that requires verbal articulation. Although the untalkative nurse might be comfortable with silence, this mode of communication might make the client feel like a fountain of information to be drained dry. Moreover, without feedback, clients have no way of knowing whether what they said was understood.

In naturally evolving interviews, open-ended techniques are interwoven with empathetic and facilitatory statements and closed-ended statements, all of which serve to clarify issues and demonstrate the interviewer's interest (Shea, 1998).

## Active Listening

People want more than just physical presence in human communication. Most people are looking for the other person to be there for them psychologically, socially, and emotionally (Egan, 1994). Active listening includes:

- Observing and paraphrasing the client's nonverbal behaviors

- Listening to and seeking to understand clients in the context of the social setting of their lives
- Listening for the "false notes" (e.g., inconsistencies or things the client says that need more clarification)

We have already noted that effective interviewers need to become accustomed to silence. It is just as important, however, for effective interviewers to learn to become active listeners when the client is talking, as well as when the client becomes silent. During active listening, nurses carefully note what the client is saying verbally and nonverbally, as well as monitoring their own nonverbal responses (Parsons and Wicks, 1994). Using silence effectively and learning to listen on a deeper, more significant level to both the client and your own thoughts and reactions are key ingredients in effective communications. Both these skills take time, profit from guidance, and can be learned.

Here is a word of caution about listening. It is important for all of us to recognize that it is impossible to listen to people in an unbiased way. In the process of socialization, we develop cultural filters through which we listen to ourselves, others, and the world around us (Egan, 1994). Cultural filters are a form of cultural bias or cultural prejudice.

One of the functions of culture is to provide a highly selective screen between us and the outside world. In its many forms, culture, therefore, designates what we pay attention to and what we ignore. This screening provides structure for the world. (Hall, 1997, p. 85)

Egan (1994) states that we need these cultural filters to provide structure for ourselves and to help us interpret and interact with the world. However, unavoidably, these cultural filters also introduce various forms of bias in our listening, because they are bound to influence our personal, professional, familial, and sociologic values and interpretations.

Active listening helps strengthen the client's ability to solve personal problems. By giving the client undivided attention, the nurse communicates that the client is not alone; rather, the nurse is working along with the client, seeking to understand and help. This kind of intervention enhances self-esteem and encourages the client to direct energy toward finding ways to deal with problems. Serving as a "sounding board," the nurse listens as the client tests thoughts by voicing them aloud. This form of interpersonal interaction often enables the client to clarify thinking, link ideas, and tentatively decide what should be done and how best to do it.

# TECHNIQUES TO MONITOR AND AVOID

Some techniques health care workers might employ are not useful and can negatively affect the interview and threaten rapport between the nurse and client. Using ineffective techniques that set up barriers to communication is something we all have done, and will do again. However, with thoughtful reflection, and appropriate alternative therapeutic behaviors and methods, communication skills will become more effective, and confidence in interviewing abilities will be gained. Most importantly, the ability to work with clients will be improved, even those clients who present the greatest challenges. Supervision and peer support are immensely valuable in identifying techniques to target and change.

Some of the most common approaches that can cause problems and are especially noticeable in the nurse who is new to psychosocial nursing are (1) asking excessive questions, (2) giving advice, (3) giving false reassurance, (4) requesting an explanation, and (5) giving approval.

## Asking Excessive Questions

Excessive questioning, especially *closed-ended* questions, puts the nurse in the role of interrogator, demanding information without respect for the client's willingness or readiness to respond. This approach conveys lack of respect and sensitivity to the client's needs. Excessive questioning controls the range and nature of response, and can easily result in a therapeutic stall or a shut-down interview. It is a controlling tactic and might reflect the interviewer's lack of security in letting the client tell his or her own story. It is better to ask more openended questions and follow the client's lead. For example:

*Excessive questions:*
"Why did you leave your wife?" "Did you feel angry at her?" "What did she do to you?" "Are you going back to her?"

*Better to say:*
"Tell me about the situation between you and your wife."

## Giving Advice

When a nurse offers clients "solutions," they eventually begin to think that the nurse does not view them as capable of making effective decisions. Giving people advice undermines their feelings of adequacy and competence. It can foster dependence on the advice giver, and shifts the problem from client to nurse. Giving constant advice to clients (or others for that matter) devalues the other individual and prevents the other person from working through and thinking through other options either on their own or with the nurse. It keeps the "advice giver" in control and feeling like the strong one, although this might be unconscious on the nurse's part. This is very different from giving information to people. People need information to make informed decisions.

*Giving advice:*

*Client:* "I don't know what to do about my brother. He is so lost."

*Nurse:* "You should call him up today and explain to him you can't support him any longer, and he will have to go on welfare." (If I were you . . . Why don't you . . . It would be best . . .)

*Better to say:*

*Client:* "I don't know what to do about my brother. He is so lost."

*Nurse:* "What do you see as some possible actions you can take?" (encourages problem solving)

OR

*Nurse:* "Have you thought about discussing this with the rest of your family?" (offers alternatives the client can consider) Clients often ask nurses for solutions. It is best to avoid this trap.

## Giving False Reassurance

Giving false reassurance underrates a person's feelings and belittles a person's concerns. This usually causes people to stop sharing feelings because they feel they are not taken seriously, or are being ridiculed. Therefore, the person's real feelings remain undisclosed and unexplored. False reassurance in effect invalidates the client's experience and can lead to increased negative affect.

*False reassurance:*

"Everybody feels that way."

"Don't worry, things will get better."

"It's not that bad."
"You're doing just fine."

*Better to say:*
"What specifically are you worried about?"
"What do you think could go wrong?"
"What do you see as the worst thing that could happen?"

## Requesting an Explanation: "Why" Questions

A "why" question from a person in authority (nurse, doctor, teacher) can be experienced as intrusive and judgmental. "Why" questions might put people on the defensive, and serve to close down communication. It is much more useful to ask, "What is happening?" rather than why it is happening. People often have no idea why they did something, although almost everyone can make up a ready answer on the spot. Unfortunately, the answer is mostly defensive and not useful for further exploration.

*Why questions:*
"Why don't you leave him if he is so abusive?"
"Why didn't you take your medications?"
"Why didn't you keep your appointment?"

*Better to say:*
"What are the main reasons you stay in this relationship?"
"Tell me about the difficulties you have regarding taking your medications."
"I notice you didn't keep your appointment even though you said that was a good time for you. What's going on?"

## Giving Approval

We often give our friends and family approval when we believe they have done something well. Even when what they have done is not *that* great, we make a big point of it. It is natural to bolster up friends' and loved ones' egos when they are feeling down.

You might wonder what is wrong with giving a person a pat on the back once in a while. The answer is nothing, as long as it is done without involving a judgment (positive or negative) by the nurse. Giving approval in the nurse-client relationship is a much more complex matter than giving approval or "a pat on the back" to one's friends or colleagues. Often people coming into the psychiatric setting are feeling overwhelmed and alienated, and might be down on themselves. During this time, clients are vulnerable and might be needy for recognition, approval, and attention. Yet, when people are feeling vulnerable, a value comment can be misinterpreted. For example:

*Value judgment:*

"You did a great job of holding your temper when Sally started screaming at you. You are really getting good at maintaining your 'cool.'"

Implied in this message is that the nurse was pleased by the way the client kept his temper in a volatile situation. In many instances, the client might see this as a way to please the nurse, or get recognition from others. Therefore, the behavior becomes a way to gain approval. This can be a much healthier and more useful behavior for the client, but, when the motivation for any behavior starts to focus on getting recognition and approval from others, it stops coming from the individual's own volition or conviction. In addition, when the people the client wants approval from are not around, the motivation for the new behavior might not be there, either. Therefore, it is not really a change in behavior as much as a ploy to win approval and acceptance from others.

*Better to say:*

"I notice that you kept your temper when Sally screamed at you. You seem to be acting more even-tempered lately. How does it feel to be more in control of your emotions?"

This response opens the door to finding out how the client is feeling. Is this new behavior becoming easier? Was this situation of holding back anger difficult? Does the client want to learn more assertiveness skills? Was it useful for the client? Is there more about this situation that the client wants to discuss? The response by the nurse also makes it clear that this was a self-choice the client made. The client is given recognition for the change in behavior, and the topic is also open for further discussion.

## ASSESSING YOUR COMMUNICATIONS SKILLS

Gaining communication and counseling skills is a process that takes time. Self-assessment over time and noting areas of improvement and areas to target for the future might be helpful. Table 2-3 is a communication self-assessment checklist. It is helpful to check yourself frequently over time and note your progress.

Table 2-3 **Nurse's Communication Self-Assessment Checklist**

*Instructions:* Periodically during your clinical experience, use this checklist to identify areas needed for growth and progress made. Think of your clinical patient experiences. Indicate the extent of your agreement with each of the following statements by marking the scale: SA, strongly agree; A, agree; NS, not sure; D, disagree; SD, strongly disagree.

| | | | | | |
|---|---|---|---|---|---|
| 1. I maintain appropriate eye contact. | SA | A | NS | D | SD |
| 2. Most of my verbal comments follow the lead of the other person. | SA | A | NS | D | SD |
| 3. I encourage others to talk about feelings. | SA | A | NS | D | SD |
| 4. I ask open-ended questions. | SA | A | NS | D | SD |
| 5. I restate and clarify a person's ideas. | SA | A | NS | D | SD |
| 6. I paraphrase a person's nonverbal behaviors. | SA | A | NS | D | SD |
| 7. I summarize in a few words the basic ideas of a long statement made by a person. | SA | A | NS | D | SD |
| 8. I make statements that reflect the person's feelings. | SA | A | NS | D | SD |
| 9. I share my feelings relevant to the discussion when appropriate to do so. | SA | A | NS | D | SD |
| 10. I give feedback. | SA | A | NS | D | SD |
| 11. At least 75% or more of my responses help enhance and facilitate communication. | SA | A | NS | D | SD |
| 12. I assist the person in listing some available alternatives. | SA | A | NS | D | SD |
| 13. I assist the person in identifying some goals that are specific and observable. | SA | A | NS | D | SD |
| 14. I assist the person in specifying at least one next step that might be taken toward the goal. | SA | A | NS | D | SD |

Adapted from Myrick, D., & Erney, T. (1984). *Caring and sharing.* Educational Media Corporation, p. 154; reprinted by permission. Copyright 1984 by Educational Media Corporation

# INTERNET SITES

**Transcultural Nursing Society**
http://www.tcns.org

**JAMARDA Resources, Inc.**
Cultural diversity in the health care field
http://www.jamardaresources.com

**Natural Health Village**
Alternative systems of health practice
http://www.naturalhealthvillage.com

# CHAPTER 3

# Guidelines for the Clinical Interview: Responsibilities of Nurses Who Counsel Clients

The foundation of nursing practice is the ability of the nurse to engage in interpersonal interactions in a goal-directed manner for the purpose of assisting clients with their emotional or physical health needs (Hagerty, 1984). This relationship between the nurse and client is a professional relationship, and, as such, implies certain responsibilities. Responsibilities inherent in the nurse-client relationship for all levels of nursing include:

- **Accountability**—The nurse assumes responsibility for the conduct and consequences of the assignment and for the nurse's actions.
- **Focus on client needs**—The interest of the client, *not* that of other health care workers or the institution, is given first consideration. *The nurse's role is that of client advocate.*
- **Clinical competence**—The nurse bases his or her conduct on the principles of knowledge of and appropriateness to the specific situation. This involves awareness and incorporation of the latest knowledge made available from research.
- **Supervision**—Validation of performance quality is through regularly scheduled supervisory sessions. Supervision is conducted either by a more experienced

clinician or through discussion with the nurse's peers in professionally conducted supervisory sessions.

# PHASES OF THE COUNSELING PROCESS

Many disciplines describe the phases of a therapeutic relationship during counseling. These phases are the same for all disciplines, although different disciplines might have their own names for these phases. We will use the names that are generally recognized in the practice of nursing, which are (1) the orientation phase, (2) the working phase, and (3) the termination phase.

In some situations, the nurse might only meet with the client once, or for only a few sessions. Although the time spent together might be brief, the relationship or encounters can be substantial, useful, and important to the client. This limited relationship is often referred to as a *therapeutic encounter*. Many of the following principles and practices apply to even a limited encounter (e.g., issues of confidentiality, goals, tasks), although the working phase is brief and adapted to the brief encounter. Termination per se might not apply; however, the nurse might want to find out what the client thought was helpful or if there is an issue the client wishes to pursue that was discussed during the encounter, and might refer the client to appropriate staff or to members of the treatment team.

There are certain tasks and phenomena that are specific to each phase, although they might overlap. For example, the issue of confidentiality, first addressed in the orientation phase, can be discussed and reiterated throughout all phases of the nurse-client relationship. The following discussion highlights important aspects and responsibilities of the nurse during each phase.

## Orientation Phase

The orientation phase can last for a few meetings or can extend for a longer period of time. The first time the nurse and client meet, they are strangers to each other. When strangers meet for the first time, they interact according to their own backgrounds, standards, values, and experiences. This fact underlies the need for self-assessment and self-awareness on the part of the nurse.

## Goals of the Orientation Phase

1. **To establish trust.** Establishing trust is essentially establishing a sound engagement with the client in a therapeutic alliance. Trust is something that will or will not develop between the two parties. Establishing an atmosphere in which trust can grow is the responsibility of the nurse. Trust is nurtured by demonstrating genuineness (congruence) and empathy, developing a positive regard for the client, demonstrating consistency, and offering assistance in alleviating the client's emotional pain or problems.
2. **To effect some degree of anxiety reduction in the client.**
3. **To instill hope and ensure that the client will remain compliant with treatment.**
4. **To develop an assessment from which nursing diagnoses can be formulated,** if a nursing assessment has not already been done.
5. **To develop appropriate treatment goals (outcome criteria) and a plan of care.**

## Tasks of the Orientation Phase

During the orientation phase, the nurse addresses four specific issues: (1) the parameters of the relationship, (2) the formal or informal contract, (3) confidentiality, and (4) termination.

**Parameters of the Relationship** Clients have the right to know about the nurse or counselor with whom they will be working. For example, who is this nurse and what is the *nurse's background?* They also need to know the stated purpose of the meetings. For a student, this information-giving might be conveyed thus.

"Hello, Mrs. Gonzalas, I am Sylvia Collins from Sullivan College. I am in my senior year, and I am doing my psychiatric rotation. I will come to City College for the next eight Thursdays, and I would like to meet with you each Thursday, if you are still here. I am here to be a support person for you as you work on your treatment goals."

*or*

"Hello, Mrs. Gonzalas. I am Jim Santos from Ohio State College. I am here only once this week, so we will have today to discuss your most important issues."

For an RN working in the clinical setting, the parameters might be altered.

"Hello, Mrs. Gonzalas, I am John Horton. I am an advanced-practice psychiatric nurse, and I have been counseling clients for about 4 years now. Dr. Sharp referred you to me and stated that you wished to work out some issues in counseling/therapy."

**Formal or Informal Contract**   A contract emphasizes the client's participation and responsibilities. It implies that the nurse does something *with* the client, not just for the client. The contract, either stated or written, includes the time, place, date, and duration of the meetings as well as mutual agreement as to goals. If a fee is to be paid, the client is told how much it will be and when the fee is due.

For a student, the statement of the contract might sound something like the following.

"Mr. Snyder, we will meet at 10:00 AM each Monday in the consultation room at the clinic for 45 minutes from September 15th to October 27th. We can use that time to further discuss your feelings of loneliness, and explore some things you could do to make things better for yourself."

For a psychiatric advanced practice nurse working in the clinical setting, the contract might be:

"Mrs. Lang, we will meet on Thursdays at 10:00 AM in my office at the clinic. Our sliding-scale fee is $45 per session. Our policy states that, if you can't make a session, it is important to let us know 24 hours in advance, otherwise we will charge you for the session. We can use our time together to explore further your feelings of loneliness and anger with your husband and any other issues you wish to work on."

**Confidentiality**   The client has the right to know who else knows about the information being shared with the nurse. He or she needs to know that the information might be shared with specific people, such as a clinical supervisor, the physician, the treatment team, or other students in conference. The client also needs to know that the information will *not* be shared with the client's family, friends, or others outside the treatment team, except in extreme situations. Extreme situations include:

- When the client reveals information that might be harmful to the client or others (child abuse, elder abuse)
- When the client threatens self-harm
- When the client does not intend to follow through with the treatment plan

When information must be given to others, it is usually done by the physician according to legal guidelines. The nurse must be aware of the client's right to confidentiality, and must not violate that right. Refer to Box 3-1 for guidelines for confidentiality.

A student might phrase the issue of confidentiality something like:

"Mrs. Martin, I will be sharing some of what we discuss with my nursing instructor, and at times I might discuss certain concerns with my peers in conference, or with the staff. However, I will not share this information with your husband or any other members of your family or your friends without your permission."

For a psychiatric nurse specialist, the issue can be broached in the following manner:

"Mr. Shapero, I might share some of what we discuss with Dr. Lean during bimonthly supervision or in peer-group supervision here at the clinic. I will not discuss this information outside of the clinic setting, or with any members of your family or friends, without your permission, unless I am concerned that your life or someone else's life is in danger."

---

### Box 3-1 Ethical Guidelines for Confidentiality

1. Keep all client records secure.
2. Consider carefully the content to be entered into the record.
3. Release information only with written consent and full discussion of the information to be shared, except when release is required by law.
4. Use professional judgment deliberately regarding confidentiality when the client is a danger to self or others.
5. Use professional judgment deliberately when deciding how to maintain the confidentiality of a minor. The rights of the parent/guardian must also be considered deliberately.
6. Disguise clinical material when used professionally for teaching and writing.
7. Maintain confidentiality in consultation and peer review situations.
8. Maintain anonymity of research subjects.
9. Safeguard the confidentiality of the student in teaching/learning situations.

---

From Colorado Society of Clinical Specialists in Psychiatric Nursing. (1990), Ethical guidelines for confidentiality. *J Psychosocial Nurs* 28, 42-44; reprinted with permission.

**Termination** The issue of termination is always discussed in the first interview. It can also be brought up during the working phase. In some cases, the termination date is known, such as in a student rotation, or short-term therapy, in which sessions are specifically limited, or when insurance issues dictate only a specific number of sessions. At other times, when the nurse-client relationship is open-ended, the termination date might not be known. A student can address termination by saying:

"Mrs. Tacinelli, as I mentioned earlier, our last clinical day is October 27th. We will have three more meetings after today."

A clinical specialist can broach termination by saying something like:

"Mr. Middelstaedt, you are here to work on your phobia of using public transportation. Many people become more comfortable with their phobias in 12 to 14 sessions. At the end of 14 sessions, we can evaluate your goals and/or see if there is anything else you want to work on."

**In summary**, the initial interview includes the following elements:
1. The nurse's role is clarified, and the responsibilities of both the client and the nurse are defined.
2. The contract containing the time, place, date, and duration of the meetings is discussed.
3. Confidentiality is discussed and assumed.
4. The terms of termination are introduced.

## Working Phase

During the working phase, the nurse and client together identify and explore areas in the client's life that are causing problems. Some of the specific tasks of the working phase of the nurse-client relationship include (Moore & Hartman, 1988):
1. Maintaining the relationship
2. Gathering additional data
3. Promoting the client's problem-solving ability
4. Facilitating behavior change
5. Overcoming resistance
6. Evaluating problems and goals, and redefining them as necessary
7. Practicing and experiencing alternative adaptive behaviors

It is important, however, to keep in mind that chronically ill clients, particularly those with schizophrenia, frequently are unable to define problem areas or goals. The illness impairs their cognitive functioning and ability to establish relationships. It is important to recognize that establishing trust with a chronically ill client, and even temporarily relieving the client's feelings of isolation and social withdrawal that accompany the illness, are significant goals to pursue.

During the orientation and working phase, clients often unconsciously employ "testing behaviors" to test the nurse. The client might want to know if the nurse will:

- Be able to set limits
- Still show concern if the client gets angry, babyish, unlikable, or dependent
- Still be there if the client is late, leaves early, refuses to speak, or is angry

Table 3-1 gives examples of common testing behaviors clients employ, and some suggested nursing responses.

## Termination Phase

Termination has been discussed in the first interview; it might also have been broached during the working phase of the relationship. Reasons for terminating include:

- Symptom relief
- Improved social functioning
- Greater sense of identity
- More adaptive behaviors in place
- Accomplishment of the client's goals
- An impasse in therapy
- End of student rotation
- End of health-maintenance organization contract
- Discharge or death

Termination is an integral part of the nurse-client relationship, and without it, the relationship remains incomplete. Summarizing the goals and objectives achieved in the relationship is part of the termination process. Reviewing situations that occurred during the time spent together and exchanging memories can help validate the experience for both the nurse and the client, and can facilitate closure of the relationship.

During the termination process, old feelings of loss, abandonment, or loneliness might be reawakened in the client.

Table 3-1 **Testing Behaviors Used by Clients**

| Client Behavior | Client Example | Nurse Response | Rationale |
|---|---|---|---|
| Shifts focus of interview *to* the nurse, *off* the client. | "Do you have any children?" or "Are you married?" | "This time is for you." If appropriate, the nurse should add: 1. "Do you have any children?" or "What about your children?" 2. "Are you married?" or "What about your relationships?" | The nurse refocuses back to the client and client's concerns. The nurse sticks to the contract. |
| Tries to get the nurse to take care of him or her. | "Could you tell my doctor . . ." | "I'll leave a message with the ward clerk that you want to see him." or "You know best what you want him to know. I'll be interested in what he has to say." | 1. The nurse validates that the client can do many things for him- or herself. This aids in increasing self-esteem. |
| | "Should I take this job?" | "What do you see as the pros and cons of this job?" | 2. The nurse always encourages the person to function at the highest level, even if he or she does not want to. |
| Makes sexual advances toward the nurse, e.g., touching the nurse's arm, wanting to hold hands or kiss nurse. | "Would you go out with me? . . . Why not? or "Can I kiss you? . . . Why not?" | "I am not comfortable having you touch (kiss) me." The nurse briefly reiterates the nurse's role: "This time is for you to focus on your problems and concerns." | 1. The nurse needs to set clear limits on expected behavior. 2. Frequently restating the nurse's role throughout the relationship can help maintain boundaries. |

| Continues to arrive late for meetings. | "I'm a little late because (excuse)." | If the client stops: "I wonder what this is all about?"<br>1. Is the client afraid the nurse will not like him or her?<br>2. Is the client trying to take the focus off of problems?<br>If the client continues: "If you can't cease this behavior, I'll have to leave. I'll be back at (time) to spend time with you then."<br>The nurse arrives on time and leaves at the scheduled time. (The nurse does not let the client manipulate him or her or bargain for more time.)<br><br>After a couple of times, the nurse can explore behavior (e.g., "I wonder if there is something going on you don't want to deal with?" or "I wonder what these latenesses mean to you?") | 3. Whenever possible, the meaning of the client's behavior should be explored.<br><br>4. Leaving gives the client time to gain control. The nurse returns at the stated time.<br><br>1. The nurse keeps the contract. Clients feel more secure when "promises" are kept, even though clients might try to manipulate the nurse through anger or helplessness, for example.<br>2. The nurse does not tell the client what to do, but the nurse and client need to explore what the behavior is all about. |

From Varcarolis, E. (2002). *Foundations of psychiatric mental health nursing* (4th ed.). Philadelphia, WB Saunders; p. 234; reprinted with permission.

Therefore, the termination phase should offer the client an opportunity to express these feelings, perhaps for the first time. These feelings might also be reawakened in the nurse, perhaps to a different degree or intensity, if he or she still has strong issues of loss. Nurses can benefit from discussing these feelings with more experienced nurses, supervisors, trusted instructors, and their mature peers. Because loss is an integral part of life, it is also an integral part of the human condition. Many feelings can be reawakened at termination, and, therefore, clients might feel vulnerable and at a loss. Although many clients can talk about their feelings, client behaviors vary widely. For example, a client might respond with anger toward the nurse, or demonstrate symptoms thought to be resolved. In addition, a client might withdraw from the nurse during the last session, or refuse to spend time with the nurse at all. It is always a good idea to acknowledge what seems to be going on, and explore this with the client:

"You seem very quiet today, and haven't made eye contact with me. Good-byes often stir up memories of past separations. Do you remember any past separations that were painful?"

Throughout the process (introduction, working, termination), pertinent clinical information is recorded in the client's record, and verbally passed along to members of the treatment team.

## THE CLINICAL INTERVIEW

Anxiety during the first clinical interview is to be expected, as in any meeting between strangers. Clients might be anxious about their problems, about the nurse's reaction to them, or about their treatment. Shea (1998) identifies some common client fears and concerns during the first interview:

- Who is this nurse/clinician?
- Is he or she competent?
- Is this person understanding?
- What does he or she already know about me?
- Am I going to be hurt?
- Do I have any control in this matter?

Students and clinicians new to psychosocial nursing might have other concerns:

- What should I say?
- What should I do?

- Will the client like me?
- How will the client respond to me?
- Can I help this person?
- Can I hurt the client if I say the wrong thing?
- What will the instructor/supervisor think of what I am doing?
- How will I do compared with my peers?

## How to Begin the Interview

Helping a person with an emotional or medical problem is rarely a straightforward task. The goal of assisting a client to regain psychologic or physiologic functional normality can be difficult to reach. It is extremely important in any kind of counseling to permit the client to set the pace of the interview, no matter how slow the progress might be (Parsons & Wicks, 1994).

### Setting

Effective communication can take place almost anywhere. However, because the quality of the interaction—whether in a clinic, a ward, an office, or the client's home—depends on the degree to which the nurse and client feel safe, establishing a setting that enhances feelings of security can be important to the relationship. A health care setting, a conference room, or a quiet part of the unit that has relative privacy but is within view of others is ideal. Home visits offer the nurse a valuable opportunity to assess the person in the context of everyday life.

### Seating

In all settings, chairs need to be arranged so that conversation can take place in normal tones of voice, and eye contact can be comfortably maintained, or avoided. For example, a nonthreatening physical environment for nurse and client would involve:
- Assuming the same height—either both sitting or both standing.
- Avoiding a face-to-face stance when possible—a 90-degree angle or side-by-side might be less intense.
- Leaving plenty of space between client and nurse.

- Making sure that the door is easily accessible to both client and nurse. This is particularly important if the client is paranoid or has a history of violence.
- Avoiding a desk barrier between nurse and client.

## Introductions

In the orientation phase, nurses tell the client who they are, the purpose of the meetings, and how long and at what time they will be meeting with the client. The issue of confidentiality is also covered at some point during the initial interview. The nurse can then ask the client how he or she would like to be addressed. This question accomplishes a number of tasks (Shea, 1998); for example:

- It conveys respect.
- It gives the client direct control.

## How to Start

Once introductions have been made, the nurse can turn the interview over to the client by using one of a number of open-ended statements:

"Where should we start?"

"Tell me a little about what has been going on with you."

"What are some of the stresses you have been coping with recently?"

"Tell me a little about what has been happening in the past couple of weeks."

"Perhaps you can begin by letting me know what some of your concerns have been recently."

"Tell me about your difficulties."

The appropriate use of offering leads (e.g., "Go on"), statements of acceptance (e.g., "Uh-huh"), or other conveyances of the nurse's interest can facilitate communication.

## Tactics to Avoid

The nurse needs to avoid some behaviors (Moscato, 1988):

- Do not argue with, minimize, or challenge the client.
- Do not praise the client or give false reassurance.
- Do not verbally interpret the client or speculate on the dynamics of the client's problem.
- Do not question the client about sensitive areas until trust is established.

- Do not try to "sell" the client on accepting treatment.
- Do not join in attacks the client launches on his or her mate, parents, friends, or associates.
- Do not participate in criticism of another nurse or any other staff member with the client.
- Do not barrage the client with many questions, especially closed-ended questions.

## Helpful Guidelines

Some guidelines for conducting the initial interviews are offered by Meier and Davis (1989):

- Speak briefly.
- When you do not know what to say, say nothing.
- When in doubt, focus on feelings.
- Avoid advice; rather, look at how the client feels about the situation and what he or she wants to change.
- Avoid relying on questions.
- Pay attention to nonverbal cues.
- Keep the focus on the client.

## Guidelines for Specific Client Behaviors

There are a number of common client behaviors that arise during the process of the nurse-client relationship in mental health settings. New nurses might not know how best to handle these situations. These behaviors include clients who (1) cry, (2) ask the nurse to keep a secret, (3) leave before the session is over, (4) say they want to kill themselves, (5) do not want to talk, (6) seek to prolong the interview, (7) give the nurse a present, and (8) ask personal questions. Table 3-2 identifies common nursing reactions to these situations and offers the nurse useful responses.

Table 3-2 **Common Client Behaviors and Nurse Responses**

| Client Behavior | Possible Reactions by Nurse | Useful Responses by Nurse |
|---|---|---|
| **The client cries.** | The nurse might feel uncomfortable and experience increased anxiety or feel somehow responsible for making the person cry. | The nurse should stay with the client and reinforce that it is all right to cry. Often, it is at that time that feelings are closest to the surface and can be best identified. "You seem ready to cry." "What are you thinking right now?" The nurse offers tissues when appropriate. |
| **The client asks the nurse to keep a secret.** | The nurse might feel conflict because he/she wants the client to share important information but is unsure about making such a promise. | The nurse *cannot* make such a promise. This information might be important to the health and safety of the client or others. "I cannot make that promise. It might be important for me to share it with other staff." The client then decides whether to share the information or not. |
| **Another client interrupts during time with your selected client.** | The nurse might feel a conflict. The nurse does not want to appear rude. Sometimes the nurse tries to engage both clients in conversation. | The time the nurse had contracted with a selected client is that client's time. By keeping their part of the contract, nurses demonstrate that they mean what they say and that they view the sessions as important. "I am with Mr. Rob for the next 20 minutes. At 10 AM, after our time is up, I can talk to you for 5 minutes." |

| The client says he wants to kill himself. | The nurse might feel overwhelmed or responsible to "talk the client out of it." The nurse might pick up some of the client's feelings of hopelessness. | The nurse tells the client that this is serious, that he or she does not want harm to come to the client, and that this information needs to be shared with other staff.<br>"This is very serious, Mr. Lamb. I do not want any harm to come to you. I will have to share this with the other staff."<br>The nurse can then discuss with the client the feelings and circumstances that led up to this decision. (Refer to Chapter 16 for strategies in suicide intervention.) |
| The clients says she does not want to talk. | A nurse who is new to this situation might feel rejected or ineffective. | At first, the nurse might say: "It's all right. I would like to spend time with you. We don't have to talk." The nurse might spend short, frequent periods (e.g., 5 minutes) with the client throughout the day. "Our 5 minutes are up. I'll be back at 10 AM and stay with you 5 more minutes."<br>This gives the client the opportunity to understand that the nurse means what he or she says and is back on time consistently. It also gives the client time between visits to assess the nurse and perhaps feel less threatened. |

From Varcarolis, E. (2002). *Foundations of psychiatric mental health nursing* (4th ed.). Philadelphia, WB Saunders; pp. 246–247; reprinted with permission.

*Continued*

Table 3-2 **Common Client Behaviors and Nurse Responses—cont'd**

| Client Behavior | Possible Reactions by Nurse | Useful Responses by Nurse |
|---|---|---|
| **The client gives the nurse a present.** | The nurse might feel uncomfortable when offered a gift. The meaning needs to be examined. Is the gift:<br>1. A way of getting better care?<br>2. A way to maintain self-esteem?<br>3. A way to make the nurse feel guilty?<br>4. A sincere expression of thanks?<br>5. A cultural expectation? | *Possible guidelines:*<br>If the gift is expensive, the best policy is to perhaps graciously refuse.<br>If it is inexpensive and<br>1. given *at the end* of hospitalization when a relationship has developed, graciously accept.<br>2. given *at the beginning* of hospitalization, graciously refuse and explore the meaning behind the present.<br>"Thank you, but it is our job to care for our clients. Are you concerned that some aspect of your care will be overlooked?"<br>If the gift is money, it might be best to graciously refuse. |

| The client asks you a personal question. | The nurse might think it is rude not to answer the client's question. | The nurse may or may not answer the client's query. If the nurse decides to answer a natural question, he or she answers in a word or two, then refocuses back on the client. |
| | *or* | P: Are you married? |
| | A new nurse might feel relieved to put off the start of the interview. | N: Yes, do you have a spouse? |
| | *or* | P: Do you have any children? |
| | The nurse might feel embarrassed and want to leave the situation. | N: This time is for you—tell me about yourself. |
| | New nurses are often manipulated by a client to change roles. This keeps the focus off the client and prevents the building of a relationship. | P: You can tell me if you have any children. |
| | | N: This is your time to focus on your concerns. Tell me something about your family. |

# PART II

# DIAGNOSIS AND CARE PLANNING

# CHAPTER 4

# Selected Disorders of Childhood and Adolescence

## OVERVIEW

The risk factors for mental disorders in childhood or adolescence are genetic, biochemical, and pre- and post-natal influences; individual temperament; and personal psychosocial development. The vulnerability to risk factors is the result of a complex interaction among many factors (e.g., constitutional endowment, trauma, disease, and interpersonal experiences). Vulnerability changes over time as children/adolescents grow, and as the emotional and physical environment changes. As children and adolescents mature, they develop competencies that enable them to communicate, remember, test reality, solve problems, make decisions, control drives and impulses, modulate affect, tolerate frustration, delay gratification, adjust to change, establish satisfying interpersonal relationships, and develop healthy self-concepts. These competencies reduce the risk for developing emotional, mental, or health problems. Children and adolescents who are missing any of these competencies, or are "at risk" for other reasons, should be monitored so that early detection and intervention can help eradicate or at least minimize developing problems.

The following disorders, most commonly seen in children and adolescents, are discussed in this chapter:

(1) attention-deficit disorders, (2) disruptive behavior disorders, and (3) pervasive developmental disorders. Anxiety disorders, are covered in Chapter 5; however, currently accepted psychopharmacologic agents used in the treatment of anxiety disorders in children and adolescents are included in Table 4-2.

## Initial Assessment

The observation/interaction part of a mental health assessment begins with a semistructured interview in which the child or adolescent is asked about life at home with parents and siblings, and life at school with teachers and peers. Because the interview is not structured, children are free to describe their current problems and give information about their own developmental history. Play activities, such as games, drawing, puppets, and free play, are used for younger children who cannot respond to a direct approach. An important part of the first interview is observing interactions among the child, the caregiver, and the siblings (if possible).

### Assessment Tools

Nurse's working with children and adolescents need to have a good grasp of growth and development. A chart comparing and contrasting the psycho-sexual stages of development between Erickson, Freud, and Sullivan is found in Appendix D-1C.

The **developmental assessment** D-1A provides information about the child's current maturational level. This can help the nurse identify current lags or deficits. The **Mental Status Assessment** (Appendix D-1B) provides information about the child's/adolescent's current mental state. The developmental and mental status assessments have many areas in common, and for this reason any observation and interaction will provide data for both assessments.

# Attention-Deficit and Disruptive Behavior Disorders

Most children and adolescents receiving treatment for mental disorders have behaviors that disrupt their lives at home and at school. The distinguishing characteristics for these disorders—**attention-deficit/hyperactivity disorder, oppositional defiant disorder**, and **conduct disorder**—are presented in the following sections.

## ASSESSMENT

## Attention-Deficit/Hyperactivity Disorder

Attention-deficit/hyperactivity disorder (**ADHD**) is a persistent pattern of inattention and/or hyperactivity-impulsivity that is *more frequently displayed* and *more severe* than that typically observed in individuals at a comparable level of development (American Psychiatric Association [APA], 2000). ADHD occurs in 3% to 7% of school-age children. ADHD children might have a higher incidence of problems with temper outbursts, bossiness, stubbornness, labile moods, poor school performance, rejection by peers, low self-esteem, and enuresis and/or encopresis. It is important to note that 50% to 65% of children with ADHD continue to have symptoms of the disorder in adulthood (Korn and Weiss, 2003). Because ADHD may be inherited, it is important to screen for ADHD in parents or relatives while a child presents with the disorder (Korn and Weiss, 2003).

ADHD is often dually diagnosed with **oppositional defiant disorder** or **conduct disorder** (APA, 2000).

## Presenting Signs and Symptoms

### Inattention

- Has difficulty paying attention in tasks or play.
- Does not seem to listen, follow through, or finish tasks.
- Does not pay attention to details and makes careless mistakes.
- Dislikes activities that require sustained attention.
- Is easily distracted, loses things, and is forgetful in daily activities (with symptoms worsening in situations requiring sustained attention).

### Hyperactivity

- Fidgets or is unable to sit still or stay seated in school.
- Runs and climbs excessively in inappropriate situations.

- Has difficulty playing in leisure activities quietly.
- Acts as though "driven by a motor" and is constantly "on the go."
- Talks excessively.

*Impulsivity*

- Blurts out an answer before question is completed.
- Has difficulty waiting for turns.
- Interrupts or intrudes in others' conversations and games.

*Other*

- Some hyperactivity, impulsiveness, or inattention present before age 7.
- Clear evidence of impairment in social, academic, or occupational functioning.
- Impairment from symptoms in at least two settings (home, school, work).

# Oppositional Defiant Disorder

Oppositional defiant disorder is a recurrent pattern of negativistic, disobedient, hostile, defiant behavior toward authority figures without the serious violations of the basic rights of others (APA, 2000). The behavior is usually evident before age 8 years and no later than early adolescence. It is more common in males until puberty, when the male-to-female ratio might become equal. The behavior is evident at home and might not be evident elsewhere. The behavior persists for at least 6 months and might be a precursor of a **conduct disorder**.

*Presenting Signs and Symptoms*

- Often loses temper.
- Often argues with adults.
- Often actively defies or refuses to comply with requests.
- Deliberately annoys others and is easily annoyed by others.
- Blames others for his or her mistakes.
- Is often angry, resentful, spiteful, and vindictive.
    Other behaviors that often accompany this disorder are low self-esteem; labile moods; low frustration tolerance;

swearing; early use of alcohol and illicit drugs; and conflicts with parents, teachers, and peers.

# Conduct Disorder

Conduct disorder is a persistent pattern of behavior in which the rights of others and age-appropriate societal norms or rules are violated (APA, 2000). The prevalence of conduct disorders appears to have increased during the past decade. The onset of this disorder might be as early as pre-school years, but is usually noted from middle adolescence through middle adulthood.

**Childhood-onset type** occurs prior to age 10 and mainly in males who are physically aggressive, have poor peer relationships with little concern for others, and lack guilt or remorse. Although they try to project a "tough" image, they have low self-esteem, low frustration tolerance, irritability, and temper outbursts. They are more likely to have their conduct disorder persist through adolescence and develop into **antisocial personality disorder**.

In the **adolescent-onset type**, no conduct problems occurred prior to age 10. These children are less likely to be aggressive, have more normal peer relationships, and act out their misconduct with their peer group. Males are more apt to fight, steal, vandalize, and have school discipline problems, whereas girls lie, are truant, run away, abuse substances, and engage in prostitution.

Complications associated with conduct disorders are school failures, suspension and dropout, juvenile delinquency, and the need for the juvenile court system to assume responsibility for youths who cannot be managed by their parents. Psychiatric disorders that frequently coexist with conduct disorder are anxiety, depression, ADHD, and learning disabilities.

## Presenting Signs and Symptoms

### Aggression toward People and Animals

- Often bullies, threatens, and intimidates others.
- Often initiates physical fights.
- Has used a weapon that could cause serious injury.
- Has been physically cruel to others and/or animals.

- Has stolen while confronting a victim.
- Has forced someone into sexual activity.

### Destructive of Property

- Has deliberately set fires intending to cause damage.
- Has deliberately destroyed another's property.

### Deceitfulness or Theft

- Has broken into a house, building, or car.
- Often lies to obtain goods or favors.
- Has stolen items of trivial value (shoplifting).

### Serious Violations of Rules

- Often stays out at night despite parental prohibition before age 13.
- Has run away from home at least twice, or once for a lengthy period of time.
- Often truant from school before age 13.

## Assessment Questions

### Attention Deficit and Disruptive Behavior Disorders (for the Parent or Caregiver)

*The nurse uses a variety of therapeutic techniques to obtain the answers to the following questions. Use your discretion and decide which questions are appropriate to complete your assessment.*

1. Describe the child's temperament. (easy, highly reactive, difficult)
2. Describe the child's overall activity level. (high energy, hyperactive)
3. Who is/was the primary caregiver? Any disruptions in that relationship?
4. Problems going to sleep or staying asleep? (nightmares, sleepwalking)
5. Describe the child's adjustment to feeding schedules or new foods. (food refusal, food fetishes)
6. Any difficulty separating from you if left in the care of others?
7. How does the child show affection toward you, siblings, peers?

8. What comforts the child when stressed?
9. Does the child express concern when others are injured or distressed? Express remorse or guilt when hurtful to others?
10. How does the child respond to limits? Being told 'no'? Having to wait, share, or end a favorite activity? (protests, tantrums)
11. How motivated is the child to learn new skills? (persistence, patience, response to frustration)
12. How long will the child attend to an activity? Easily distracted?
13. Can the child follow 1-, 2-, and 3-part directions?
14. Does the child have difficulty organizing or completing tasks? Lose personal belongings?
15. Does the child have friends? How well do they play together?
16. Does the child frequently seek attention? Talk a lot? Interrupt or intrude on other's activities or body space?
17. At what grade level is the child? How is the child's academic progress?
18. Describe any problematic behaviors. (acts impulsively or recklessly, is physically aggressive, is hostile, is cruel to people and animals, is manipulative, lies and cheats, steals, destroys property, sets fires, swears, skips school, runs away from home, uses drugs or alcohol, sexually acts out)

## Assessment Guidelines

### Attention-Deficit and Disruptive Behavior Disorders

1. Assess the quality of the relationship between the child and parent/caregiver for evidence of bonding, anxiety, tension, and difficulty-of-fit between the parents' and the child's temperament, which can contribute to the development of disruptive behaviors.
2. Assess the parent/caregiver's understanding of growth and development, parenting skills, and handling of problematic behaviors, because lack of knowledge contributes to the development of these problems.
3. Assess cognitive, psychosocial, and moral development for lags or deficits, because immature developmental competencies result in disruptive behaviors.

*Attention-Deficit/Hyperactivity Disorder*

1. Observe the child for level of physical activity, attention span, talkativeness, and the ability to follow directions and control impulses. Medication is often needed to ameliorate these problems.
2. Assess for difficulty in making friends and performing in school. Academic failures and poor peer relationships lead to low self-esteem, depression, and further acting out.
3. Assess for problems with enuresis and encopresis.

*Oppositional Defiant Disorder*

1. Identify issues that result in power struggles, when they began, and how they are handled.
2. Assess the severity of the defiant behavior and its impact on the child's life at home, at school, and with peers.

*Conduct Disorder*

1. Assess the seriousness of the disruptive behavior, when it started, and what has been done to manage it. Hospitalization or residential placement might be necessary, as well as medication.
2. Assess the child's levels of anxiety, aggression, anger, and hostility toward others, and the ability to control destructive impulses.
3. Assess the child's moral development for the ability to understand the impact of the hurtful behavior on others, to empathize with others, and to feel remorse.

# Nursing Diagnoses With Interventions

## Discussion of Potential Nursing Diagnoses

Children and adolescents with attention-deficit/hyperactivity disorder, oppositional defiant disorder, and conduct disorder have disruptive behaviors that are impulsive, angry/aggressive, and often dangerous **(Risk for Violence)**. These children and adolescents are often in conflict with parents and authority figures, refuse to comply with requests, do not follow age-appropriate social norms, or have inappropriate ways of getting needs met **(Defensive Coping)**. When their behavior is disruptive or aggressive and hostile, they have difficulty making or keeping friends **(Impaired Social Interaction)**. Their problematic behaviors can impair learning and result in academic failure. Interpersonal and academic problems lead to high levels of anxiety, low self-esteem, and blaming others for one's troubles **(Chronic Low Self-Esteem)**. Parents/caregivers have difficulty handling disruptive behaviors and being effective parents, so their participation in the therapeutic program is essential **(Impaired Parenting)**.

## Overall Guidelines for Nursing Interventions
## *Attention-Deficit and Disruptive Behavior Disorders*

Help the child reach his or her full potential by fostering developmental competencies and coping skills:

1. Protect the child from harm and provide for biologic and psychosocial needs while acting as a parental surrogate.
2. Increase the child's ability to trust, control impulses, modulate the expression of affect, tolerate frustration, concentrate, remember, reality test, recognize cause and effect, make decisions, problem solve, use interpersonal skills to maintain satisfying relationships, form a realistic self-identity, and play with enjoyment and creativity.
3. Foster the child's identification with positive role models so that positive attitudes and moral values can develop that enable the child to experience feelings of empathy, remorse, shame, and pride.
4. Provide support, education, and guidance for the parents/caregivers.

## Selected Nursing Diagnoses and Nursing Care Plans

### RISK FOR VIOLENCE: SELF-DIRECTED OR OTHER-DIRECTED

At risk for behaviors in which an individual demonstrates that he/she can be physically, emotionally, and/or sexually harmful to self or to others

*Related To (Etiology)*

- ▲ Impaired neurologic development or dysfunction
- ▲ Cognitive impairment (e.g., learning disabilities, attention-deficit disorder, decreased intellectual functioning)
- ● Birth temperament
- ● Disturbance or immaturity in the competencies of normal growth and development result in lack of impulse control, poor frustration tolerance, and lack of empathy toward others
- ● Disturbances in attachment or bonding with the parent/caregiver
- ● Identification with aggressive and abusive role models

*As Evidenced By*
*(Assessment Findings/Diagnostic Cues)*

- ▲ Bullying, threatening, and having physical fights with others
- ▲ Physical cruelty to people and animals
- ▲ Setting fires and/or destroying property
- ● Forcing someone into sexual activity (attempted rape, rape, sexual molestation)
- ● History of aggressive behavior (e.g., mugs or robs others)

*Outcome Criteria*

- ● Control aggressive, impulsive behaviors
- ● Demonstrate respect for the rights of others

*Long-Term Goals*

Child/adolescent will:
- ● Demonstrate the ability to control aggressive impulses and delay gratification within 3 months

*Short-Term Goals*

Child/adolescent will:
- ● Respond to limits on aggressive and cruel behaviors within 2 to 4 weeks
- ● Identify at least three situations that trigger violent behaviors within 1 to 2 months

---

▲ NANDA International accepted; ● In addition to NANDA International

- Channel aggression into constructive activities and appropriate competitive games within 2 to 4 weeks
- State the effects of his or her behavior on others within 2 to 4 weeks
- Demonstrate the ability to control aggressive impulses and delay gratification within 2 to 8 weeks

## Interventions and Rationales

| Intervention | Rationale |
|---|---|
| 1. Use one-on-one or appropriate level of observation to monitor rising levels of anxiety; <u>determine</u> emotional and situational triggers. | 1. External controls are needed for ego support and to prevent acts of aggression and violence. |
| 2. Intervene early to calm the client and defuse a potential incident. | 2. Learning can take place before the client loses control; new ways to cope can be discussed and role modeled. |
| 3. Use graduated techniques for managing disruptive behaviors (Table 4-1) | 3. Techniques such as signals/warnings, proximity and touch control, humor, and and attention might be all that is needed. |
| 4. Set clear, consistent limits in a calm, nonjudgmental manner; remind client of consequences of acting out. | 4. A child gains a sense of security with clear limits and calm adults who follow through on a consistent basis. |
| 5. Avoid power struggles and repeated negotiations about rules and limits. | 5. When limits are realistic and enforceable, manipulation can be minimized. |
| 6. Use strategic removal if the client cannot respond to limits (time out, quiet room, therapeutic holding). | 6. Removal allows the client to express feelings and discuss problems without losing face in front of peers. |

| Intervention | Rationale |
|---|---|
| 7. Process incidents with the client to make it a learning experience. | 7. Reality testing, problem solving, and testing new behaviors are necessary to foster cognitive growth. |
| 8. Use a behavior modification program that rewards the client for seeking help with handling feelings and controlling impulses to act out. | 8. Rewarding the client's efforts can increase positive behaviors and foster development of self-esteem. |
| 9. Redirect expressions of disruptive feelings into non-destructive, age-appropriate behaviors; channel excess energy into physical activities. | 9. Learning how to modulate the expression of feelings and use anger constructively is essential for self-control. |
| 10. Help the client see how acting out hurts others; appeal to the child's sense of "fairness" for all. | 10. These children are insensitive to the feelings of others. However, they can understand the concept of "fairness" and generalize it to other persons. |
| 11. Encourage feelings of concern for others and remorse for misdeeds. | 11. Development of empathy is a therapeutic goal with these children. |
| 12. Use medication if indicated to reduce anxiety and aggression or to modulate moods. | 12. A variety of medications are effective in children who experience behavioral dyscontrol. |

## Table 4-1 Techniques for Managing Disruptive Behaviors in Children*

| | |
|---|---|
| 1. Planned ignoring | 1. Evaluate surface behavior and intervene when the intensity is becoming too great. |
| 2. Use of signals or gestures | 2. Use a word, gesture, or eye contact to remind child/adolescent to use self-control. |
| 3. Physical distance and touch control | 3. Move closer to the child/adolescent for a calming effect—maybe put arm around child/adolescent. |
| 4. Increase involvement in the activity | 4. Redirect child/adolescent's attention to the activity and away from a distracting behavior by asking a question. |
| 5. Additional affection | 5. Ignore the provocative content of the behavior and give the child emotional support for the current problem. |
| 6. Use of humor | 6. Use well-timed kidding as a diversion to help the child/adolescent save face and relieve feelings of guilt or fear. |
| 7. Direct appeals | 7. Appeal to the child/adolescent's developing self-control (e.g., "Please, . . . not now") |
| 8. Extra assistance | 8. Give early help to the child/adolescent who "blows up" and is easily frustrated when trying to achieve a goal; do not overuse this technique. |
| 9. Clarification as intervention | 9. Help child/adolescent understand the situation and his or her own motivation for the behavior. |
| 10. Restructuring | 10. Change the activity in ways that will lower the stimulation or the frustration (e.g., shorten a story or change to a physical activity). |

Adapted from Redl, F., & Wineman, D. (1957). *The aggressive child.* Glencoe, IL: The Free Press; reprinted with permission.

*Although an old reference, it is valid, useful, and reflects current practice. *Continued*

Table 4-1 **Techniques for Managing Disruptive Behaviors in Children*—cont'd**

| 11. Regrouping | 11. Use total or partial changes in the group's composition to reduce conflict and contagious behaviors. |
| --- | --- |
| 12. Strategic removal | 12. Remove child/adolescent who is disrupting or acting dangerously, but consider whether it gives too much status or makes the child a scapegoat. |
| \13. Physical restraint | 13. Use "therapeutic holding" to control, give comfort, and assure a child that he or she is protected from his or her own impulses to act out. |
| ↖14. Setting limits and giving permission | 14. Use sharp, clear statements about what behavior is not allowed and give permission for the behavior that is expected. |
| 15. Promises and rewards | 15. Use very carefully and very infrequently to avoid situations in which the child/adolescent bargains for a reward. |
| 16. Threats and punishment | 16. Use very carefully; the child/adolescent needs to internalize the frustration generated by the punishment and use it to control impulses rather than externalizing the frustration in further acting out. |

Adapted from Redl, F., & Wineman, D. (1957). *The aggressive child*. Glencoe, IL: The Free Press; reprinted with permission.

*Although an old reference, it is valid, useful, and reflects current practice.

## DEFENSIVE COPING

Repeated projection of falsely positive self-evaluation based on a self-protective pattern that defends against underlying perceived threats to positive self-regard

## Related To (Etiology)

▲ Disturbance in pattern of tension release (problems in impulse control and frustration tolerance)

● Impaired neurologic development or dysfunction

● Birth temperament (highly reactive, difficult to comfort, high motor activity)

● Disturbed relationship with parent/caregiver (lack of trust, abuse, neglect, conflicts, inadequate role models, disorganized family system)

## As Evidenced By
## (Assessment Findings/Diagnostic Cues)

▲ Uses forms of coping that impede adaptive behavior (defiant, negative, and/or hostile toward authority figures)

● Refuses to follow directions or comply with limits set on behaviors

● Tests limits persistently

● Is argumentative, stubborn, and unwilling to give in or negotiate

● Exhibits temper tantrums and rage reactions when unable to get his or her way

● Refuses to accept responsibility for misbehavior, often blames others

## Outcome Criteria

● Complies with requests and limits on behaviors in the absence of arguments, tantrums, or other acting-out behaviors

## Long-Term Goals

Child/adolescent will:

● Question the requests or limits that seem unreasonable and negotiate a settlement within 2 to 3 months

---

▲ NANDA International accepted; ● In addition to NANDA International

## Short-Term Goals

Child/adolescent will:
- Demonstrate increased impulse control within 2 weeks using a scale of 1 to 10 (1 being the most controlled)
- Demonstrate the ability to tolerate frustration and delay gratification within 6 weeks
- Demonstrate an absence of tantrums, rage reactions, or other acting-out behaviors within 4 to 8 weeks
- Discuss requests and behavioral limits and understand their rationale with the authority figure within 4 to 6 weeks
- Accept responsibility for misbehaviors within 2 to 6 weeks

## Interventions and Rationales

| Intervention | Rationale |
| --- | --- |
| 1. Use one-on-one or appropriate level of observation to monitor rising levels of frustration; determine emotional and situational triggers. | 1. External controls are needed for emotional support and to prevent tantrums and rage reactions. |
| 2. Intervene early to calm the client, problem solve, and defuse a potential outburst. | 2. Learning can take place before the client loses control; new solutions and compromises can be proposed. |
| 3. Avoid power struggles and "no-win" situations. | 3. Therapeutic goals are lost in power struggles. |
| 4. Use a behavior modification program to reward tolerating frustration, delaying gratification, and responding to requests and behavioral limits. | 4. Rewarding the client's efforts will increase the positive behaviors and help with development of self-control. |

| Intervention | Rationale |
|---|---|
| 5. Allow the client to question the requests or limits *within reason;* give simple, understandable rationale for requests or limits. | 5. Discussion allows the client to maintain some sense of autonomy and power. (Rationale is tailored to the developmental age and promotes socialization.) |
| 6. When feasible, negotiate an agreement on the expected behaviors. Avoid giving bribes or allowing the client to manipulate the situation. | 6. An agreement on expected behavior will result in better compliance. However, constant negotiations can result in increased manipulation and testing of limits. |
| 7. Use medication if indicated to reduce anxiety, rage, and aggression, and to modulate moods. | 7. A variety of medications are effective in children who experience behavioral and emotional dyscontrol. |

## IMPAIRED SOCIAL INTERACTION

Insufficient or excessive quantity or ineffective quality of social exchange

### *Related To (Etiology)*

- Impaired neurologic development or dysfunction
- Disturbance in the development of impulse control, frustration tolerance, or empathy for others
- Disturbed relationship with parents/caregiver (lack of trust, abuse, neglect, conflicts, disorganized family system)
- Lack of appropriate role models and/or identification with aggressive/abusive models
- Loss of friendships due to disruptions in family life and living situations

---

▲ NANDA International accepted; ● In addition to NANDA International

## As Evidenced By
### (Assessment Finding/Diagnostic Cues)

- Dysfunctional interaction with peers (teases, taunts, bullies, and fights with others)
- Difficulty making friends because of immature, disruptive, destructive, cruel, or manipulative behaviors
- Isolated, having few or no friends, and/or poor sibling relationships
- Blames others for poor peer relationships
- Sad/depressed about not being liked by peers
- Low self-esteem, or unrealistic, inflated esteem as the aggressor

## Outcome Criteria

- Use age-appropriate interpersonal skills to establish genuine and equal-status friendship with at least one person

## Long-Term Goals

Child/adolescent will:
- Interact with others using age appropriate and acceptable behavior within 4 months

## Short-Term Goals

Child/adolescent will:
- Participate in one-on-one and group activities without attempts to interrupt, intimidate, or manipulate others within 4 to 6 weeks
- Use age-appropriate skills in play activities and interpersonal exchanges within 4 to 8 weeks
- Describe a realistic sense of self using feedback from adults and peers within 4 to 8 weeks

---

▲ NANDA International accepted; ● In addition to NANDA International

## Interventions and Rationales

| Intervention | Rationale |
|---|---|
| 1. Use one-on-one relationship to engage the client in a working relationship. | 1. The client needs positive role models for healthy identification. |
| 2. Monitor for negative behaviors and identify maladaptive interaction patterns. | 2. Negative behaviors are identified and targeted to be replaced with age-appropriate social skills. |
| 3. Intervene early, give feedback and alternative ways to handle the situation. | 3. Children learn from feedback; early intervention prevents rejection by peers and provides immediate ways to cope. |
| 4. Use therapeutic play to teach social skills such as sharing, cooperation, realistic competition, and manners. | 4. Learning new ways to interact with others through play allows the development of satisfying friendships and self-esteem. |
| 5. Use role playing, stories, therapeutic games, and the like to practice skills. | 5. Solidifies new skills in safe environment. |
| 6. Help client find and develop a special friend; set up one-on-one play situations; be available for problem-solving peer relationship conflicts; role model social skills. | 6. The abilities to reality test, problem solve, and resolve conflicts in peer relationships are important competencies needed for interpersonal skills. |
| 7. Help the client develop equal-status peer relationships with reciprocity for honest, appropriate expression of feelings and needs. | 7. When people can identify personal feelings and needs, they are better prepared to use more direct communication rather than manipulation and/or intimidation. |

## CHRONIC LOW SELF-ESTEEM

Long-standing negative self-evaluation/feelings about self or self-capabilities

### Related To (Etiology)

- Disturbances in development of self-concept formation
- Disturbed relationship with parent/caregiver (lack of trust, abuse, neglect, conflicts, inadequate role models, disorganized family system)
- Negative feedback for failure to perform expected roles (academic, work-related, interpersonal) or achieve desired skills
- Being targeted by peers for rejection or abuse

### As Evidenced By
### (Assessment Findings/Diagnostic Cues)

- ▲ Self-negating verbalization.
- ▲ Lacks initiative to try new things and is fearful in new situations.
- ▲ Expresses feelings of shame, doubt, and/or guilt.
- Has unrealistic, overvalued appraisal of self-worth (grandiosity).
- Uses defense mechanisms (denial, rationalization, projection, reaction formation) to protect against threats to self-esteem.
- Uses manipulation or intimidation.
- Presents self as dependent and/or helpless.
- Discounts positive feedback.
- Overly sensitive to negative feedback

### Outcome Criteria

- Develop cognitive and emotional competencies needed for self-concept development

---

▲ NANDA International accepted; • In addition to NANDA International

## Long-Term Goals

Child/adolescent will:
- Participate in three new activities and new situations with relative comfort
- Identify four positive personal attributes
- Develop genuine, positive self-regard based on a more realistic appraisal of personal abilities/talents within 2 months

## Short-Term Goals

Child/adolescent will:
- Recognize when feeling threatened in unfamiliar situations and seek adult help in reducing anxiety and enhancing self-esteem within 2 to 4 weeks
- Demonstrate ways to cope with new situations using reality testing, problem solving, and positive affirmations within 4 to 8 weeks
- Identify realistic goals and start to develop desired skills/abilities that will increase self-esteem within 2 to 8 weeks
- Name two things he/she likes about self within 1 week
- Use social skills to develop rewarding peer relationships within 4 to 8 weeks

## Interventions and Rationales

| Intervention | Rationale |
|---|---|
| 1. Give "unconditional positive regard" without reinforcing negative behaviors. | 1. The client often sets up situations in which the behavior brings rejection and further confirms the lack of self-worth. |
| 2. Reinforce the client's self-worth with time and attention. | 2. Giving one-on-one time or attention in group activity confirms the client's self-worth. |
| 3. Help the client identify positive qualities and accomplishments. | 3. An accurate appraisal of accomplishments can help dispel unrealistic expectations. |
| 4. Help the client identify behaviors needing changing and set realistic goals. | 4. To change, the client needs goals and knowledge of new behaviors. |

| Intervention | Rationale |
|---|---|
| 5. Use a behavior modification program that rewards the client for trying new behaviors and evaluates results. | 5. Rewarding the client's efforts will increase the positive behaviors and foster the development of self-esteem. |

## IMPAIRED PARENTING

Inability of the primary caregiver to create, maintain, or regain an environment that promotes the optimum growth and development of the child

### Related To (Etiology)

▲ Physical illness (impaired neurologic development or dysfunction)
▲ Attention-deficit/hyperactivity disorder
▲ Lack of parent/caregiver fit with child
▲ Lack of knowledge about parenting or the special needs of the child
▲ Role strain or overload (multiple stressors)
▲ Mental or physical illness
● Constraints of child's birth temperament
● Disturbance in parent/care-giver attachment or bonding with the child

### As Evidenced By
### (Assessment Findings/Diagnostic Cues)

● Behavioral disorder
● Poor cognitive development
● Inability to control child
● Disturbed relationship between parent/caregiver and child (lack of trust, abuse, neglect, conflicts, inadequate role models, disorganized family system)
● Unrealistic expectations of self or the child

---

▲ NANDA International accepted; ● In addition to NANDA International

## Outcome Criteria

• Parent/caregiver has the resources to help client reach his or her age-related potential

## Long-Term Goals

Parent/caregiver will:
• Learn the appropriate parenting skills to deal with the client's individual problematic behavior within 3 months

## Short-Term Goals

Parent/caregiver will:
• Participate in the client's therapeutic program within 1 to 2 weeks
• Increase knowledge of normal growth and development, the client's diagnosis, medications, and parenting skills needed within 2 to 6 weeks
• Set realistic, age-appropriate behavioral goals for client when at home within 4 weeks
• Learn at least four new skills that will help provide client's biologic and psychosocial needs when at home within 2 to 4 weeks
• Learn the skills necessary to facilitate the development of client's competencies and coping skills when at home within 4 to 6 weeks
• Develop a support system to assist them with parenting within 4 to 6 weeks
• Use available resources to advocate for the client's needs within 2 to 4 weeks

## Interventions and Rationales

| Intervention | Rationale |
|---|---|
| 1. Explore the impact of the problematic behavior on the life of the family. | 1. Helps nurse understand the parent/caregiver situation. Feeling understood and supported can help foster an alliance. |
| 2. Assess the parent/caregiver's level of knowledge of growth and development, and parenting skills. | 2. Problem identification and analysis of learning needs is necessary before intervention begins. |

| Intervention | Rationale |
|---|---|
| 3. Assess the parent/caregiver's understanding of the diagnosis, treatment, and medications. | 3. Knowledge will increase the parent/caregiver participation, motivation, and satisfaction. |
| 4. Help the parent/caregiver identify the client's biologic and psychosocial needs. | 4. Adequate parenting involves being able to identify client's actual age-appropriate needs. |
| 5. Involve the parent in identifying a realistic plan for how these needs will be met when the client is at home. | 5. Parents/caregivers have the opportunity to learn the skills necessary to meet the client's needs. |
| 6. Work with the parent/caregiver to set behavioral goals; help set realistic goals for when the client is at home. | 6. Mutually set goals provide continuity and keep the client from using splitting or manipulation to sabotage treatment. |
| 7. Teach behavior modification techniques; give parent/caregiver support in using them and evaluating effectiveness. | 7. Education and follow-up support is the key to a successful treatment program. |
| 8. Assess the parent/caregiver support system; use referrals to establish additional supports. | 8. Self-help groups and special programs such as respite care can increase the caregiver ability to cope. |
| 9. Give information on legal rights and available resources that can assist in advocating for child services. | 9. Parent/caregiver frequently lacks information on how to secure services for the child. |

# Pervasive Developmental Disorders

Pervasive developmental disorders are characterized by their severe and pervasive impairment in reciprocal social interaction and communication skills. The four subtypes of pervasive developmental disorders are autistic, Asperger's, Rett's, and childhood disintegrative disorders. These disorders are usually evident in the first years of life and might be associated with some degree of mental retardation (APA, 2000).

## ASSESSMENT

### Autistic Disorder

Predominant features include markedly abnormal or impaired development in social interaction and communication. The impairment in reciprocal social interaction and communication skills is gross and sustained (APA, 2000).

Autistic disorder is usually recognized before the age of 3. What is most notable is the restrictive, repetitive, and stereotypic patterns of behavior, interests, and activities.

The prognosis is generally poor. Few can live and work independently; approximately 33% can achieve partial independence.

### Presenting Signs and Symptoms

*Impairment in Social Interactions*

- Lack of responsiveness to and interest in others
- Lack of eye-to-eye contact and facial responses
- Indifference to or aversion to affection and physical contact
- Failure to cuddle or be comforted
- Lack of seeking or sharing enjoyment, interest, or achievement with others
- Failure to develop cooperative play or imaginative play with peers
- Lack of friendships

*Impairment in Communication and Imaginative Activity*

- Language delay or total absence of language
- Immature grammatic structure; pronoun reversal; inability to name objects

- Stereotyped or repetitive use of language (echolalia, idio-syncratic words, inappropriate high-pitched squealing/giggling, repetitive phrases, sing-song speech quality)
- Lack of spontaneous make-believe play or imaginative play
- Failure to imitate

### Markedly Restricted, Stereotyped Patterns of Behavior, Interests, and Activities

- Rigid adherence to routines and rituals with catastrophic reactions to minor changes in them or changes made in the environment (moving furniture)
- Stereotyped and repetitive motor mannerisms (hand/finger flapping, clapping, rocking, dipping, swaying, spinning, dancing around and walking on toes, head banging, or hand biting)
- Preoccupation with certain objects (buttons, parts of the body, wheels on toys) that is abnormal in intensity or focus
- Preoccupation with certain repetitive activities (pouring water/sand, spinning wheels on toys, twirling string) that is abnormal in intensity or focus

## Asperger's Disorder

This disorder differs from autistic disorder in that it appears to have a later onset and there is no significant delay in cognitive and language development (APA, 2000). Mental retardation is not usually observed. This is a continuum and a lifelong disorder.

### Presenting Signs and Symptoms

- Recognized later than autistic disorder.
- No significant delays in cognitive and language development.
- Severe and sustained impairment in social interactions.
- Development of restricted, repetitive patterns of behavior, interests, and activities resembling autistic disorder.
- Might have delayed motor-development milestones with clumsiness noted in preschool.
- Social interaction problems more noticeable when child enters school.
- Problems with empathy and modulating social relationships might continue into adulthood.

# Rett's Disorder

This disorder differs from autistic and Asperger's disorders in that it has been observed only in females, with the onset before the age of 4 (APA, 2000). Rett's disorder is usually associated with profound mental retardation.

## Presenting Signs and Symptoms

- Development of multiple deficits after a normal prenatal and postnatal period of development
- Head circumference is normal at birth but growth rate slows between the 5th and 48th months of life
- Persistent and progressive loss of previously acquired hand skills between the 5th and 30th months of life
- Development of stereotyped hand movements (hand-wringing and hand-washing)
- Problems with coordination of gait and trunk movements
- Severe psychomotor retardation
- Severe problems with expressive and receptive language
- Loss of interest in social interactions but might develop this interest later in childhood or adolescence

# Childhood Disintegrative Disorder

This disorder is marked by regression in multiple areas of functioning following a period of at least 2 years of normal development (APA, 2000). The onset can be abrupt or insidious. This disorder is usually associated with severe mental retardation.

## Presenting Signs and Symptoms

- Marked regression in multiple areas of function after at least 2 years of normal development
- Loss of previously acquired skills in at least two areas (communication, social relationships, play, adaptive behavior, motor skills, and bowel/bladder control)
- Deficits in communication and social interactions (same as autistic disorder)
- Stereotyped behaviors (same as autistic disorder)
- Loss of skills reaches a plateau followed by limited improvement

## Assessment Questions

### *Pervasive Developmental Disorders (for the Parent or Caregiver)*

*The nurse uses a variety of therapeutic techniques to obtain the answers to the following questions. Use your discretion and decide which questions are appropriate to complete your assessment.*

1. Describe the child's temperament and adjustment as a newborn.
2. Describe any unusual responses to stimuli. (sounds, lights, or being touched)
3. When did the child develop a social smile? Become responsive to words and physical contact?
4. Can the child be comforted? How does the child comfort self?
5. Does the child show interest in others? Concern when others are hurt?
6. When did speech develop? Unusual characteristics? (in rate, rhythm, tone, inflection pattern, echolalia, made-up words)
7. Describe any unusual behaviors. (hand/finger flapping, clapping, rocking, dipping, swaying, spinning, dancing around, and walking on toes)
8. What, if any, behaviors cause self-injury? (head banging, slapping, or hand biting)
9. What are the child's favorite toys? Any preoccupation with round or shiny objects, objects that can spin or move, or parts of the body?
10. What is the child's favorite activity? Any preoccupation with repetitive activities? (pouring water/sand, spinning/twirling objects, chewing or eating inedible items)
11. How does the child respond to limit setting? Tantrum behaviors?
12. How does the child respond to changes? (routines, schedules, activities or rituals, changes in furniture arrangements)
13. How well does the child do at self-care activities? (dressing, toileting, eating)
14. Have previously learned skills or abilities changed or been lost?

### Assessment Guidelines
*Pervasive Developmental Disorders*

1. Assess for developmental spurts, lags, uneven development, or loss of previously acquired abilities. (Use baby books/diaries, photographs, films/videotapes. First-time mothers might not be aware of development lags, and family members might need to be consulted.)
2. Assess the quality of the relationship between the child and parent/caregiver for evidence of bonding, anxiety, tension, and difficulty-of-fit between the parents' and child's temperaments.
3. Be aware that children with behavioral and developmental problems are at risk for abuse.

# NURSING DIAGNOSES WITH INTERVENTIONS

## Discussion of Potential Nursing Diagnoses

The child with pervasive developmental disorders has severe impairments in social interactions and communications skills. Often these are accompanied by stereotyped behavior, interests, and activities. The severity of the impairment is demonstrated by the child's lack of responsiveness to or interest in others, lack of empathy or sharing with peers, and lack of cooperative or imaginative play with peers. Therefore, **Impaired Social Interaction** is almost always present. Language delay or absence of language and the unusual stereotyped or repetitive use of language is another area for nursing interventions. Therefore, **Impaired Verbal Communication** and **Delayed Growth and Development** (language delay) are useful nursing diagnoses. Stereotyped and repetitive motor behaviors can include behaviors such as head banging, face slapping, and hand biting. The child's apparent indifference to pain can result in serious self-injury, and, therefore, **Risk for Self-Mutilation** and/or **Risk for Injury** can become a priority. If the child's rigid adherence to specific routines and rituals is disrupted, the child might have a catastrophic reaction, such as severe temper tantrums or rage reactions, leading to **Risk for**

**Self-Directed Violence or Risk for Other-Directed Violence**. The child's lack of interest in activities outside of self and the frequent disregard for bodily needs interfere with the development of a personal identity, and, therefore, **Disturbed Personal Identity** might be an appropriate nursing diagnosis.

## Overall Guidelines for Nursing Interventions
### Pervasive Developmental Disorders

Help the child reach his or her full potential by fostering developmental competencies and coping skills:

1. Increase the child's interest in reciprocal social interactions.
2. Foster the development of social skills.
3. Facilitate the expression of appropriate emotional responses, including the development of trust, empathy, shame, remorse, anger, pride, independence, joy, and enthusiasm.
4. Foster the development of reciprocal communication, especially language skills.
5. Provide for the development of psychomotor skills in play and activities of daily living (ADLs).
6. Facilitate the development of cognitive skills (attention, memory, cause and effect, reality testing, decision making, and problem solving).
7. Foster the development of self-concepts (identity, self-awareness, body image, and self-esteem).
8. Foster the development of self-control, including controlling impulses and tolerating frustration and the delay of gratification.

## Selected Nursing Diagnoses and Nursing Care Plans

### IMPAIRED SOCIAL INTERACTION

Insufficient or excessive quantity or ineffective quality of social exchange

## Related To (Etiology)

▲ Self-concept disturbance (immaturity or developmental deviation)
▲ Absence of available significant others/peers
● Impaired neurologic development or dysfunction
● Disturbance in response to external stimuli
● Disturbance in attachment/bonding with the parent/caregiver

## As Evidence By
## (Assessment Findings/Diagnostic Cues)

▲ Dysfunctional interaction with peers
● Lack of responsiveness to or interest in others (eye contact, facial expressions, verbalizations)
● Lack of bonding or affectional ties to parental figures (indifference or aversion to physical contact)
● Lack of interest or ability to play and share with peers
● Lack of empathy or concern for others

## Outcome Criteria

• Child initiates actions with peers and trusted friends

## Long-Term Goals

Child will:
• Participate in at least four activities that reflect reciprocal social interactions within 1 year

## Short-Term Goals

Child will:
• Seek out nurse/caregiver for activities/ADLs and for comfort when distressed within 1 to 3 months
• Show interest and begin to participate in play activities with others, especially peers, within 2 to 6 months
• Use at least two social skills to initiate contact with peers at the same developmental level within 6 to 12 months

---

▲ NANDA International accepted; ● In addition to NANDA International

*Interventions and Rationales*

| Intervention | Rationale |
|---|---|
| 1. Use one-on-one interaction to engage the client in a working alliance. | 1. Assigning the same primary nurse who will be a parental surrogate can promote attachment. |
| 2. Monitor for signs of anxiety/distress. Intervene early to provide comfort. | 2. Anticipating need for help in managing stress enhances the client's feelings of security. |
| 3. Provide emotional support and guidance for ADLs and other activities; use a system of rewards for attempts and successes. | 3. Learning occurs through meaningful social interactions involving imitation, modeling, feedback, and reinforcement. |
| 4. Set up play situations starting with play with parallel peers and moving toward cooperative play. | 4. Learning to play with peers is sequential. |
| 5. Help the client find a special friend. | 5. Having a special friend enhances learning experience. |
| 6. Role model social interaction skills (interest, empathy, sharing, waiting, and required language). | 6. Facilitates the development of needed social/emotional skills. |
| 7. Reward attempts to interact and play with peers and the use of appropriate emotional expressions. | 7. Behaviors that are rewarded are repeated. |
| 8. Role play situations that involve conflicts in social interactions to teach reality testing, cause and effect, and problem solving. | 8. These cognitive skills are needed for successful social/emotional reciprocity. |

## IMPAIRED VERBAL COMMUNICATION

Decreased, delayed, or absent ability to receive, process, transmit, and use a system of symbols

### Related To (Etiology)

▲ Physiologic conditions
▲ Alteration of central nervous system
● Impaired neurologic development or dysfunction
● Disturbance in attachment/bonding with the parent/caregiver

### As Evidenced By
(Assessment Findings/Diagnostic Cues)

● Language delay or total absence of language
● Immature grammatic structure; pronoun reversal; inability to name objects
● Stereotyped or repetitive use of language (echolalia, idiosyncratic words, inappropriate high-pitched squealing/giggling, repetitive phrases, sing-song speech quality)
● Lack of response to communication attempts by others

### Outcome Criteria

● Communicate in words/gestures that are understood by others

### Long-Term Goals

Child will:
● Communicate to parent/caregiver and peers at least four basic needs (hunger, thirst, fatigue, pain), verbally and/or through gestures and body language

---

▲ NANDA International accepted; ● In addition to NANDA International

## Short-Term Goals

Child will:
- Communicate through eye contact, facial expressions, and other nonverbal gestures within 1 month
- Attempt to use language and begin to communicate with words within 5 to 6 months
- Increase language skills needed for social and emotional reciprocal interactions within 6 to 8 months
- Use language or gestures to identify self, others, objects, feelings, needs, plans, and desires within 12 months

## Interventions and Rationales

| Intervention | Rationale |
|---|---|
| 1. Use one-on-one interactions to engage the client in nonverbal play. | 1. The nurse enters the client's world in a nonthreatening interaction to form a trusting relationship. |
| 2. Recognize subtle cues indicating the client is paying attention or attempting to communicate. | 2. Cues are often difficult to recognize (glancing out of the corner of the eye). |
| 3. Describe for the client what is happening, and put into words what the client might be experiencing. | 3. Naming objects and describing actions, thoughts, and feelings helps the client to use symbolic language. |
| 4. Encourage vocalizations with sound games and songs. | 4. Children learn through play and enjoyable activities. |
| 5. Identify desired behaviors and reward them (e.g., hugs, treats, tokens, points, or food). | 5. Behaviors that are rewarded will increase in frequency. Desire for food is a powerful incentive in modifying behavior. |
| 6. Use names frequently, and encourage the use of correct pronouns (e.g., I, me, he). | 6. Problems with self-identification and pronoun reversal are common. |

| Intervention | Rationale |
|---|---|
| 7. Encourage verbal communication with peers during play activities using role modeling, feedback, and reinforcement. | 7. Play is the normal medium for learning in a child's development. |
| 8. Increase verbal inter-action with parents and siblings by teaching them how to facilitate language development. | 8. Education and emotional support help parents and siblings to become more therapeutic in their inter-actions with the client. |

## RISK FOR SELF-MUTILATION

At risk for deliberate self-injurious behavior causing tissue damage with the intent of causing nonfatal injury to attain relief of tension

### Related To (Etiology)

- Impaired neurologic development or dysfunction
- Need for painful stimuli to increase opiate levels and reduce tension
- Rage reactions and aggression turned toward self
- Lack of impulse control and the ability to tolerate frustration

### As Evidenced By
### (Assessment Findings/Diagnostic Cues)

- History of self-injuries (head banging, biting, scratch-ing, hair pulling) when frustrated or angry
- Old scars or new areas of tissue damage
- Self-injurious tantrums when changes are made in routines, rituals, or the environment, or when asked to end a pleasurable activity

---

▲ NANDA International accepted; ● In addition to NANDA International

## Outcome Criteria

- Demonstrate new behaviors and skills to cope with anxiety and feelings

## Long-Term Goals

Child will:
- Be free of self-inflicted injury

## Short-Term Goals

Child will:
- Respond to a parent or surrogate's limits on self-injurious behaviors within 1 to 6 months
- Seek help when anxiety and tension rise within 1 to 6 months
- Express feelings and describe tensions verbally and/or with noninjurious body language within 6 months to 1 year
- Use appropriate play activities for the release of anxiety and tension within 1 to 6 months

## Interventions and Rationales

| Intervention | Rationale |
|---|---|
| 1. Monitor the client's behavior for cues of rising anxiety. | 1. Behavioral cues signal increasing anxiety. |
| 2. Determine emotional and situational triggers. | 2. Knowledge of triggers is used in planning ways to prevent or manage outbursts. |
| 3. Intervene early with verbal comments or limits and/or removal from the situation. | 3. Potential outbursts can be be defused through early recognition, verbal interventions, or removal. |
| 4. Give plenty of notice when having to change routines or rituals or end pleasurable activities. | 4. Children often react to change with catastrophic reactions and need time to adjust. |
| 5. Provide support for the recognition of feelings, reality testing, impulse control. | 5. These competencies are often underdeveloped in these children. |

| Intervention | Rationale |
|---|---|
| 6. If the client does not respond to verbal interventions, use therapeutic holding. Some might need special restraints (helmets, mittens, special padding). | 6. Therapeutic holding reassures the client that the adult is in control; feelings of security can become feelings of comfort and affection. |
| 7. Help the client connect feelings and anxiety to self-injurious behaviors. | 7. Self-control is enhanced through understanding the relationship between feelings and behaviors. |
| 8. Help the client develop ways to express feelings and reduce anxiety verbally and through play activities. Use various types of motor and imaginative play (e.g., swinging, tumbling, role playing, drawing, singing). | 8. Methods for modulating and directing the expression of emotions and anxiety must be learned to control destructive impulses. |

## DISTURBED PERSONAL IDENTITY

Inability to distinguish between self and nonself

*Related To (Etiology)*

- ▲ Biochemical imbalance
- ● Impaired neurologic development or dysfunction
- ● Failure to develop attachment behaviors resulting in fixation at autistic phase of development
- ● Interrupted or uncompleted separation/individuation process resulting in extreme separation anxiety

▲ NANDA International accepted; ● In addition to NANDA International

## As Evidenced By
## (Assessment Findings/Diagnostic Cues)

- Seemingly unaware of or uninterested in others or their activities
- Unable to identify parts of the body or bodily sensations (enuresis, encopresis)
- Fails to imitate others or not able to stop imitating other's actions or words (echolalia, echopraxis)
- Fails to distinguish parent/caregiver as a whole person, instead relates to body parts (e.g., takes person's hand and places it on doorknob)
- Becomes distressed by bodily contact with others
- Spends long periods of time in self-stimulating behaviors (self-touching, sucking, rocking)
- Needs ritualistic behaviors and sameness to control anxiety
- Has extreme distress reactions to changes in routines or the environment
- Cannot tolerate being separated from parent/caregiver

## Outcome Criteria

- Demonstrate recognition of self-boundaries and being separate from others

## Long-Term Goals

Child will:
- Adjust to changes in activities and the environment within 9 months

## Short-Term Goals

Child will:
- Seek comfort and physical contact from others within 1 to 2 months
- Relate to caregiver by name with eye contact and verbal requests within 6 months
- Recognize body parts, body boundaries, and sexual identity within 6 months

---

▲ NANDA International accepted; ● In addition to NANDA International

- Show an interest in the activities of others and tolerate their presence within 3 to 6 months
- Spend more time in purposeful activities rather than rituals and self-stimulating activities in 2 to 6 months
- Recognize body sensations (pain, hunger, fatigue, elimination needs) within 2 to 6 months
- Express a full range of feelings within 4 to 6 months
- Recognize the feelings and activities of others as separate within 6 months
- Adjust to changes in activities and the environment within 5 to 9 months

## Interventions and Rationales

| Intervention | Rationale |
|---|---|
| 1. Use one-on-one interaction to engage the client in a safe relationship with nurse/caregiver. | 1. A consistent caregiver provides for the development of trust needed for a sense of safety and security. |
| 2. Use names and descriptions of others to reinforce their separateness. | 2. Consistent reinforcement will help break into the client's autistic world. |
| 3. Draw the client's attention to the activities of others and events that are happening in the environment. | 3. Interrupts the client's self-absorption and stimulates outside interests. |
| 4. Limit self-stimulating and ritualistic behaviors by providing alternative play activities or by providing comfort when stressed. | 4. Redirecting the client's attention to favorite or new activities, or giving comfort, reduces anxiety. |
| 5. Foster self-concept development; reinforce identity, sexual identity, and body boundaries through drawing, stories, and play activities. | 5. Learning body parts and sexual identity is necessary and fun in play activities. |

| Intervention | Rationale |
|---|---|
| 6. Help client distinguish body sensations and how to meet bodily needs by picking up on cues and using ADLs to teach self-care. | 6. The lack of self-awareness contributes to problems with self-care, especially toileting. |
| 7. Provide play opportunities for the client that identify the feelings of others (stories, puppet play, peer interactions). | 7. Consistent feedback about the feelings of others helps with self-differentiation and the development of empathy. |

# MEDICAL TREATMENTS

## Psychopharmacology

Most likely, the majority of emotional suffering experienced by children and adolescents is related to situational stress and best treated through a variety of therapeutic modalities. However, it is also becoming increasingly apparent that many major mental diseases have their origin in childhood (Preston, et al 2005).

Medications that target specific symptoms can make a decided difference in the family's ability to cope and their quality of life, and can enhance the child's or adolescent's optimal potential for growth. Medication use should be closely supervised, especially SSRIs and those used to treat ADHD (Table 4-2).

## Psychosocial Treatment for Child and Adolescent Disorders

Treatment of childhood and adolescent disorders requires a multimodal approach in most instances. Close work with schools, the availability of remediation services, and the incorporation of behavior modification techniques should all be part of the intervention.

Table 4-2 **Psychopharmacology of Child and Adolescent Disorders and Symptoms**

| Disorder and/or Symptoms | Type of Drug | Examples and Comments |
|---|---|---|
| Pervasive developmental disorders | • Antipsychotics | Risperidone (Risperdal) can help with tantrums, aggression, and self-injurious behavior. |
| | • Selective serotonin reuptake inhibitors (SSRIs) | |
| Autistic disorder (AD) | • Antipsychotics | Haloperidol (Haldol) can reduce irritability and labile affect. |
| | • Propranolol | Inderal reduces rage outbursts, aggression, and severe anxiety. |
| | • SSRI | Clomipramine (Anafranil) might help treat anger and compulsive behavior. |
| Attention-deficit/hyper-activity disorder (ADHD) | • Stimulants (first line) | **Methylphenidate**<br>• Short-acting (Ritalin, Methylin) (used less often than in the past)<br>• Intermediate-acting (Ritalin SR/LA Metadate ER)<br>• Long-acting (Concerta, Methadate CD)<br>**Amphetamine**<br>• Short-acting (Dexedrine, Dextrostat)<br>• Intermediate-acting (Adderall, Dexedrine Spansule)<br>• Long acting (Adderall-XR*) |
| | • Antidepressants (second line) | Bupropion (Wellbutrin), and atomoxetine (Strattera) |
| | • Alpha-adrenergic agonists | For example, Clonidine (Catapres) can be used for aggressive-ness, impulsivity, and hyperactivity in ADHD clients. |

*Continued*

* Not yet FDA approved

Table 4-2 **Psychopharmacology of Child and Adolescent Disorders and Symptoms—cont'd**

| Disorder and/or Symptoms | Type of Drug | Examples and Comments |
|---|---|---|
| **Conduct disorders** | Antipsychotics<br>Stimulants<br>Antidepressants<br>Mood stabilizers<br>Alpha-adrenergic agonists | Carbamazepine (Tegretol)<br>Clonidine (Catapres) might help with impulsive and disordered behaviors. |
| **Anxiety disorders**<br>• Panic and school phobia | Antidepressants (TCAs, monoamine oxidase inhibitors [MAOIs], SSRIs)<br>Benzodiazepines | TCA: imipramine (Tofranil) commonly used.<br><br>Alprazolam for short-term use. |
| • Obsessive-compulsive disorder (OCD) | Antidepressants (SSRIs)<br>Atypical anxiolytic | Clomipramine (Anafranil)<br>Buspirone (BuSpar) used as adjunct treatment in refractory OCD |

| | | |
|---|---|---|
| • Separation anxiety disorder | Antidepressants (TCAs, SSRIs) | TCA: imipramine (Tofranil), protriptyline (Vivactil) |
| • Social phobia | TCAs | SSRI: fluoxetine (Prozac) |
| | | Protriptyline (Vivactil) |
| | Antianxiety | Buspirone (BuSpar) |
| | Antianxiety | Buspirone (BuSpar) |
| • Posttraumatic stress disorder (PTSD) | Atypical antipsychotic SSRIs | Risperidone (Risperdal) being used to control the flashbacks and aggression in PTSD |
| **Anxiety symptoms** | | |
| • Insomnia | Antihistamines | Diphenhydramine (Benadryl) |
| **Depressive symptoms** | Major depression and dysthymia | |
| | • SSRIs | |
| | • Atypical antidepressants | Venlafaxine |
| With: | | |
| Sleep disorders | | Trazodone |
| Bipolar depression | | Bupropion |
| **Psychotic symptoms** | Antipsychotics | Risperdal, Zyprexa |

Therapies include cognitive-behavioral therapies. Effective behavioral techniques for supporting desirable behaviors include:
- Positive reinforcement
- Time out
- Token economy—earning points for privileges/rewards
- Response costs—withdrawing privileges based on undesirable behavior

Other therapies including social skills groups, family therapy, parent training in behavioral techniques, and individual therapy focused on esteem issues have all been found to be useful. Skills training might focus on a variety of areas, depending on the child's or adolescent's presenting symptoms. For example, some children need to learn basic ADLs, others have difficulty with their impulse control and frustration tolerance, and those with anxiety disorders might benefit from anxiety-reduction skills. Many children and adolescents benefit from a variety of social skills (problem solving, decision making, initiating and maintaining contacts with peers) that will help them negotiate satisfying and productive relationships and friendships in the outside world. Many young people suffer from severe symptoms of depression, and although medication might be immediately useful, family and individual therapies should be made a pivotal part of the patient's treatment. Rarely, if ever, is medication alone treatment of choice.

## NURSE AND PARENT/CAREGIVER RESOURCES

## BOOKS FOR PARENTS

Barkley, R.A. (1995). *Taking charge of ADHD: The complete authoritative guide for parents.* New York: Guilford Press.

Barkley, R.A., & Benton, C.M. (1998). *Your defiant child: 8 Steps to better behavior.* New York: Guilford Press.

Burt, S., & Perlis, L. (1998). *Parents as mentors.* Rocklin, CA: Prima Publishing.

Gardner, R.A. (1997). *Understanding children.* Northvale, NJ: Jason Aronson.

Greenspan, S.J., & Salmon, J. (1995). *The challenging child: Understanding, raising and enjoying five different types of children*. Reading, PA: Perseus Books.

Maurice, C., Green, G., & Luce, S. (1996). *Behavioral interventions for your children with autism: A manual for parents and professionals*. Austin, TX: PRO-ED.

Powers, M.D. (Ed.). (1993). *A parent's guide to autism*. Rockville, MD: Woodbine House.

Schaefer, C.E. (1991). *Teach your child to behave*. New York: Penguin.

Witkin, G. (1999). *Kid stress: Effective strategies parents can teach kids for school, family, peers, the world and everything*. New York: Viking Penguin.

## REFERENCES FOR NURSES

Cittone, R.A, & Madonna, J.M. (1997). *Play therapy with sexually abused children*. New York: Jason Aronson.

Greenspan, S.I., & Wiedet, S. (1998). *The child with special needs: Encouraging intellectual and emotional growth*. Reading, PA: Perseus Books.

Kaduson, H. (1997). Play therapy for children with attention-deficit hyperactivity disorder. In H. Kaduson, D. Cangelosi, & C.E. Schaefer (Eds.). *The playing cure: Individualized play therapy for specific childhood problems*. New York: Jason Aronson.

Kaduson, H., & Schaefer, C.E. (1997). *101 Favorite play therapy techniques*. New York: Jason Aronson.

King, N.J; & Ollendick, T.H. (1997). Treatment of childhood phobias. *J Child Psychol Psychiatr 38*, 389–400.

Maurice, C., Green, G., & Luce, S. (1996). *Behavioral interventions for your children with autism: A manual for parents and professionals*, Austin, TX: PRO-ED.

Pfefferbaum, B. (Ed.). (1998). Stress in children. *Child Adolesc Psychiatr Clin North Am 7*(1).

Shelby, J.S. (1997). Rubble, disruption, and tears: Helping young survivors of natural disasfer. In H. Kaduson, D. Cangelosi, & C.E. Schaefer (Eds.), *The playing cure: Individualized play therapy for specific childhood problems*. New York: Jason Aronson.

Tait, D., & Depta, T. (1997). Play group therapy for bereaved children. In N.B. Webb (Ed.), *Helping bereaved children*. New York: Guilford Press.

## INTERNET SITES

**Autism Society of America Home Page**
http://www.autism-society.org

**Autism Resources**
http://www.autism-resources.com

**Children and Adults with Attention
  Deficit/Hyperactivity Disorder**
http://www.chadd.org

**ADD Medical Treatment Center of Santa Clara Valley**
http://www.addmtc.com

**Conduct Disorders Support Site**
http://www.conductdisorders.com

**Anxiety Disorders in Children and Adults**
http://www.algy.com/anxiety/children.html

**American Academy of Child & Adolescent Psychiatry**
http://www.aacap.org

**Association of Child and Adolescent Psychiatric Nurses**
http://www.ispn-psych.org/html/acapn.html

# CHAPTER 5

# Anxiety and Anxiety Disorders

## OVERVIEW

### Anxiety

Anxiety is a normal response to threatening situations. Anxiety can be a positive motivating factor in our lives. For example, the anxiety a student experiences before taking a test gives the student help with awareness and sharpens focus. Anxiety *does* become a problem when it:

- Interferes with adaptive behavior
- Causes physical symptoms
- Becomes intolerable to the individual

**Anxiety** is conceptualized on four levels, mild (+), moderate (++), severe (+++), and panic (++++). When working with people who are anxious, it is helpful to distinguish between these levels of anxiety, primarily because the interventions are different for mild to moderate levels of anxiety versus severe to panic levels of anxiety. Integral to all discussions of anxiety are some of the defenses against anxiety. Please refer to Appendix E.

Following a discussion of the various anxiety disorders and nursing assessment of symptoms seen in anxiety disorders, nursing interventions are presented that are effective for clients with moderate levels of anxiety, and for clients with severe to panic levels of anxiety. The rest of the chapter is devoted to targeting common problem areas (nursing diagnoses) and identifying useful nursing actions for these problem areas.

## Anxiety Disorders

Anxiety disorders are often the most common of all psychiatric disorders and result in considerable distress and functional impairment. Anxiety disorders are a group of disorders that have as their primary symptom anxiety levels that are so high that they interfere with personal, occupational, or social functioning. Anxiety disorders produce symptoms that range from mild to severe, and they tend to be persistent and are often disabling. People often suffer from more than one anxiety disorder and anxiety and depression often occur together. Physicians and nurses need to be alerted to the fact that anxiety can be a symptom of a physical disease, medical problem, or substance use problem. **Therefore, medical causes and drug-induced anxiety must be ruled out before a diagnosis of anxiety disorder can be made.**

People who have anxiety disorders are usually treated in the community setting. Rarely is hospitalization needed unless the client is suicidal or the symptoms are severely out of control (e.g., client is employing self-mutilating behaviors). The best treatment for anxiety disorders is often a combination of medication and therapy (cognitive/behavioral). In the last section of this chapter, we discuss medications and therapies that seem to prove most effective for each of the anxiety disorders. Anxiety disorders include panic disorder (with or without agoraphobia), phobias, obsessive-compulsive disorder (OCD), generalized anxiety disorder (GAD), and stress disorders.

*Panic Disorder (with or without Agoraphobia)* A diagnosis of panic disorder is made in the presence or history of recurrent, unexpected panic attacks that do not have an underlying medical or chemical etiology. A **panic attack** involves extreme apprehension or fear, usually associated with feelings of impending doom or terror. During an attack, normal functioning is suspended, the peripheral field of vision is severely limited, and misinterpretations of reality might occur. Individuals experiencing panic attacks often have the terrifying belief that they are having a heart attack. These signs and symptoms can be mistaken for a heart attack by hospital personnel because the symptoms of a panic attack can be similar to those of a myocardial infarction (shortness of breath, chest pain, feelings of impending doom). Box 5-1 provides the signs and symptoms of a panic attack. Panic attacks can also be present in other anxiety disorders, including social phobia, simple phobia, and posttraumatic stress disorder (PTSD). Box 5-2 presents the *Diagnostic and Statistical Manual of Mental Disorders* (4th edition, text revision) (DSM-IV-TR) diagnost ic criteria for panic disorder.

**Agoraphobia** is frequently seen with panic disorder. Individuals who are agoraphobic avoid places or situations from which escape might be difficult or embarrassing, or where help might not be available if a panic attack occurred. Agoraphobia is a phobia and is discussed further under phobias. Approximately 67% of panic clients lose or quit their jobs because they can no longer tolerate traveling to their place of business. Approximately 20% of people with panic disorder attempt suicide (Weissman et al., 1989).

## Phobias

Phobias are irrational fears of an object or situation that persist although the person recognizes them as unreasonable. There are three categories of phobias: agoraphobia, social phobia, and specific phobia. See Box 5-3 for DSM-IV-TR diagnostic criteria for phobias.

## Obsessive-Compulsive Disorder

People with OCD have either *obsessions* (intrusive thoughts, impulses, or images) that break into their conscious awareness and are perceived as senseless and intrusive, *compulsions* (repetitive behaviors or mental acts that the person feels driven to perform in order to reduce distress or prevent a dreaded event or situation), or both. Common compulsions involve touching, counting, cleaning, and arranging things. People with OCD often present in a physician's office with a complaint of compulsive hand washing, compulsive cleanliness, or alopecia resulting from pulling out their hair (trichotillomania). Box 5-4 presents the DSM-IV-TR diagnostic criteria for OCD.

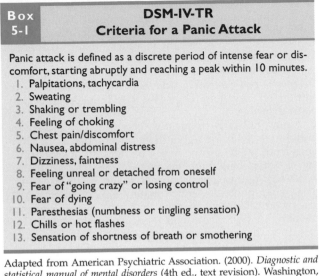

Box 5-1

# DSM-IV-TR
## Criteria for a Panic Attack

Panic attack is defined as a discrete period of intense fear or discomfort, starting abruptly and reaching a peak within 10 minutes.
1. Palpitations, tachycardia
2. Sweating
3. Shaking or trembling
4. Feeling of choking
5. Chest pain/discomfort
6. Nausea, abdominal distress
7. Dizziness, faintness
8. Feeling unreal or detached from oneself
9. Fear of "going crazy" or losing control
10. Fear of dying
11. Paresthesias (numbness or tingling sensation)
12. Chills or hot flashes
13. Sensation of shortness of breath or smothering

Adapted from American Psychiatric Association. (2000). *Diagnostic and statistical manual of mental disorders* (4th ed., text revision). Washington, DC: American Psychiatric Association, p. 432; reprinted with permission.

Box 5-2

# DSM-IV-TR
## Criteria for a Panic Disorder

1. Both a and b
   a. Recurrent episodes of panic attacks
   b. At least one of the attacks has been followed by 1 month (or more) of the following:
      • Persistent concern of having additional attacks
      • Worry about consequences ("going crazy," having a heart attack, losing control)
      • Significant change in behavior
2. Absence of agoraphobia = **Panic disorder without agoraphobia**
3. Presence of agoraphobia = **Panic disorder with agoraphobia**
4. Panic attacks are not due to a drug of abuse or medication, a general medical condition or another mental disorder such as a phobia, or posttraumatic stress disorder.

Adapted from American Psychiatric Association. (2000). *Diagnostic and statistical manual of mental disorders* (4th ed., text revision). Washington, DC: American Psychiatric Association, p. 440; reprinted with permission.

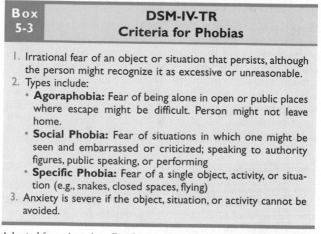

| Box 5-3 | DSM-IV-TR Criteria for Phobias |
| --- | --- |

1. Irrational fear of an object or situation that persists, although the person might recognize it as excessive or unreasonable.
2. Types include:
   • **Agoraphobia:** Fear of being alone in open or public places where escape might be difficult. Person might not leave home.
   • **Social Phobia:** Fear of situations in which one might be seen and embarrassed or criticized; speaking to authority figures, public speaking, or performing
   • **Specific Phobia:** Fear of a single object, activity, or situation (e.g., snakes, closed spaces, flying)
3. Anxiety is severe if the object, situation, or activity cannot be avoided.

Adapted from American Psychiatric Association. (2000). *Diagnostic and statistical manual of mental disorders* (4th ed., text revision). Washington, DC: American Psychiatric Association, pp. 449–450; reprinted with permission.

| Box 5-4 | DSM-IV-TR Criteria for Obsessive-Compulsive Disorder |
| --- | --- |

1. Either obsessions or compulsions:
   • Preoccupation with persistent, intrusive thoughts, impulses, or images (obsession) that cannot be ignored or suppressed, *or*
   • Repetitive behaviors or mental acts that the person feels driven to perform in order to reduce distress or prevent a dreaded event or situation (**compulsion**), but are not connected in a realistic way with what they are designed to neutralize or prevent.
2. Person knows the obsessions/compulsions are excessive and unreasonable.
3. The obsession/compulsion can cause increased distress and is time-consuming.

Adapted from American Psychiatric Association. (2000). *Diagnostic and statistical manual of mental disorders* (4th ed., text revision). Washington, DC: American Psychiatric Association, p. 462; reprinted with permission.

## Generalized Anxiety Disorder

People are diagnosed with GAD when they have chronic and excessive anxiety or worry most of the time during a 6-month period of time. Other symptoms include restlessness, fatigue, difficulty concentrating, irritability, muscle tension, and sleep problems. The symptoms cause the individual to have significant distress, and these individuals tend to have impairment in their social and occupational functioning. Box 5-5 presents the DSM-IV-TR diagnostic criteria for GAD.

## Stress Disorders

Two other disorders that are included in the anxiety disorders are **posttraumatic stress disorder (PTSD)** and **acute stress disorder (ASD)**. Both of these disorders follow exposure to an extremely traumatic event, usually outside of the range of normal experiences (e.g., natural disasters, crime-related events, prisoner of war, diagnosis of a life-threatening disease, rape). They also share similar symptoms:

- Reexperiencing the symptoms through dreams or images
- Reliving the event through flashbacks, illusions, hallucinations
- Marked symptoms of anxiety
  - Difficulty falling/staying asleep
  - Irritability/outbursts of anger
  - Difficulty concentrating
- Avoidance of stimuli associated with the trauma that could arouse memory of the trauma

The main difference is one of time. ASD lasts from 2 days to 4 weeks, and occurs within 4 weeks of the traumatic event. PTSD lasts for *more* than 1 month and might last for years. Boxes 5-6 and 5-7 present DSM-IV-TR diagnostic criteria for these two stress responses.

| Box 5-5 | **DSM-IV-TR Criteria for Generalized Anxiety Disorder** |
|---|---|

1. Excessive anxiety or worry that has predominated for a period of 6 months.
2. Uncontrollable worrying.
3. Anxiety and worry associated with three or more of the following symptoms **(only one item is required in children):**
   - Restlessness, keyed-up
   - Easily fatigued
   - Difficulty concentrating, mind goes blank
   - Irritability
   - Muscle tension
   - Sleep disturbance
4. Anxiety or worry or physical symptoms cause significant impairment in social, occupational, or other areas of important functioning.
5. The disturbance is not due to a substance, medical condition, or exclusively during a mood disorder, a psychotic disorder, or pervasive developmental disorder.

Adapted from American Psychiatric Association. (2000). *Diagnostic and statistical manual of mental disorders* (4th ed., text revision). Washington, DC: American Psychiatric Association, p. 476; reprinted with permission.

## ASSESSMENT

### Presenting Signs and Symptoms

- Might state they feel as though they are going to die or have a sense of impending doom
- Narrowing of perceptions, difficulty concentrating, problem solving inefficient
- Increased vital signs (blood pressure, pulse, respirations), increased muscle tension, sweat glands activated, pupils dilated
- Palpitations, urinary urgency/frequency, nausea, tightening of throat, unsteady voice
- Complaints of fatigue, difficulty sleeping, irritability, disorganization

| Box 5-6 | DSM-IV-TR Criteria for Posttraumatic Stress Disorder |
|---|---|

1. The person experienced, witnessed, or was confronted with an event that involved actual or threatened death to self or others **and** responded in fear, helplessness, or horror.
2. The event is persistently re-experienced:
   * Recurring, distressing recollections of the event including thoughts or perceptions
   * Distressing dreams or images
   * Reliving the event through flashbacks, illusions, hallucinations
   * Intense psychologic distress to exposure to internal or external cues that symbolize or resemble an aspect of the traumatic event
3. Persistent avoidance of stimuli associated with trauma and numbing of general responsiveness as indicated by three or more of the following:
   * Efforts to avoid thoughts, feelings, conversations that trigger trauma
   * Efforts to avoid people, places, activities that trigger trauma
   * Inability to recall aspects of trauma
   * Decreased interest in usual activities
   * Feelings of detachment, estrangement from others
   * Restriction in feelings (love, enthusiasm, joy)
   * Sense of shortened feelings
4. Persistent symptoms of increased arousal (two or more):
   * Difficulty falling/staying asleep
   * Irritability/outbursts of anger
   * Difficulty concentrating
   * Hypervigilance
   * Exaggerated startle response
5. **Duration more than 1 month:**
   * *Acute:* Duration less than 3 months
   * *Chronic:* Duration 3 months or more
   * *Deloyed:* Onset of symptoms is at least 6 months after stress

Adapted from American Psychiatric Association. (2000). *Dingnostic and statistical manual of mental disorders* (4th ed., text revision). Washington, DC: American Psychiatric Association, p. 468; reprinted with permission.

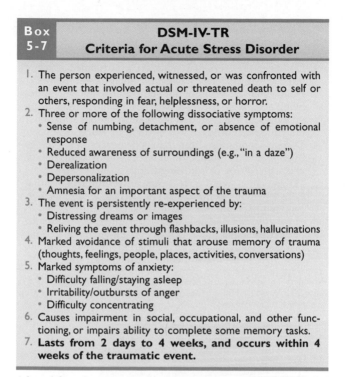

| Box 5-7 | DSM-IV-TR Criteria for Acute Stress Disorder |
|---|---|

1. The person experienced, witnessed, or was confronted with an event that involved actual or threatened death to self or others, responding in fear, helplessness, or horror.
2. Three or more of the following dissociative symptoms:
   • Sense of numbing, detachment, or absence of emotional response
   • Reduced awareness of surroundings (e.g., "in a daze")
   • Derealization
   • Depersonalization
   • Amnesia for an important aspect of the trauma
3. The event is persistently re-experienced by:
   • Distressing dreams or images
   • Reliving the event through flashbacks, illusions, hallucinations
4. Marked avoidance of stimuli that arouse memory of trauma (thoughts, feelings, people, places, activities, conversations)
5. Marked symptoms of anxiety:
   • Difficulty falling/staying asleep
   • Irritability/outbursts of anger
   • Difficulty concentrating
6. Causes impairment in social, occupational, and other functioning, or impairs ability to complete some memory tasks.
7. **Lasts from 2 days to 4 weeks, and occurs within 4 weeks of the traumatic event.**

Adapted from American Psychiatric Association. (2000). *Diagnostic and statistical manual of mental disorders* (4th ed., text revision). Washington, DC: American Psychiatric Association; p. 471–472; reprinted with permission.

## Assessment Tools

There are a number of tools that help the health care worker assess for anxiety symptoms. The Hamilton Rating Scale for Anxiety helps the clinician to identify a client's level of anxiety. Refer to Appendix D-2 for this tool. Box 5-8 presents a simple screening guide that can be done quickly and can elicit specific anxiety symptoms that the client might not offer without being asked. Any positive answers alert the nurse clinician that more detailed assessment is needed.

---

### Box 5-8 Sample Questions for Assessing Anxiety Symptoms

1. Do you ever experience a sudden, unexplained attack of intense fear, anxiety, or panic for no apparent reason?
2. Have you been afraid of not being able to get help or not being able to escape in certain situations, such as being on a bridge, in a crowded store, or in similar situations?
3. Do you find it difficult to control your worrying?
4. Do you spend more time than is necessary doing things over and over again, such as washing your hands, checking things, or counting things?
5. Do you either avoid or feel very uncomfortable in situations involving people, such as parties, weddings, dating, dances, or other social events?
6. Have you ever had an extremely frightening, traumatic, or horrible experience such as being a victim of a crime, being seriously injured in a car accident, being sexually assaulted, or seeing someone injured or killed?

---

Provided by Screening for Mental health, Inc, 1 Washington Street, Suite 304, Welksky Hills, MA, 20481-1706; (701) 239-0071; *http://www.mental-healthscreening.org.*

## Assessment Guidelines

### Anxiety Disorders

1. A sound **physical and neurologic examination** helps to determine if the anxiety is primary or secondary to another psychiatric disorder, medical condition, or substance.
2. Assess for **potential for self-harm**, because it is known that people suffering from high levels of intractable anxiety might become desperate and attempt suicide.
3. Many people with anxiety disorder greatly benefit from **cognitive and behavioral techniques**, as well as certain **medications. Assess client's community for appropriate clinics, groups, and counselors who offer these techniques**. Table 5-1 identifies which approaches and medications seem to be the most effective for each of the anxiety disorders.
4. Be aware that differences in culture can affect how anxiety is manifested.

# NURSING DIAGNOSES WITH INTERVENTIONS

## Discussion of Potential Nursing Diagnoses

Several nursing diagnoses target symptoms for people with high levels of anxiety and anxiety disorders. The nursing diagnosis **Anxiety** is most often used. When using the nursing diagnosis of Anxiety, the nurse needs to clarify the level of anxiety, because different levels of anxiety call for different intervention strategies. For example, the diagnosis should be stated **Anxiety—Moderate Level**, or **Anxiety—Severe-Panic Level**.

**Ineffective Coping** is another frequently used diagnosis, because high levels of anxiety lead to interference in ability to work, disruptions in relationships, and changes in ability to interact satisfactorily with others. For example, people with phobias often develop avoidance behaviors, and people with obsessions and compulsions make it difficult for others to relate to them other than under rigid circumstances.

People with anxiety disorders often have **Disturbed Thought Processes**. Individuals with OCD are preoccupied with their obsessive thoughts, and people with panic disorder are filled with fear and terror during anxiety attacks when their ability to problem solve, use sound judgment, or understand directions is totally impaired. Individuals with PTSD and ASD suffer from intrusive thoughts and memories that increase levels of anxiety so that their ability to function and think clearly is greatly hampered for brief periods of time. They would then qualify for **Posttrauma Syndrome**. Most people with anxiety disorders also suffer from **Disturbed Sleep Pattern**. Sleep deprivation can lead to the inability to function at work or school, and in social situations.

The nursing diagnoses **Anxiety, Ineffective Coping, Disturbed Thought Processes, Posttrauma Syndrome, and Disturbed Sleep Pattern** are presented here with suggested nursing interventions for each diagnosis.

## Overall Guidelines for Nursing Interventions
### Anxiety Disorders

1. Identify community resources that can help the client develop skills that have been proven to be highly effective for people with a variety of anxiety disorders:
   - Cognitive restructuring
   - Relaxation training
   - Modeling techniques
   - Systematic desensitization/graduated exposure
   - Flooding (implosion therapy)
   - Behavior therapy
2. Identify community support groups for people with specific anxiety disorders.
3. Assess need for interventions with families and significant others (support groups, family therapy) and help with issues that might lead to relationship stress and turmoil.
4. When medications are used in conjunction with therapy, clients and their significant others will need thorough teaching. Written information and instructions should be given to client/family/partner.
5. Refer to Table 5-1 for the accepted treatment for psychopharmacologic and therapeutic modalities for selected anxiety disorders.

## Selected Nursing Diagnoses and Nursing Care Plans

### ANXIETY

Vague uneasy feeling of discomfort or dread accompanied by an autonomic response (the source often nonspecific or unknown to the individual); a feeling of apprehension caused by anticipation of danger; it is an alerting signal that warns of impending danger and enables the individual to take measures to deal with the threat

*Related To (Etiology)*

▲ Perceived threat to self-concept, health status, socioeconomic status, role function, interaction patterns, or environment
▲ Perceived threat of death
▲ Unconscious conflict
▲ Unmet needs
● Exposure to phobic object or situation
● Cessation of ritualistic behavior
● Traumatic experience
● Fear of panic attack
● Intrusive unwanted thoughts
● Flashbacks

*As Evidenced By*
*(Assessment Findings/Diagnostic Cues)*

▲ Autonomic signs and symptoms (tachycardia, rapid breathing, palpitations, muscle tension, diaphoresis)
▲ Narrowing focus of attention
▲ Perceptual focus shattered
▲ Restlessness to purposeless activity to immobilization
▲ Feelings of dread, apprehension, nervousness, or concern
● Increase in symptoms (compulsions, phobias, obsessions, nightmares/flashbacks)
● Inability to complete tasks

*Outcome Criteria*

■ ● Controls anxiety response
● Reports absence of physical manifestations of anxiety
● Behavioral manifestations of anxiety absent
▲ Uses effective coping strategies

*Long-Term Goals*

Client will:
• Demonstrate three anxiety-reducing skills that work for him or her by (date)

---

▲ NANDA International accepted; ● In addition to NANDA International; ■ NOC Outcomes for Anxiety Control

- State that he or she feels comfortable and physical symptoms of anxiety are reduced
- Electively solve problems without assistance much of the time by (date)
- Identify negative "self-talk" and reframe thoughts successfully by (date)
- Demonstrate ability to reframe problems in solvable terms by (date)
- Demonstrate ability to get needs met using assertive communication skills by (date)
- Decrease time spent in ritualistic behaviors by (date)

## Short-Term Goals

Client will:
- Demonstrate skills at reframing anxiety-provoking situations with aid of nurse/clinician (date).
- Demonstrate one relaxation technique that works well for him or her (date).
- Role play with the nurse two behavioral techniques that help reduce feelings of anxiety to tolerable levels by (date).
- Decrease anxiety level from severe (+++) to moderate (++) within 2 hours on (date).
- Role play assertive communication skills with nurse.
- Attend a support group if warranted (e.g., PTSD)

## Interventions and Rationales

| Intervention | Rationale |
|---|---|
| 1. Provide a safe, calm environment:<br>a. Decrease environmental stimuli.<br>b. Listen to and reassure client that he or she can feel more in control. | 1. When people feel fearful and vulnerable, being heard in an atmosphere of calm helps to foster a sense of connectedness with someone and control over what will happen. |
| 2. Encourage client to talk about feelings and concerns. | 2. When concerns are stated out loud, problems can be discussed and feelings of isolation decreased. |
| 3. Reframe the problem in a way that is solvable. Provide a new perspective and correct distorted perceptions. | 3. Correcting distortions increases the possibility of finding workable solutions to a realistically defined problem. |

| Intervention | Rationale |
|---|---|
| 4. Identify thoughts or feelings prior to the onset of anxiety: "What were you doing/thinking right before you started to feel anxious?" | 4. Identify triggers for escalating anxiety, and a chance to understand why these triggers are so frightening to the client. |
| 5. Identify any "self-talk" clients might use at this time (e.g., "I'll never be able to do this right." *or* "This means I'll never succeed in anything"). | 5. Identify what thoughts trigger anxious feelings. Then cognitive skills can be used to help client to reframe his or her thinking so that problems can be solved. |
| 6. Teach relaxation techniques (deep breathing exercises, meditation, progressive muscle relaxation). | 6. When clients learn to lower levels of anxiety, their ability to assess a situation and utilize their own problem-solving skills are improved. |
| 7. Refer client and significant others to support groups, self-help programs, or advocacy groups when appropriate. | 7. Clients with specific problems are known to greatly benefit from being around others who are grappling with similar issues. Provides the client with information and support and lowers feelings of isolation in stressful and difficult situations. |
| 8. Administer medications or obtain an order for medications when appropriate. | 8. Use least restrictive interventions to decrease anxiety. |

## INEFFECTIVE COPING

Inability to form a valid appraisal of the stressors; inadequate choices of practical responses; and/or inability to use available resources

## Related To (Etiology)

- Severe to panic levels of anxiety—panic attack, GAD
- Excessive negative beliefs about self—GAD, OCD, other
- Hypervigilance after a traumatic event—PTSD, ASD
- Presence of obsessions and compulsions associated with fear of contamination—OCD, phobia
- Avoidance behavior associated with phobia (list phobia)—phobia

## As Evidenced By
### (Assessment Findings/Diagnostic Cues)

- ▲ Verbalization of inability to cope or inability to ask for help
- ▲ Inability to problem solve
- ▲ Expression of anxiety
- Disturbance in vocational and social functioning related to (phobias, obsessions, compulsions, panic attacks, posttrauma symptoms)
- Panic attacks, severe obsessive acts, disturbing thoughts, disabling phobias, posttrauma symptoms

## Outcome Criteria

- Uses multiple coping strategies
- Verbalizes a sense of control
- Functions at previous level of independence without interference from phobias, compulsions, obsessions, posttrauma event, panic attacks, disabling anxiety

## Long-Term Goals

Client will:
- Verbalize ability to cope effectively with anxiety using two new stress-reducing skills by (date)
- Demonstrate new coping skills (cognitive, behavioral, relaxation techniques, insight) that allay anxiety symptoms, such as visualization, deep breathing, and thought-stopping techniques by (date)
- Report increase in psychologic comfort by (date)

## Short-Term Goals

Client will:
- Demonstrate knowledge of breathing techniques and relaxation skills by end of first/second session with nurse

---

▲ NANDA International accepted; ● In addition to NANDA International; ■ NOC Outcomes For Coping

- Describe the different therapies that are effective in treating their particular anxiety disorder (cognitive, behavioral, group) (see Table 5-1)
- Demonstrate one new anxiety reduction technique that works best for him or her within 2 weeks
- Accurately describe the desired effects, side effects, and toxic effects of any medication he or she might be given as an adjunct to therapy within 2 days

## Interventions and Rationales

| Intervention | Rationale |
|---|---|
| 1. Monitor and reinforce client's use of positive coping skills and healthy defense mechanisms. | 1. Identifies what does and does not work for client. Nurse uses client's strengths to build upon. |
| 2. Teach new coping skills to substitute for ineffective ones. | 2. Gives client options. |
| 3. At client level of understanding, explain the *fight-or-flight response* and the *relaxation response* of the autonomic nervous system. Address how breathing can be used to elicit the *relaxation response*. | 3. Understanding the physiologic aspects of anxiety, and that people have some degree of control over their physiologic responses, gives clients hope and a sense of control in their lives, and aids them in mastering relaxation techniques. |
| 4. When the client's level of anxiety is mild to moderate, teach client proper **breathing techniques** and breathe with the client. (See Box 5-9 for client instructions for abdominal breathing.) | 4. Breathing techniques can prevent anxiety from escalating. Doing exercises with client helps foster compliance. |

| Intervention | Rationale |
|---|---|
| 5. When the client's level of anxiety is mild to moderate, teach client **relaxation techniques** (such as imaging, visualization [Box 5-10]). | 5. Help the client gain some control over switching the autonomic nervous system from the fight-or-flight response to the relaxation response. |
| 6. Identify for client which therapies have been highly effective with individuals who have the same disorder (cognitive, behavioral) (see Table 5-1). | 6. Not only do cognitive and behavioral approaches work to decrease clients' anxiety and improve quality of life, they also foster chemical changes in the brain that lessen the brain's response to anxiety. |
| 7. Use a cognitive approach. | 7. Helps the client recognize that thoughts and beliefs can cause anxiety. |
| 8. Teach client proven behavioral techniques. Client can become desensitized to a feared object or situation over time. | 8. Cognitive and behavioral techniques are extremely effective interventions for treating anxiety disorders. Once they are learned, clients can draw upon these skills for the rest of their lives. |
| 9. Keep focus on manageable problems; define them simply and concretely. | 9. Concrete, well-defined problems lend themselves to intervention. |
| 10. Provide behavioral rehearsals (role play) for anticipated stressful situations. | 10. Predetermination of previous effective or new coping strategies, along with practice, increases potential for success. |
| 11. Some clients respond well to biofeedback and feel more comfortable with physiologic manipulations than one-on-one therapy. | 11. Biofeedback is extremely useful for decreasing anxiety levels. Some clients might feel less "shame" in getting help. |

| Intervention | Rationale |
|---|---|
| 12. Many anxiety disorders respond to medications along with therapy (e.g., selective serotonin reuptake inhibitors [SSRIs] for OCD, buspirone [Buspar] for GAD). Therefore, medication teaching is extremely important, especially with the anxiolytics. | 12. Clients need to know what the medications can and cannot do. They need to know that "more is not better," the side effects and toxic effects, and what to do if an untoward reaction occurs. This information should always be given to clients in writing after it is verbally explained by the nurse clinician. |

---

**Box 5-9 Teaching Abdominal Breathing**

Instruct the client to:
1. Place one hand on the abdomen beneath the rib cage.
2. Inhale slowly and deeply through the nose, sending air as far down into the lungs as possible. The hand should rise.
3. After taking the full breath, pause for a moment, then exhale slowly and fully.
4. While exhaling, allow the entire body to go limp.
5. Count each breath up to 10 by saying the appropriate number after each exhalation.
6. Do two or three "sets" of 10 abdominal breaths to produce a state of considerable relaxation.

From Varcarolis E. (1998). *Foundations of psychiatric mental health nursing* (3rd ed.). Philadelphia: WB Saunders, p. 472; reprinted with permission.

---

## DISTURBED THOUGHT PROCESSES

Disruption in cognitive operations and activities

---

**Box 5-10 Script for Visualizing a Peaceful Scene**

Imagine releasing all the tension in your body . . . letting it go.

Now, with every breath you take, feel your body drifting down deeper and deeper into relaxation . . . floating down . . . deeper and deeper.

Imagine your peaceful scene. You're sitting beside a clear, blue mountain stream. You are barefoot, and you feel the sun-warmed rock under your feet. You hear the sound of the stream tumbling over the rocks. The sound is hypnotic, and you relax more and more. You see the tall pine trees on the opposite shore bending in the gentle breeze. Breathe the clean, pine-scented air, each breath moving you deeper and deeper into relaxation. The sun warms your face.

You are very comfortable. There is nothing to disturb you. You experience a feeling of well-being.

You can return to this peaceful scene by taking time to relax. The positive feelings can grow stronger and stronger each time you choose to relax.

You can return to your activities now, feeling relaxed and refreshed.

---

## Related To (Etiology)

- ▲ Severe levels of anxiety
- ● Distorted perceptions
- ● Intrusive, obsessive thoughts
- ● Anticipatory anxiety

## As Evidenced By
### (Assessment Findings/Diagnostic Cues)

- ▲ Hypervigilance
- ▲ Distractibility
- ▲ Inaccurate interpretation of the environment
- ● Flashbacks
- ● Intrusive, obsessive thinking

---

▲ NANDA International accepted; ● In addition to NANDA International

## Outcome Criteria

- Identifies effective coping patterns
- Demonstrates increase in concentration and attentiveness
- Demonstrates control over selected events and situtions
- ■ Maintains focus without being distracted

## Long-Term Goals

Client will:
- Recognize when anxiety begins to escalate and link anxiety to precipitating thoughts or feelings by (date)
- Demonstrate techniques that can distract and distance self from thoughts and feelings that are anxiety producing by (date)
- Reframe automatic thoughts and self-judgments that lead to increase in anxiety and lowering of self-worth by (date)

## Short-Term Goals

Client will:
- Identify two thoughts or feelings that precede increases in anxiety and will discuss with the nurse within 1 week or (date)
- Share daily journal with counselor/nurse regarding thoughts/feelings preceding anxiety (date)
- Rate the anxiety on a scale from 1 to 10, then re-rate anxiety after using breathing, relaxation, cognitive, behavioral, or other anxiety-reducing skills
- Demonstrate one cognitive or behavioral technique after 1 week (date)

## Interventions and Rationales

| Intervention | Rationale |
|---|---|
| 1. Explore with client the thoughts that lead up to client's anxious feelings and relief behaviors. | 1. Recognition of precipitating thoughts or feelings leading to anxiety behaviors might give clues about how to arrest escalating anxiety. |

● In addition to NANDA International; ■ NOC Outcomes for Concentration

| Intervention | Rationale |
|---|---|
| 2. Link client's relief behaviors to thoughts and feelings. | 2. Client becomes aware of how anxiety can be the result of thoughts, and realizes that people can have some control over their thoughts and, therefore, their anxiety levels, with practice. |
| 3. Teach cognitive principles.<br>a. Anxiety is the result of dysfunctional appraisal of a situation.<br>b. Anxiety is the result of automatic thinking. | 3. Again, introduces the concept to clients that they can have some control over their thoughts and feelings, instills hope, and stimulates compliance to try new ways of thinking. |
| 4. Teach some brief **cognitive techniques** that the client can try out right away (Box 5-11). | 4. Increases self-awareness while distancing self from own anxiety. In a sense, helps distract client from feelings of anxiety, and allows him or her to be more of an observer. |
| 5. Teach client **behavioral techniques** that can interrupt intrusive, unwanted thoughts (Box 5-12). | 5. Can help distract client and interrupt escalating anxiety. During this time, alternative coping skills can be employed. |
| 6. Role play and rehearse with client alternative coping strategies that can be used in threatening or anxiety-provoking situations. | 6. Gives client chance to be proactive, giving client a choice of alternatives instead of client employing usual unsatisfactory automatic reactions. |
| 7. Encourage client to keep a daily journal of thoughts and situations that seem to precede anxiety, and coping strategies used. | 7. Allows client to monitor "triggers" and evaluate useful coping strategies over time. |

| Intervention | Rationale |
|---|---|
| 8. Teach client to rate his or her anxiety levels on a scale from 1 to 10, where 1 is the least and 10 the highest. Have client document situations and anxiety levels in the journal. | 8. Allows client to evaluate effectiveness of coping strategies and monitor decrease in anxiety levels over time. |
| 9. Review journal with client and identify which strategies worked and which did not work. Review with client progress made and give credit for the client's hard work. | 9. Helps client see what seems to be working and what does not and encourages compliance when going through phases of feeling discouraged. |
| 10. Teach client to recognize triggers of anxiety. | 10. Gives client opportunity to use alternative responses and skills. |
| 11. Refer client to support groups in the community in which people are dealing with similar issues. | 11. Groups can foster a sense of belonging and diminish feelings of isolation and alienation. Positive feedback from others helps foster compliance and enhances self-esteem. |
| 12. Review **stress reduction techniques** with client, family, and significant others during family and client teaching (Box 5-13). Encourage client and family members members to practice relaxation techniques; give handouts and references. | 12. Everyone around the client might be tense. Sometimes simple steps make big differences in people's lives. |

| Intervention | Rationale |
|---|---|
| 13. Refer family members and significant others to appropriate resources in the community. Resources might include family therapy, couples counseling, financial counseling, support groups, or classes in meditation and other relaxation techniques. | 13. Family and others close to the client might need a great deal of support. They might benefit from learning new coping strategies that can lessen conflicts and stress on the whole family unit. |

---

**Box 5-11 Brief Cognitive Techniques**

1. Instruct client to refer to self by first name and comment on own anxiety or thoughts (e.g., "Mary's heart is beating fast"; "Ted thinks everyone is looking at him now").
2. Work with the client to recognize his or her automatic thinking, and how certain words can trigger anxiety (e.g., *should, never, always*). Help client use words that are more objective and neutral; for example:
   - *Change* "I should have gone to college." *to* "I would have benefited from going to college, and, if I still wish to go, I can."
   - *Change* "I always use poor judgment when it comes to money; I'll never get it right!" *to* "Although I have made mistakes regarding money in the past, it would be useful for me to get some advice and check out my ideas more thoroughly in the future."

---

**Box 5-12 Thought Stopping: Brief Behavioral Techniques**

- Have client wear a rubber band around his or her wrist. When intrusive repetitive thoughts start to occur (as in obsessive compulsive disorder), have client snap the rubber band hard on his or her wrist.
- When client is experiencing intrusive painful memories, clap your hands loudly in front of client, then teach client and family to do the same thing.

## POSTTRAUMA SYNDROME

Sustained maladaptive response to a traumatic, overwhelming event

---

### *Related To (Etiology)*

▲ Wars
▲ Sexual assault/abuse
▲ Terrorism
▲ Military combat
▲ Physical and psychologic abuse
▲ Serious accidents
▲ Witnessing violent death or mutilations
▲ Motor vehicle and industrial accidents
▲ Being held prisoner of war
▲ Natural disasters and man-made disasters

### *As Evidenced By*
### *(Assessment Findings/Diagnostic Cues)*

▲ Difficulty concentrating
▲ Intrusive thoughts
▲ Anger and/or rage
▲ Hopelessness
▲ Panic attacks
▲ Depression
▲ Anxiety
▲ Fear
▲ Detachment
▲ Numbing
▲ Compulsive behavior
▲ Flashbacks
▲ Headaches
▲ Avoidance
▲ Regression
▲ Nightmares
▲ Exaggerated startle response

---

▲ NANDA International accepted; ● In addition to NANDA International

## Outcome Criteria

- Diminished symptoms of PTSD (e.g., nightmares, flashbacks, depression, isolation, headaches, confusion, difficulty concentrating)
- ■ ● Maintains self-control without supervision
- Satisfaction with coping ability
- Satisfaction with close relationships
- Use of available social supports
- Increased psychologic comfort

## Long-Term Goals

Client will:
- Report feelings of support and comfort within support group of people sharing similar experiences by (date)
- Use three new effective relaxation strategies to help reduce tension and anxiety by (date)
- Talk about a traumatic event, fears, terrors, and experiences and demonstrate congruent feelings within ___ weeks
- Participate in social skills training targeting specific previously identified behaviors
- Demonstrate a new sense of control over certain situations or events by (date)
- Agree to continue with treatment goals and management strategies by (date)

## Short-Term Goals

Client will:
- Identify one person or group that client is willing to talk to or spend time with working on issues of PTSD
- Identify three coping skills client believes would improve his/her sense of well being and functioning and agree to work on them with (nurse/staff/clinician) within 1 week
- Identify two problems that, if addressed, would improve client's quality of life and those of family/friends/coworkers/boss (e.g., impulse control, assertiveness, social skills)

---

● In addition to NANDA International; ■ NOC Outcome for Impulse Self-Control

## Interventions and Rationales

| Intervention | Rationale |
|---|---|
| 1. Assess for any suicidal or homicidal thoughts and feelings. (See Chapters 16 and 17 for nursing care plans related to suicide behaviors and anger and aggression.) | 1. Priority of concern and nursing measures would be for client and other safety. |
| 2. Assess the client's anxiety level. | 2. Identify what level of intervention might be needed to minimize further escalation of anxiety. |
| 3. Assess for alcohol or drug abuse. If yes, assess readiness for substance use abuse therapies (e.g., support groups, counseling). Offer referrals if client is ready. | 3. Most clients cannot participate in learning coping skills, reliving traumatic memories, and making positive changes while impaired. |
| 4. Identify the client's symptoms and clarify that they are anxiety related and not the product of a physiologic condition (e.g., chest tightness, headaches, dizziness, numbness). | 4. Physical causes of symptoms need to be ruled out before assumptions of psychologic causes are made. (A client might well have PTSD along with a cardiac problem, etc.) |
| 5. Identify and document the psychologic response the client is experiencing (e.g., shock, anger, withdrawal, panic, confusion, psychotic episodes, emotional instability, nightmares, flashbacks). | 5. The psychologic symptoms are often many, and different ones might require different intervention strategies. When the symptoms begin to diminish, you know that goals are being reached. |

| Intervention | Rationale |
|---|---|
| 6. Identify if client has been or is exposed to groups in which others deal with similar traumatic issues. If not, offer referrals to groups in the client's community. | 6. Support groups of people with similar experiences are perhaps pivotal to healing. Allows for expressing similar feelings in a safe environment. |
| 7. Spend time with client, allowing client to go at own speed regarding describing present or past traumatic events. | 7. Often feelings and memories of trauma are buried. It often takes time and trust for a person to open up to a "stranger" or discuss a topic he/she might not have shared with anyone. |
| 8. Monitor your own feelings in response to your client's experience. | 8. Many of the stories clients tell are horrifying and difficult to listen to. |
| 9. Refrain from interrupting or minimizing the horror, or overidentifying with the events. | 9. Venting with other staff or supervisor helps nurse process feelings and discharge tensions. |
| 10. Remain nonjudgmental in your interactions. | 10. Avoid reinforcing blame, shame, guilt, and so on. |
| 11. Listen attentively to client's description of the event. | 11. Although it might be difficult to listen to the trauma, sharing the pain with others can be the beginning of healing. |
| 12. Encourage the expression of feelings through talking, writing, crying, role playing, or other ways the client is comfortable with. | 12. The description of the events and the expression of feelings associated with the event is paramount to the healing process. |

| Intervention | Rationale |
|---|---|
| 13. Teach the client adaptive cognitive and behavioral strategies to manage symptoms of emotional and physical reactivity:<br>  a. Deep breathing (see Box 5-9)<br>  b. Relaxation exercises (see Box 5-10)<br>  c. Cognitive techniques (see Box 5-11)<br>  d. Desensitization<br>  e. Assertive behaviors<br>  f. Thought-stopping techniques (see Box 5-12)<br>  g. Stress reduction techniques (see Box 5-13) | 13. Once repressed areas are opened up, accompanying, often unbearable, feelings will emerge. |
| 14. Assess family and social support system. Is there a need for family interventions or counseling? | 14. Often family and friends become confused, afraid, hurt, angry, or feel hopeless and depressed over time. |
| 15. Instruct client and family on the signs and symptoms of PTS. | 15. Often when actions and behaviors that seemed totally chaotic and unrelated are viewed in terms of an identifiable syndrome, relief is experienced, especially when treatment is available. |

| Intervention | Rationale |
|---|---|
| 16. Assess if the client found comfort in religious or spiritual activities in the past. Are they still practicing? Do they wish to resume practice or contact with supportive spiritual persons? | 16. Deep spiritual convictions, when activated, can provide a sense of hope and meaning for clients struggling with feelings of helplessness and hopelessness. |
| 17. Offer the client access to coping skills training when client is ready and when appropriate (e.g., anger management, assertive skills, anxiety reduction techniques, coping skills training, social skills training). | 17. Clients might need to learn or relearn a variety of coping skills once they begin to function again. |
| 18. Identify the need for social services (e.g., employment, legal issues, living arrangements) and give client referrals. | 18. Some clients might have multiple social needs related to long-term, entrenched behaviors. |

## DISTURBED SLEEP PATTERN

Time limited disruption of sleep (natural, periodic suspension of consciousness), amount, and quality

*Related To (Etiology)*

▲ Depression
▲ Fear
▲ Anxiety
▲ Fear of insomnia

---

▲ NANDA International accepted; ● In addition to NANDA International

▲ Fatigue
▲ Inadequate sleep hygiene
▲ Biochemical agents
● Nightmares
● Obsession thoughts
● Fears (e.g., dark, intrusion, death)
● Adrenaline rush related to high levels of anxiety
● Panic attacks

## As Evidenced By
## (Assessment Findings/Diagnostic Cues)

▲ Early morning awakenings
▲ Arising earlier or later than desired
▲ Verbal complaints of difficulty falling asleep
▲ Verbal complaints of not feeling well-rested
▲ Three or more nighttime awakenings
▲ Decreased ability to function

## Outcome Criteria

● Develops an uninterrupted sleep pattern 5 to 8 hours per night
■ ● Reports feelings of being rejuvinated after sleep
■ ● Establishes an effective sleep routine

## Long-Term Goals

Client will:
• State he/she begins to see improvement in quality of sleep and pattern of sleep after 2 weeks
• State that the relaxation exercises (tapes) are useful sleep aids by (date)
• Work with nurse to review and revise plan if sleep pattern has not improved after 2 weeks

## Short-Term Goals

Client will:
• Identify personal habits that disrupt sleep pattern and those things that could augment quality of sleep after first interview

---

▲ NANDA International accepted; ● In addition to NANDA International; ■ NOC Outcome For Sleep

- Form a "sleep plan" with nurse that the client is willing to try within 2 days
- Identify any other issues that might need attention that are contributing to sleep pattern disturbance, and be open for referrals

## Interventions and Rationales

| Intervention | Rationale |
|---|---|
| 1. Assess client and family usual sleep pattern, any changes that have occurred, and what was happening at the time. Identify if there was a precipitating event around onset of sleep problem or if it is chronic. | 1. Information from both client and family clarifies specific sleep disturbance. |
| 2. Identify the client's usual sleep patterns including the following: <ul><li>Bedtime rituals</li><li>Time of rising, time of retiring</li><li>Use of alcohol and/or caffeine before sleep</li><li>Use of sleep aids (prescribed or over-the-counter medications)</li></ul> | 2. Establish a baseline and help identify problems: <ul><li>Sleeping medications and alcohol interfere with rapid eye movement (REM) sleep.</li><li>Caffeine and exercise before retiring can interfere with sleep.</li></ul> |
| 3. Review sleep hygiene measures with the client. Determine if the client does any of the following: refrains from naps, alcohol and caffeine at night; follow a regular retiring and arising schedule; exercise pattern. | 3. Identifying baseline helps target needed interventions. |

| Intervention | Rationale |
|---|---|
| 4. Develop a sleep relaxation program with client (e.g., self-hypnosis, progressive muscle relaxation, imagery). | 4. Employing both physical and mental relaxation can help minimize anxiety and promote sleep. |
| 5. Demonstrate and rehearse these techniques with client until client feels relaxed and is able to practice them at bedtime. | 5. Have client practice chosen relaxation method with nurse. Allow time for client to begin to feel results of relaxation. |
| 6. Suggest use of relaxation tapes. | 6. If client has racing thoughts or is troubled by a problem, tapes can help the client focus on relaxation. |
| 7. Encourage client to: <br>• Use decaffeinated beverages until sleep pattern improves. <br>• Limit fluid intake 3 to 5 hours before retiring. <br>• Increase physical activity during the day, even if fatigued. <br>• Avoid daytime naps. <br>• Establish regular times of retiring and waking. | 7. These are known sleep aids. |
| 8. Establish with client a sleep program that incorporates the elements of good sleep hygiene and relaxation tools. | 8. Client is more likely to follow plan if he/she is involved with the incorporation of known effective techniques. |

| Intervention | Rationale |
|---|---|
| 9. Suggest to client that if he/she does not feel drowsy after 20 minutes, get up and engage in a quiet activity that is "boring"—*not* stimulating. | 9. Waiting for sleep that will not come can increase anxiety and frustration. Doing something monotonous at bedtime might help the client become drowsy. |
| 10. Encourage client to practice the agreed-upon bedtime routine for 2 weeks even if there does not seem to be a benefit. | 10. It might take 2 weeks or longer for habits to settle in. |
| 11. Encourage client to simultaneously work on any issues that might be adversely affecting sleep (e.g., anxiety disorders, social or personal problems, job related issues, interpersonal difficulties). Offer referrals when appropriate. | 11. Disturbances in sleep are often secondary to other issues, either emotional or physical. If such issues are present, they need to be addressed. |

## MEDICAL TREATMENTS

### Psychopharmacology

Although psychopharmacology is often an important adjunct to treating anxiety disorders, it is important to be aware of the therapeutic modalities that are proven effective for these disorders and might be superior in the long run because they can teach clients coping skills and behavior that might enhance their quality of life. Refer to the psychosocial interventions for more on useful therapies.

At one time, the predominant treatment for anxiety disorders was antianxiety medications, or *anxiolytics*, as they are currently referred to. The benzodiazepines were often the treatment of choice and still are used for severe anxiety. However, there are currently many groups of medications that can be used effectively for clients with anxiety disorders. Each group seems to be helpful for specific disorders. For example, the tricyclic antidepressants (TCAs) (e.g., *imipramine*) seem to be effective in targeting **panic attacks**. The monoamine oxidase inhibitor (MAOI) antidepressants seem to have **antiagoraphobic effects**. Although the benzodiazepiness are useful in **GAD**, they are best used for a short time because they can become addicting. Benzodiazepines might also cause "rebound anxiety" when they are stopped. Clinicians might prefer to start with *buspirone*, which is not addicting nor does the client develop a tolerance for the drug. The downside of buspirone (Buspar) is that it can take a long time to work (3 weeks or much longer for some). The client can be maintained with buspirone for a long time. Although anxiolytics might be the most widely used treatment for GAD, the World Federation of Societies of Biological Psychiatry (2002) recently recommended SSRIs as first-line therapy. The SSRI antidepressants (e.g., fluvoxamine [Luvox], fluoxetine [Prozac]) have also been found to be very effective for people with **OCD**.

Table 5-1 gives a good example of effective drugs for each of the anxiety disorders. Note that it is best when these drugs are given as an adjunct to therapy. Drugs are not a cure. Therapy gives clients options on how to assess situations and how to deal with situations in ways that are appropriate and effective, and, in doing so, enhances the client's quality of life. Drugs cannot do that. Refer to Chapter 21 for the neurotransmitters targeted, the negative side effects related to receptor-blocking activity, and client and family teaching to optimize compliance and drug safety and effectiveness. Table 5-2 offers a more comprehensive list of specific antianxiety medications, their trade names, and usual daily range. Refer to Appendix G for medication monographs.

## Psychosocial Treatment for Anxiety Disorders

Among the variety of psychosocial methods that have been used in the treatment of anxiety disorders, those that are **behavioral and cognitive-behavioral are those with the strongest empirical support**. In fact, cognitive-behavioral and behavioral are the treatments of choice for these disorders.

Table 5-1 **Accepted Treatment for Selected Anxiety Disorders**

| Disorder | Pharmacotherapy | Therapeutic Modality | Comments |
|---|---|---|---|
| Panic disorder | Antidepressants<br>a. TCAs (imipramine)<br>b. SSRIs<br>c. MAOIs (second-line because of dietary restrictions)<br>**Benzodiazepines (short-term)**<br>a. Alprazolam (Xanax)<br>b. Lorazepam (Ativan)<br>c. Clonazepam (Klonopin) | Cognitive-behavioral therapy (CBT)<br>Behavioral therapy<br>Relaxation techniques<br>Breathing techniques | Current CBT emphasizes:<br>a. Information on anxiety and the panic cycle<br>b. Symptom management (relaxation-breathing)<br>c. Cognitive restructuring<br>d. Systematic desensitization<br>e. In vivo exposure aimed at elementary avoidance behavior<br>f. Coping skills aquisition |
| **Agoraphobia** | a. Treatment of panic attacks (above) if present<br>b. Phenelzine (Nardil) an MAOI, might have anti-agoraphobic effects | Behavioral therapy<br>Cognitive therapy<br>Insight-oriented psychotherapy<br>Social skills training | Systematic desensitization<br>Deep-muscle relaxation<br>Rebreathing techniques<br>Self-hypnosis<br>Biofeedback<br>Recognition of irrational beliefs<br>Stopping irrational thoughts<br>Replacing irrational thoughts with new thoughts or activities<br>Especially for agoraphobia without history of panic disorder |

| Generalized anxiety disorder | a. SSRIs (paroxetine [Paxil]) b. Benzodiazepines—short-term only c. Buspirone d. TCAs, especially imipramine e. Gabapentin (antiseizure drug) | Cognitive therapy Behavioral therapy Stress Management Relaxation Training Aerobic level exercises | |
| Posttraumatic stress disorder | a. MAOIs (especially phenelzine) b. TCAs (imipramine and amitriptyline) and SSRIs for depressive symptoms might diminish nightmares and flashbacks c. Tiagabine (Gabitril) (anticonvulsant) found useful in clinical trials | Psychotherapy Family therapy Vocational rehabilitation Group therapy Relaxation techniques | **More than one treatment modality should be used\*** a. Establish support. b. Focus on abreaction, survivor guilt or shame, anger, and helplessness. |
| Obsessive-compulsive disorder | a. SSRIs (fluvoxamine [Luvox] and fluoxetine [Prozac]) b. Clomipramine (Anafranil) (TCA) | Cognitive-Behavioral therapy | Effective and necessary in addition to serotonergic medications Exposure in vivo plus response prevention are the crucial essential factors |

From Varcarolis E. (2002). *Foundations of psychiatric mental health nursing* (4th ed.). Philadelphia: WB Saunders, p. 331; reprinted with permission; and Preston and associates, 2005.

\*The sooner treatment begins, the more successful recovery is likely to be.

*MAOI,* Monoamine oxidase inhibitor; *SSRI,* selective serotonin reuptake inhibitor; *TCA,* tricyclic antidepressant.

Table 5-2 **Medications for Anxiety Disorders**

| Generic Name | Trade Name | Usual Daily Dosage (mg/day) | Action and Indication |
|---|---|---|---|
| **Benzodiazepines** | | | Anxiolytic effects result from depressing neurotransmission in the limbic system and cortical areas. Useful for **short-term treatment of anxiety; dependence and tolerance can develop.** |
| Alprazolam | Xanax | 0.5–6 | |
| Clonazepam | Klonopin | 0.5–2 | |
| Diazepam | Valium | 4–40 | |
| Lorazepam | Ativan | (1.5–6) | |
| Oxazepam | Serax | 30–90 | |
| Chlordiazepoxide | Librium | 15–100 | |
| Halazepam | Paxipam | 20–60 | |
| Clorazepate | Tranxene | 7.5–60 | |
| Prazepam | Centrax | 10–60 | |
| **Antihistamines** | | | |
| Hydroxyzine hydrochloride zine | Atarax/Vistaril | 30–200 | Depress subcortical centers. Produce **no dependence, tolerance, or intoxication.** Can be used for anxiety relief for indefinite periods. |
| Diphenhydramine | Benadryl | 75–200 | |
| **Nonbenzodiazepine Antianxiety Agents** | | | |
| Buspirone hydrochloride | BuSpar | 10–40 | Alleviates anxiety, but works best **before** benzodiazepines have been tried. Less sedating than the benzodiazepines. **Does not appear to produce physical or psychologic dependence.** Requires 3 weeks or more to be effective. |

| **Beta Blockers** | | | |
|---|---|---|---|
| Propranolol | Inderal | 20–160 | Used to relieve physical symptoms of anxiety, as in stage fright. Acts by attaching to sensors that detect arousal messages. |
| Atenolol | Tenormin | 25–100 | |
| **Tricyclics** | | | |
| Clomipramine | Anafranil | 50–125 | Used to prevent panic attacks, phobias, and PTSD. Act by regulating brain's reactions to serotonin. Clomipramine helpful for some in lowering obsessions in OCD. |
| Imipramine | Tofranil | 150–500 | |
| Nortriptyline | Aventyl, Pamelor | 75–125 | |
| Desipramine | Norpramin | 150–200 | |
| **MAOIs** | | | |
| Phenelzine | Nardil | 30–90 | Used to treat panic disorders, phobias, and PTSD. Acts by blocking reuptake of norepinephrine and serotonin in central nervous system. |
| **SSRIs** | | | |
| Sertraline | Zoloft | 50–200 | Used to treat OCD, panic, agoraphobia, generalized anxiety disorder; **effective with mild anxiety and depression.** |
| Fluoxetine | Prozac | 20–80 | |

Adapted from Varcarolis E. (2002). *Foundations of psychiatric mental health nursing* (4th ed.). Philadelphia, WB Saunders, p. 329; and Preston and associates, 2005

*MAOI,* Monoamine oxidase inhibitor; *OCD,* obsessive-compulsive disorder; *PTSD,* posttraumatic stress disorder; *SSRI,* selective serotonin reuptake inhibitor.

*Continued*

Table 5-2 **Medications for Anxiety Disorders—cont'd**

| | | |
|---|---|---|
| Paroxetine | Paxil | 20–60 |
| Fluvoxamine | Luvox | 100–150 |
| Citalopram | Celexa | 20–40 |
| Escitalopram | Lexapro | 20–40 |

Adapted from Varcarolis E. (2002). *Foundations of psychiatric mental health nursing* (4th ed.). Philadelphia, WB Saunders, p. 329; and Preston and associates, 2005

Cognitive strategies focus on altering the perception of the anxiety-producing stimuli. These interventions often make use of "coping skills," which involve teaching people various ways to help manage anxiety or fear. Coping skills are any behaviors that help people feel more secure; these often involve the use of self-statement.

Cognitive-behavioral interventions include:
- Cognitive therapy
- Cognitive restructuring
- Focus cognitive therapy
- Focal cognitive therapy
- Anxiety-management training

In addition to these general cognitive-behavioral strategies, several specific behavioral and cognitive-behavioral interventions have been developed for certain anxiety disorders. These involve:
- Panic control therapy for panic disorders
- Social effectiveness therapy for social phobia
- Applied relaxation for blood or injury phobia
- Flooding and response prevention for OCD

Table 5-1 identifies useful medications and therapies for each of the anxiety disorders. Brief stress reduction techniques that can be used during health teaching are outlined in Box 5-13.

---

### Box 5-13 Selected Stress Reduction Techniques

**Relaxation Techniques**

1. Induce a relaxation state more physiologically refreshing than sleep
2. Neutralize stress energy, producing a calming effect

**Reframing**

1. Changes the way we look and feel about things
2. There are many ways to interpret the same reality (seeing the glass as half full rather than half empty).
3. Reassess situation. We can learn from most situations. Ask:
   - "What positive thing came out of the situation/experience?"
   - "What did you learn in this situation?"
   - "What would you do differently next time?"

**Box 5-13 Selected Stress Reduction Techniques—cont'd**

4. Walking in another person's shoes can help dissipate tension and help us step outside of ourselves. We might even feel some compassion toward the person.
   - "What might be going on with your (spouse, boss, teacher, friend) that would cause him/her to (say, do) that?"
   - "Is he/she having problems? Feeling insecure? Under pressure?"

**Sleep**

1. Chronically stressed people are often fatigued.
2. Go to sleep 30 to 60 minutes earlier each night for a few weeks.
3. If still fatigued, try going to bed another 30 minutes earlier.
4. Sleeping later in the morning is not helpful and can throw off body rhythms.

**Exercise (Aerobic)**

1. Exercise can dissipate chronic and acute stress.
2. Recommended at least for 30 minutes, three times a week.

**Lower/Eliminate Caffeine Intake**

1. Such a simple thing can lead to more energy, and fewer muscle aches, and help people feel more relaxed.
2. Wean off coffee, tea, colas, and chocolate drinks.

**Stress Lowering Tips For Living**

1. Engage in meaningful, satisfying work.
2. Don't let work dominate your entire life.
3. Associate yourself with gentle people who affirm your personhood.
4. Guard your personal freedom, your freedom to:
   - Choose your friends
   - Live with and/or love whom you choose
   - Think and believe as you choose
   - Structure your time as you see fit
   - Set your own life's goals

# INTEGRATED APPROACHES (CAM)

A general caveat for all herbal and dietary supplements is that they are not subjected to rigorous testing and not required to be uniform, and problems can occur with their interaction with other substances. That said, **Kava** is one drug that has proved promising in the treatment of anxiety. Kava has also been used to reduce pain and relax muscles, and it has anticonvulsant effects as well. In clinical trials, kava has been found to be roughly equivalent to the benzodiazepines in its ability to decrease anxiety. **When taken in normal doses** of 50 to 75 mg three times a day, kava seems to have a better side effect profile than the benzodiazepines and seems to have a low tolerance for dependence. Kava might have adverse effects that include gastrointestinal complaints, headache, dizziness, and allergic skin reactions (Limon, 2000). Kava products might be beneficial in the management of anxiety and tension of nonpsychotic origin, and do not adversely affect cognitive function, mental acuity, or coordination, in contrast with the benzodiazepines. Kava should not be taken with other substances that act on the central nervous system, such as alcohol, barbiturates, antidepressants, and antipsychotics . . . or those with liver disease. The FDA (2002) states that hepatic toxicity is possibly associated with kava containing products. Check consumerLab.com for reputable brands.

# Nurse, Client, and Family Resources

## ASSOCIATIONS

**Anxiety Disorders Association of America**
8730 Georgia Avenue, Suite 600
Silver Spring, MD 20910
(240) 485-1001
http://www.adaa.org

**Obsessive-Compulsive Foundation, Inc.**
337 Notch Hill Road
North Branford, CT 06471
(203) 315-2190
http://www.ocfoundation.org

## INTERNET SITES

**Panic/Anxiety Disorders Guide**
http://www.panicdisorder.about.com

**Panic Disorder**
www.nlm.nih.gov/medlineplus/panicdisorder.html

**David Baldwin's Trauma Information Pages**
http://www.trauma-pages.com
Site focuses on emotional trauma and traumatic stress,
    including PTSD

**National Center for PTSD**
http://www.ncptsd.org

**Mental Help Net**
http://mentalhelp.net

# CHAPTER 6

# Depressive Disorders

## OVERVIEW

Happiness and unhappiness are appropriate responses to life events. When sadness, grief, or elation is extremely intense and the mood unduly prolonged, a mood disorder results. Depressive symptoms often coexist in people with alcohol or substance abuse problems. **Depressive symptoms are common in people who have other psychiatric disorders or behaviors** (anorexia nervosa, borderline disorders, phobias, and schizophrenia), or **people who have been physically or mentally abused** (posttrauma behaviors). **Depression might also be a critical symptom of many medical disorders or conditions** (hepatitis, mononucleosis, multiple sclerosis, dementia, cancer, diabetes, chronic pain). **Depression might also be directly related to the intake of many commonly prescribed medications** (antihypertensive medications, steroids, hormones, digitalis, stimulants). Therefore, mood disorders can be caused by a medical condition, psychoactive drugs, and medications, as well as a host of psychiatric conditions. However, specific nursing diagnoses and interventions for depression can be helpful, regardless of the etiology. **Risk for Suicide** is an essential component of a thorough assessment, regardless of the cause of depression. Refer to Chapter 16.

## Major Depressive Disorder

In major depressive disorder, a severely depressed mood, usually recurrent, causes clinically significant distress or impairment in social, occupational, or other important areas of the person's life. The depressed mood can be distinguished from the person's usual functioning and might occur suddenly or gradually. Major depression is considered to be a "severe biologically based mental illness" as determined by medical science in conjunction with the *Diagnostic and Statistical Manual of Mental Disorders* (4th edition, text revision) (DSM-IV-TR) (National Alliance for the Mentally Ill [NAMI], 1999).

Major depression might be characterized by certain features. For example:

- **Psychotic features**—delusions or hallucinations
- **Seasonal affective disorder (SAD)**—most prominent during certain seasons (e.g., winter or summer); SAD is more prevalent in climates with longer periods of darkness in a 24-hour cycle
- **Catatonic features**—for example, peculiarities of voluntary movement, motor immobility, purposeless motor activity, echolalia, or echopraxia
- **Melancholic features**—severe symptoms, loss of feelings of pleasure, worse in morning, early morning awakening, significant weight loss, excessive feelings of guilt
- **Postpartum onset**—within 4 weeks of delivery

Box 6-1 presents the DSM-IV-TR diagnostic criteria for a major depressive disorder.

## Dysthymic Disorder

Dysthymic disorder (dysthymia) is characterized by less severe, usually chronic depressive symptoms that have been present for at least 2 years (1 year for children or adolescents). Although dysthymia is not as severe as a major depression, the symptoms can cause significant distress or impairment in major areas of the person's life.

Box 6-2 provides a summary of the DSM-IV-TR diagnostic criteria for dysthymia.

# ASSESSMENT

## Presenting Signs and Symptoms

- Depressed mood (or irritability in children or adolescents)
- Diminished interest in or pleasure in almost all activities (anhedonia)

| Box<br>6-1 | **DSM-IV-TR**<br>**Criteria for Major Depressive Episode** |
| --- | --- |

1. Represents a change in previous functions.
2. Symptoms cause clinically significant distress or impair social, occupational, or other important areas of functioning.
3. **Five or more** of the following occur nearly every day for most waking hours during the same 2-week period. At least one of the symptoms is either a (1) depressed mood or (2) loss of interest or pleasure (anhedonia).
   - Depressed mood
   - Anhedonia
   - Significant weight loss or gain (more than 5% of body weight in 1 month)
   - Insomnia or hypersomnia nearly every day
   - Increased or decreased motor activity
   - Anergia (fatigue or loss of energy)
   - Feelings of worthlessness or inappropriate guilt (might be delusional)
   - Decreased concentration, indecisiveness, or inability to think clearly
   - Recurrent thoughts of death or suicidal ideation (with or without pain)
4. Symptoms are not due to (1) psychologic effects of substance, (2) a general medical condition, or (3) recent bereavement.

Adapted from American Psychiatric Association. (2000). *Diagnostic and statistical manual of mental disorders* (4th ed., text revision). Washington, DC: American Psychiatric Association p. 356; reprinted with permission.

- Alterations in eating, sleeping, activity level (fatigue), and libido
- Feelings of worthlessness or guilt
- Difficulty with concentration, memory, and making decisions
- Recurrent thoughts of death and/or self-harm

## Assessment Tools

There are many useful assessment tools available. See Appendix D-3 for an initial assessment guide.

| Box 6-2 | DSM-IV-TR Criteria for Dysthymia |
|---|---|

1. Depressed mood for most of the day during a 2-year period (1 year for children and adolescents), presence of depressed mood. **Note:** In children or adolescents, mood can be irritable and duration must be at least 1 year.
2. Symptoms cause clinically significant distress in social, occupational, and other important areas of functioning.
3. Presence of two or more of the following:
   - Decreased or increased appetite
   - Insomnia or hypersomnia
   - Anergia or chronic fatigue
   - Anhedonia
   - Poor concentration or difficulty making decisions
   - Feelings of hopelessness and despair
4. The symptoms are not related to a major depressive episode, a bipolar disorder, a psychotic disorder, the physiologic effects of any substances, or general medical condition.

Adapted from American Psychiatric Association. (2000). *Diagnostic and statistical manual of mental disorders* (4th ed., text revision). Washington, DC: American Psychiatric Association, p. 380; reprinted with permission.

## Assessment Guidelines

### Depression

1. A thorough physical and neurologic examination helps to determine if the depression is primary or secondary to another disorder. Depression is a mood that can be secondary to a host of medical or other psychiatric disorders, as well as drugs/medications. Essentially, the nurse evaluates if:
   - The client is psychotic
   - The client has taken drugs or alcohol
   - Medical conditions are present
2. Always evaluate the client's risk of harm to self or others. Overt hostility is highly correlated with suicide.

# NURSING DIAGNOSES WITH INTERVENTIONS

## Discussion of Potential Nursing Diagnoses

There are many areas in a person's life that can be severely affected by depression. **Risk for Self-Directed Violence** is the number one priority for assessment and intervention. **Risk for Suicide** is a concern with people who have a variety of psychiatric disorders (schizophrenia, bipolar disorder, substance abuse, borderline personality disorder) as well as medical disorders and syndromes. See Chapter 16 for a broader discussion.

Depression drastically affects a person's life and often affects cognitive ability. Poor concentration, lack of judgment, and difficulties with memory can all affect cognitive abilities **(Disturbed Thought Processes)**. Feelings of self-worth plummet **(Chronic Low Self-Esteem)**, and ability to gain strength from their usual religious activities dwindles **(Spiritual Distress)**. Feelings of hopelessness are common. Most noticeably, the ability to interact and gain solace from others is markedly reduced **(Impaired Social Interaction)**.

The vegetative signs of depression can lead to physical complications such as lack of sleep **(Disturbed Sleep Pattern)**, change in eating patterns **(Imbalanced Nutrition)**, and change in elimination (most often **Constipation**, although diarrhea can also occur in agitated clients). Therefore, **Self-Care Deficit** is often an obvious occurrence.

Table 6-1 identifies some potential nursing diagnoses for depressed clients.

Table 6-1 **Potential Nursing Diagnoses for Depressive Disorders**

| Signs and Symptoms | Potential Nursing Diagnoses |
| --- | --- |
| Previous suicidal attempts, putting affairs in order, giving away prized possessions, suicidal ideation (has a plan and the ability to carry it out), makes overt or covert statements regarding killing self, feelings of worthlessness, hopelessness, helplessness | **Risk for Self-Directed Violence** **Risk for Self-Mutilation** **Risk for Suicide** |

*Continued*

Table 6-1 **Potential Nursing Diagnoses for Depressive Disorders—cont'd**

| Signs and Symptoms | Potential Nursing Diagnoses |
|---|---|
| Lack of judgment, memory difficulty, poor concentration, inaccurate interpretation of environment, negative ruminations, cognitive distortions | **Disturbed Thought Processes** |
| Difficulty with simple tasks, inability to function at previous level, poor problem solving, poor cognitive functioning, verbalizations of inability to cope | **Ineffective Coping** <br> **Interrupted Family Processes** <br> **Risk for Impaired Parenting** <br> **Ineffective Role Performance** |
| Difficulty making decisions, poor concentration, inability to take action | **Decisional Conflict** |
| Feelings of helplessness, hopelessness, powerlessness | **Hopelessness** <br> **Powerlessness** |
| Questions meaning of life, own existence; unable to participate in usual religious practices, conflict over spiritual beliefs, anger toward spiritual deity or religious representatives | **Spiritual Distress** <br> **Impaired Religiosity** |
| Feelings of worthlessness, poor self-image, negative sense of self, self-negating verbalizations, feels like a failure, expressions of shame or guilt, hypersensitive to slights or criticism | **Chronic Low Self-Esteem** <br> **Situational Low Self-Esteem** |
| Withdrawn, noncommunicative, speaks only in monosyllables, shies away from contact with others | **Impaired Social Interaction** <br> **Social Isolation** <br> **Risk for Loneliness** |
| Vegetative signs of depression: Changes in sleep, eating, grooming and hygiene, elimination, sexual patterns | **Self-Care Deficit (bathing/ hygiene, dressing/grooming, feeding, toileting)** <br> **Imbalanced Nutrition** <br> **Disturbed Sleep Pattern** <br> **Constipation** <br> **Sexual Dysfunction** |

The section that identifies specific nursing diagnoses, goals, and interventions is useful when working with depressed clients and targeting discrete problems. However, the following overall guidelines are important throughout your work with depressed clients.

## Overall Guidelines for Nursing Interventions

### Depression

1. Convey caring, empathy, and potential for change by spending time with the client, even in silence, anticipating client's needs.
2. **The instillation of hope is a key tool for recovery.**
3. Enhance the person's sense of self by highlighting past accomplishments and strengths.
4. Whether in the hospital or in the community:
   - Assess needs for self-care and offer support when appropriate.
   - Monitor and intervene to help maintain adequate nutrition, hydration, and elimination.
   - Monitor and intervene to help provide adequate balance of rest, sleep, and activity.
   - Monitor and record increases/decreases in symptoms and which nursing interventions are effective.
   - Involve the client's support system and find supports for the client and family members in the community that are appropriate to their needs.
5. The dysfunctional attitude or learned helplessness and hopelessness seen with depressed people can be alleviated through cognitive therapy or other psychotherapeutic interventions.
6. **Continuously assess for the possibility of suicidal thoughts and ideation throughout the client's course of recovery.** (Refer to Chapter 16 for suicide assessment and interventions.)
7. Primary depression is a medical disease. People respond well to psychopharmacology and electroconvulsive therapy (ECT). Be sure clients and those closely involved with them understand the nature of the disease and have written information about the specific medications the client is taking. **Psychoeducation and a support system are essential.**
8. Assess family's and significant others' needs for teaching, counseling, self-help groups, knowledge of community resources.

## Selected Nursing Diagnoses and Nursing Care Plans

The following section offers key nursing diagnoses, goals, and nursing interventions that can help practitioners plan care for depressed clients.

### RISK FOR SELF-DIRECTED VIOLENCE*

At risk for behaviors in which an individual demonstrates that he/she can be physically, emotionally, and/or sexually harmful to self

### Related To (Etiology)

- ▲ Severe depression/psychosis/severe personality disorder, substance abuse
- ▲ Hopelessness, helplessness, anhedonia
- ▲ Loneliness
- ▲ Social isolation

### As Evidenced By
### (Assessment Findings/Diagnostic Cues)

- ▲ Suicidal behavior (attempts, talk, ideation, plan, available means)
- ● Suicide plan (clear, specific, lethal method and available means)
- ● Previous attempts
- ● When depression begins to lift, clients may have energy to carry out a suicide plan

### Outcome Criteria

- ● Behavioral manifestations of depression are absent
- ● Satisfaction with social circumstances and achievement of life goals
- ■ Seeks help when experiencing self-destructive impulses.

---

▲ NANDA International accepted; ● In addition to NANDA International; ■ NOC Outcomes for Impulse Self-Control

*Refer to chapter 16 for more detailed intervention for *Risk For Suicide*

## Long-Term Goals

Client will:
- Demonstrate alternative ways of dealing with negative feelings and emotional stress by (date)
- Identify supports and support groups with whom he/she is in contact within 1 month
- State that he/she wants to live
- Start working on constructive plans for the future
- Demonstrate compliance with any medication or treatment plan within 2 weeks

## Short-Term Goals

Clients will:
- Not harm self or others
- Identify at least two people he/she can call for support and emotional guidance when he/she is feeling self-destructive before discharge

## Interventions and Rationales

| Intervention | Rationale |
|---|---|
| 1. Determine level of suicide precautions needed. If high, does client need hospitalizaton? If low, will client be safe to go home with supervision from a friend or family member? For example, does client:<br>• Have a suicide plan<br>• Admit previous suicide attempts<br>• Abuse substances<br>• Have no friends | 1. A high-risk client will need constant supervision and a safe environment. Appendix D has an assessment tool to help evaluate the level of suicide risk. |
| 2. Does client have more than a week's supply of medication? | 2. Usually, when a client is suicidal, medication supply should be limited to 3 to 5 days. |

| Intervention | Rationale |
|---|---|
| 3. Encourage clients to talk freely about feelings (anger, disappointments), and help client plan alternative ways to handle anger and frustration. | 3. Client can learn alternative ways of dealing with overwhelming emotions and gain a sense of control over his/her life. |
| 4. Implement a written no-suicide contract if appropriate. | 4. Reinforces action the client can take when feeling suicidal. |
| 5. Contact family, arrange for crisis counseling. Activate links to self-help groups. | 5. Clients need a network of resources to help diminish personal feelings of worthlessness, isolation, and helplessness. |
| 6. If hospitalized, follow unit protocols. | 6. Refer to Chapter 16 for detailed interventions for the suicidal client in in either the hospital or the community. |

## DISTURBED THOUGHT PROCESSES

A state in which an individual experiences a disruption in cognitive operations and activities

### *Related To (Etiology)*

- Severe anxiety or depressed mood
- Biochemical/neurophysical imbalances
- Overwhelming life circumstances
- Persistent feelings of extreme anxiety, guilt, or fear
- Biologic/medical factors
- Prolonged grief reaction

---

- In addition to NANDA International

## As Evidenced By
## (Assessment Findings/Diagnostic Cues)

▲ Memory deficit/problems
▲ Inaccurate interpretation of the environment
▲ Hypovigilance
● Impaired perception, judgment, decision making
● Impaired attention span/easily distracted
● Impaired ability to grasp ideas or order thoughts
● Negative ruminations
● Impaired insight
● Decreased problem-solving abilities

## Outcome Criteria

• Recalls recent and remote information accurately
• Processes information and makes appropriate decisions
■ Exhibits organized thought process

## Long-Term Goals

Client will:
• Give examples showing that short-term memory and concentration have improved to usual levels by (date)
• Demonstrate an increased ability to make appropriate decisions when planning with nurse by (date)
• Identify negative thoughts and rationally counter them and/or reframe them in a positive manner within 2 weeks
• Show improved mood as demonstrated by the Beck Depression Inventory (see Appendix D-3)

## Short-Term Goals

Client will:
• Remember to keep appointments, attend activities, and attend to grooming with minimal reminders from others within 1 to 3 weeks
• Identify two goals he or she wants to achieve from treatment, with aid of nursing intervention, within 1 to 2 days

---

▲ NANDA International accepted; ● In addition to NANDA International; ■ NOC Outcomes for Information Processing

- Discuss with nurse two irrational thoughts about self and others by the end of the first day
- Reframe three irrational thoughts with nurse by (date)

## Interventions and Rationales

| Intervention | Rationale |
|---|---|
| 1. Identify client's previous level of cognitive functioning (from client, family, friends, previous medical records). | 1. Establishing a baseline of ability allows for evaluation of client's progress. |
| 2. Help the client to postpone important major life decision making. | 2. Making rational major life decisions requires optimal psychophysiologic functioning. |
| 3. Minimize client's responsibilities while he/she is severely depressed. | 3. Decreases feelings of pressure and anxiety, and minimizes feelings of guilt. |
| 4. Use simple, concrete words. | 4. Slowed thinking and difficulty concentrating impair comprehension. |
| 5. Allow client plenty of time to think and frame responses. | 5. Slowed thinking necessitates time to formulate a response. |
| 6. Help client and significant others structure an environment that can help re-establish set schedules and predictable routines during severe depression. | 6. A routine that is fairly repetitive and nondemanding is easier to both follow and remember. |
| 7. Allow more time than usual for client to finish usual activities of daily living (ADL) (e.g., dressing, eating). | 7. Usual tasks might take long periods of time; demands that the client hurry only increase anxiety and slow down ability to think clearly. |

| Intervention | Rationale |
|---|---|
| 8. Work with client to recognize negative thinking and thoughts. Teach client to reframe and/or refute negative thoughts. | 8. Negative ruminations add to feelings of hopelessness and are part of a depressed person's faulty thought processes. Intervening in this process aids in healthier and more useful outlook. |

## CHRONIC LOW SELF-ESTEEM

Long-standing negative self-evaluation/feelings about self or self-capabilities

*Related To (Etiology)*

- Biochemical/neurophysiologic imbalances
- Impaired cognitive self-appraisal
- Unrealistic expectations of self
- Shame and guilt
- Repeated past failures

*As Evidenced By*
*(Assessment Findings/Diagnostic Cues)*

- ▲ Negative feedback about self
- ▲ Self-negating verbalizations
- ▲ Rejection of positive feedback
- Repeated expressions of worthlessness
- Inability to recognize own achievements
- Negative view of abilities

*Outcome Criteria*

- Expresses belief in self
- Demonstrates a zest for life and ability to enjoy the present
- ■ Maintains self-esteem

---

▲ NANDA International accepted; ● In addition to NANDA International; ■ NOC Outcome for Psychosocial Adjustment: Life Change

## Long-Term Goals

Client will:
- Give an accurate and nonjudgmental account of four positive qualities as well as identify two areas he or she wishes to improve by (date)
- Demonstrate the ability to modify unrealistic self-expectations by (date)
- Report decreased feelings of shame, guilt, and self-hate by using a scale of 1 to 10 (1 lowest, 10 highest)

## Short-Term Goals

Client will:
- Identify one or two strengths by the end of the day
- Identify two unrealistic self-expectations and reformulate more realistic life goals with nurse by the end of the day
- Keep a daily log and identify on a scale of 1 to 10 (1 lowest, 10 highest) feelings of shame, guilt, self-hate
- Identify three judgmental terms (e.g., "I am lazy") client uses to describe self, and identify objective terms to replace them (e.g., "I do not feel motivated to") by (date)

## Interventions and Rationales

| Intervention | Rationale |
|---|---|
| 1. Work with the client to identify cognitive distortions that encourage negative self-appraisal. For example: | 1. Cognitive distortions reinforce negative, inaccurate perception of self and the world. |
| a. Overgeneralizations | a. Taking one fact or event and making a general rule out of it ("He always"; "I never") |
| b. Self-blame | b. Consistent self-blame for everything perceived as negative. |
| c. Mind reading | c. Assuming others "do not like me," for example, without any real evidence that assumptions are correct |
| d. Discounting positive attributes | d. Focusing on negative qualities |

| Intervention | Rationale |
|---|---|
| 2. Teach visualization techniques that help client replace negative self-images with more positive thoughts and images. | 2. Promotes a healthier and more realistic self-image by helping the client choose more positive actions and thoughts. |
| 3. Work with client on areas that he or she would like to improve using problem-solving skills. Evaluate need for more teaching in this area. | 3. Feelings of low self-esteem can interfere with usual problem-solving abilities. |
| 4. Evaluate client's need for assertiveness training tools to pursue things he or she wants or needs in life. Arrange for training through community-based programs, personal counseling, literature, etc. | 4. People with low self-esteem often feel unworthy and have difficulty asking appropriately for what they need and want. |
| 5. Role model assertiveness. | 5. Clients can follow examples. |
| 6. Encourage participation in a support/ therapy group where others are experiencing similar thoughts, feelings, and situations. | 6. Decrease feelings of isolation and provide an atmosphere where positive feedback and a more realistic appraisal of self are available. |

## SPIRITUAL DISTRESS

Impaired ability to experience and integrate meaning and purpose in life through a person's connectedness with self, others, art, music, literature, nature, or a power greater than oneself

## Related To (Etiology)

- ▲ Self-alienation
- ▲ Sociocultural deprivation
- ▲ Death or dying of self or others
- ▲ Chronic illness of self or others
- ▲ Life changes
- ▲ Pain
- ▲ Lack of purpose and meaning in life

## As Evidenced By
## (Assessment Findings/Diagnostic Cues)

- ▲ Expresses lack of hope, meaning or purpose in life, forgiveness of self, peace/serenity, acceptance
- ▲ Questions meaning of own existence
- ▲ Refuses interactions with friends/families/religious leaders
- ▲ Expresses concern with meaning of life/death or belief systems
- ▲ Expresses being abandoned by or having anger toward God
- ▲ Unable to participate in usual religious practices
- ▲ Inability to pray
- ▲ Inability to express previous state of creativity (e.g., singing, listening to music, writing)
- ▲ No interest in art
- ▲ Expresses hopelessness and helplessness
- ▲ Searching for spiritual source of strength
- ▲ Expresses intense feelings of guilt

## Outcome Criteria

- ● Expression of purpose and meaning in life
- ■ Participates in spiritual rites and passages
- ■ Connectedness with others to share thoughts, feelings, and beliefs
- ■ Connectedness with inner self

---

▲ NANDA International accepted; ● In addition to NANDA International; ■ NOC Outcome for Spiritual Health

## Long-Term Goals

Client will:
- State that he/she gained comfort from previous spiritual practices by (date)
- State that he/she feels a sense of forgiveness by (date)
- State that he/she wants to participate in former creative activities by (date)

## Short-Term Goals

Client will:
- Talk to nurse or spiritual leader about spiritual conflicts and concerns within 3 days
- Discuss with nurse two things that gave his or her life meaning in the past within 3 days
- Keep a journal tracking thoughts and feelings for 1 week

## Interventions and Rationales

| Intervention | Rationale |
|---|---|
| 1. Assess what spiritual practices have offered comfort and meaning to the client's life when not ill. | 1. Evaluates neglected areas in the person's life that, if reactivated, might add comfort and meaning during a painful depression. |
| 2. Discuss with the client what has given meaning and comfort to the person in the past. | 2. When depressed, clients often struggle for meaning in life and reasons to go on when feeling hopeless and despondent. |
| 3. Encourage client to write in a journal every day expressing daily thoughts and reflections. | 3. Helps some to identify significant personal issues and one's thoughts and feelings surrounding spiritual issues. Journal writing is an excellent way to explore deeper meanings of life. |
| 4. If client is unable to write, have client use a tape recorder. | 4. Often speaking aloud helps a person clarify thinking and explore issues. |

| Intervention | Rationale |
|---|---|
| 5. Provide information on referrals, when needed, for religious or spiritual information (e.g., readings, programs, tapes, community resources). | 5. When hospitalized, spiritual tapes and readings can be useful; when the client is in the community, client might express other needs. |
| 6. Suggest that the spiritual leader affiliated with the facility contact client. | 6. Spiritual leaders in an institution or community are familiar with spiritual distress and might offer comfort to client. |

## IMPAIRED SOCIAL INTERACTION

Insufficient or excessive quantity or ineffective quality of social exchange

### Related To (Etiology)

▲ Self-concept disturbance (negative view of self)
▲ Absence of available significant others/peers (support system deficit)
▲ Altered thought processes
● Fear of rejection
● Feelings of worthlessness
● Anergia (lack of energy and motivation)

### As Evidenced By
### (Assessment Findings/Diagnostic Cues)

▲ Family reports change of style or patterns of interaction
▲ Verbalized or observed discomfort in social situations (e.g., inability to receive or communicate a satisfying sense of belonging, caring, interest, or shared history)
▲ Dysfunctional interaction with peers, family, and/or others
● Remains secluded, lacks eye contact, and avoids contact with others

---

▲ NANDA International accepted; ● In addition to NANDA International

## Outcome Criteria

- ■ Interacts with Family/Friends/Neighbors
- ■ Participation in community activities (e.g., church member, club officer, volunteer group, leisure activity)
- • Performance of premorbid role behaviors

## Long-Term Goals

Client will:
- • State and demonstrate progress in the resumption of sustaining relationships with friends and family members within 1 month
- • State that he/she enjoys interacting with others in activities and one-to-one interactions to the extent they did before becoming depressed by (date)

## Short-Term Goals

Client will:
- • Participate in one activity by the end of each day
- • Discuss three alternative actions to take when feeling the need to withdraw by (date)
- • Identify two personal behaviors that might discourage others from seeking contact by (date)
- • Eventually voluntarily attend individual/group therapeutic meetings within a therapeutic milieu (hospital or community) by (date)

## Interventions and Rationales

| Intervention | Rationale |
|---|---|
| 1. While client is most severely depressed, involve the client in one-to-one activity. | 1. Maximizes the potential for interactions while minimizing anxiety levels. |
| 2. Engage the client in activities involving gross motor activity that call for limited concentration (e.g., taking a walk). | 2. Physical activities can help relieve tensions and might help to elevate mood. |

■ Adapted from NOC Outcome Social Involvement

| Intervention | Rationale |
|---|---|
| 3. Initially, provide activities that require very little concentration (e.g., playing simple card games, looking through a magazine, drawing). | 3. Concentration and memory are poor in depressed people. Activities that have no "right or wrong" or "winners or losers" minimize opportunities for the client to put himself or herself down. |
| 4. Eventually increase the client's contacts with others (first one other, then two others, etc.). | 4. Contact with others distracts the client from self-preoccupation. |
| 5. Eventually involve the client in group activities (e.g., dance therapy, art therapy, group discussions). | 5. Socialization decreases feelings of isolation. Genuine regard for others can increase self-worth. |
| 6. Refer the client as well as the family to self-help groups in the community. | 6. Both client and family can gain tremendous support and insight from people sharing their experiences. |

## SELF-CARE DEFICIT (SPECIFY LEVEL)

Impaired ability to perform or complete bathing/hygiene, dressing/grooming, feeding, or toileting activities for oneself

*Related To (Etiology)*

▲ Perceptual or cognitive impairment
▲ Decreased or lack of motivation (anergia)
▲ Severe anxiety
● Severe preoccupation

---

▲ NANDA International accepted; ● In addition to NANDA International

*As Evidenced By*
*(Assessment Findings/Diagnostic Cues)*

▲ Consuming insufficient food or nutrients to meet minimum daily requirements
▲ Awakening earlier or later than desired
▲ Decreased ability to function secondary to sleep deprivation
▲ Weight loss
▲ Persistent insomnia or hypersomnia
● Body odor/hair unwashed and unkempt
● Inability to organize simple steps in hygiene and grooming
● Constipation related to lack of exercise, roughage in diet, and poor fluid intake

*Outcome Criteria*

• Performs all tasks of self-care consistently (all ADL*)
• Experiences normal elimination
• Sleeps 6 to 8 hours a night without medication

*Long-Term Goals*

Client will:
• Gradually return to weight consistent for height and age or baseline before illness by (date)
• Sleep between 6 and 8 hours per night within 1 month
• Demonstrate progress in the maintenance of adequate hygiene and be appropriately groomed and dressed (shave/makeup, clothes clean and neat)
• Experience normal elimination with the aid of diet, fluids, and exercise within 3 weeks

*Short-Term Goals*

Client will:
• Gain 1 pound a week with encouragement from family, significant others, and/or staff if significant weight loss exists.
• Sleep between 4 and 6 hours with aid of medication and/or nursing measures.

---

▲ NANDA International accepted; ● In addition to NANDA International

*ADL = Activities of daily living

- Groom and dress appropriately with help from nursing staff and/or family.
- Regain more normal elimination pattern with aid of foods high in roughage, increased fluids, and exercise daily (also with aid of medications).

## Interventions and Rationales

| Intervention | Rationale |
|---|---|
| **Imbalanced Nutrition** | |
| 1. Encourage small, high-calorie, and high-protein snacks and fluids frequently throughout the day and evening if weight loss exists. | 1. Minimize weight loss, dehydration, and constipation. |
| 2. Encourage eating with others. | 2. Increase socialization, decrease focus on food. |
| 3. Serve foods or drinks the client likes. | 3. Clients are more likely to eat the foods they like. |
| 4. Weigh the client weekly and observe the client's eating patterns. | 4. Give the information needed for revising the intervention. |
| **Disturbed Sleep Pattern** | |
| 1. Provide rest periods after activities. | 1. Fatigue can intensify feelings of depression. |
| 2. Encourage the client to get up and dress and to stay out of bed during the day. | 2. Minimizing sleep during the day increases the likelihood of sleep at night. |
| 3. Encourage relaxation measures in the evening (e.g., backrub, tepid bath, or warm milk). | 3. These measures induce relaxation and sleep. |
| 4. Reduce environmental and physical stimulants in the evening; provide decaffeinated coffee, soft lights, soft music, and quiet activities. | 4. Decreasing caffeine and epinephrine levels increases the possibility of sleep. |

| Intervention | Rationale |
|---|---|
| 5. Teach relaxation exercises (see Chapter 5). | 5. Besides deeply relaxing the body, relaxation exercises often lead to sleep. |

### Bathing/Hygiene Self-Care Deficit

| | |
|---|---|
| 1. Encourage the use of toothbrush, washcloth, soap, makeup, shaving equipment, and so forth. | 1. Being clean and well groomed can temporarily raise self-esteem. |
| 2. Give step-by-step reminders, such as "Wash the right side of your face, now the left . . ." | 2. Slowed thinking and difficulty concentrating make organizing simple tasks difficult. |

| Intervention | Rationale |
|---|---|
| **Constipation** | |
| 1. Monitor intake and output, especially bowel movements. | 1. Many depressed clients are constipated. If this condition is not checked, fecal impaction can occur. |
| 2. Offer foods high in fiber and provide periods of exercise. | 2. Roughage and exercise stimulate peristalsis and help evacuation of fecal material. |
| 3. Encourage the intake of nonalcoholic/noncaffeinated fluids, 6 to 8 glasses/day. | 3. Fluids help prevent constipation. |
| 4. Evaluate the need for laxatives and enemas. | 4. These prevent the occurrence of fecal impaction. |

# MEDICAL TREATMENTS

## Psychopharmacology

Depression is a recurring disorder. About 75% to 95% of people with a primary depression have multiple episodes. However, the discovery of effective antidepressants has resulted in depression being one of the most "treatable" disorders (Zajecka, 1995). Keller (1995) noted that:

- 65% to 75% of depression clients "respond" to antidepressant treatment.
- 25% to 35% of clients with a major depression fail to respond meaningfully to currently available treatment. However, **waiting too long to start treatment can lead to**:
- Greater morbidity
- Greater disability
- Greater expense
- Greater resistance to treatment and increased potential for relapse

All depressed individuals need to be evaluated for suicide risk, whether they are in the hospital or the community. When a depressed person is hospitalized, staff members need to check to make sure that all medications are swallowed (not placed in the cheek or under the tongue). If a client is being treated in an outpatient setting, only a week's supply of medication should be given to a severely depressed person to minimize client overdosing.

Antidepressant drugs can improve poor self-concept, degree of withdrawal, vegetative signs of depression, and activity level.

The major types of antidepressant drugs are the:

- Selective serotonin reuptake inhibitors **(SSRIs)**
- Tricyclic antidepressants **(TCAs)**
- Monoamine oxidase inhibitors **(MAOIs)**
- Novel (atypical) antidepressants

## *Selective Serotonin Reuptake Inhibitors*

SSRIs are recommended as first-line therapy in all depressions, except severe inpatient depression (in which ECT might be the first choice) or melancholic depression, or mild outpatient depression.

SSRI antidepressant drugs have a lower incidence of anticholinergic side effects (dry mouth, blurred vision, urinary retention), less cardiotoxicity, and faster onset than the TCAs. For most clients, the SSRIs are better tolerated than the TCAs. The SSRIs are also being used successfully with many individuals who have anxiety disorders and eating disorders. See Table 6-2 for a list of SSRIs and dosages. Refer to Chapter 21 for pharmacology and a guide to client and family teaching for SSRIs.

Table 6-2 **Adult Dosages for Antidepressants**

| Generic Name | Trade Name | Initial Dose*† (mg/day) | Dose after 4-8 Weeks* (mg/day) | Maximum Dose‡ (mg/day) |
|---|---|---|---|---|
| **Tricyclic Antidepressants (TCAs)** | | | | |
| Amitriptyline | Elavil | 50 | 100–200 | 300 |
| Clomipramine | Anafranil | 25 | 100–200 | 250 |
| Desipramine | Norpramin | 50 | 100–200 | 300 |
| Doxepin | Sinequan | 50 | 75–150 | 300 |
| Imipramine | Tofranil | 50 | 75–150 | 300 |
| Maprotiline | Ludiomil | 50 | 100–150 | 225 |
| Nortriptyline | Pamelor | 20 | 75–125 | 200 |
| Protriptyline | Vivactil | 10 | 15–40 | 80 |
| Trimipramine | Surmontil | 50 | 100–200 | 300 |
| Amoxapine | Asendin | 50 | 200–300 | 400 |
| **Monoamine Oxidase Inhibitors (MAOIs)** | | | | |
| Isocarboxazid | Marplan | 20 | 20–60 | 80 |
| Phenelzine | Nardil | 15 | 45–60 | 90 |
| Tranylcypromine | Parnate | 10 | 30–40 | 60 |
| **Selective Serotonin Reuptake Inhibitors (SSRIs)** | | | | |
| Citalopram | Celexa | 10 | 20–60 | 80 |
| Escitalopram | Lexapro | 10 | 10–20 | 40 |
| Fluoxetine | Prozac | 20 | 20–80 | 80 |
| Fluvoxamine | Luvox | 50 | 50–300 | 300 |
| Paroxetine | Paxil | 10 | 20–50 | 50 |
| Sertraline | Zoloft | 50 | 50–250 | 200 |
| **Atypical Antidepressants** | | | | |
| Bupropion | Wellbutrin | 150 | 50–300 | 450 |
| Trazodone | Desyrel | 50 | 150–400 | 600 |
| **Dual Action Reuptake Inhibitors (Serotonin and Norepinephrine) (SNRIs)** | | | | |
| Mirtazepine | Remeron | 15 | 15-45 | 60 |
| Duloxetine | Cymbalta | 20 | 40-60 | 120 |
| Venlafaxine | Effexor | 37.5 | 75-225 | 375 |
| **Selective Norepinephrine Reuptake Inhibitors (NRIs)** | | | | |
| Reboxetine | Vestra | 4-8 | 4-10 | 10 |

From Lehne RA. (2004). Preston et al, 2005, Preston and Johnson, 2004.
*Doses listed are total daily doses. Depending on the drug and the patient, the total dose might be given in a single dose or in divided doses.
†Initial doses are employed for 4 to 8 weeks, the time required for most symptoms to respond. Dosage is gradually increased as required.
‡Doses higher than these might be needed for some people with severe depression.

## Tricyclic Antidepressants

TCAs benefit approximately 65% to 80% of people with nondelusional depressive disorders. It can take up to 10 to 14 days before these agents start to work. The full effect might not be seen for 4 to 8 weeks. As with all drugs, side effects and toxic effects can occur. As mentioned, the SSRIs are considered the drugs of choice.

People taking TCAs can have adverse reactions to numerous other medications. For example, use of an MAOI along with a TCA is contraindicated.

Clients and families should be aware of the side effects and toxic effects of the medications as well as other relevant information. This information should be written down and given to the family and client once teaching is complete. See Table 6-2 for a list of TCAs and dosages. Refer to Chapter 21 for pharmacology and a guide to client and family teaching for the TCAs.

## Monoamine Oxidase Inhibitors

These drugs are usually *not* first-line drugs because of their serious side effects. A serious side effect of these drugs is that they interact with foods containing tyramine, a natural product of bacterial fermentation found in many cheeses, some wines, and chopped liver as well as certain medications, including sympathomimetic amines. The interaction results in a hypertensive crisis that can cause a stroke or even death.

Because these drugs have the danger of hypertensive crisis, they are usually contraindicated for people who are debilitated, elderly, or hypertensive; those who have cardiac or cerebrovascular disease; those who have severe renal and hepatic disease; and those unwilling or unable to adhere to dietary restrictions.

Client teaching is as important with these drugs as all others, perhaps even more so because of the danger of hypertensive crisis with tyramine-containing foods and with medications. Clients and their families should know these foods and drugs, and be taught to read food labels very carefully, because some of these tyramine-containing foods might be present as an ingredient. Clients should also be told that, before they take *any* over-the-counter medication, they should first check with their physician. See Table 6-2 for a list of MAOIs and dosages. Refer to Chapter 21 for pharmacology, a list of "forbidden" foods, and client and family teaching.

## Novel (Atypical) Antidepressants

Novel (atypical) antidepressants are among a group of drugs that differ structurally or in their pharmacologic action from the medications in the categories mentioned earlier. Included in this group are trazodone (Desyrel), nefazodone (Serzone), bupropion (Wellbutrin), venlafaxine (Effexor), mirtazapine (Remeron), and reboxetine (Vestra). See Table 6-2 for a list of atypical antidepressants and dosages. Refer to Chapter 21 for further discussion of the atypical antidepressants. Refer to Appendix G for monographs of these drugs.

## Electroconvulsive Therapy

Electroconvulsive therapy (ECT) is indicated when antidepressant drugs have no effect or for severely depressed suicidal clients who need rapid relief of symptoms. Typically 80% to 90% of people with a major depressive disorder will respond to ECT (American Psychiatric Association [APA], 2000b). ECT has also been found to be approximately 50% effective with clients who have not responded to antidepressant medication (APA, 2000b). ECT should be considered the first-line of treatment for severe major depressive disorder when psychotic features, catatonic stupor, severe suicidality, or self-starvation are present.

ECT can terminate an ongoing episode of depression; therefore, some people greatly benefit from "maintenance" treatments on a weekly or monthly basis to prevent recurrence. One study demonstrated a relapse rate of 73% without "maintenance" and only an 8% relapse rate among those getting maintenance treatments (Lehne, 2004).

ECT is generally considered a very safe treatment. Death from ECT has not occurred in the past 15 years (Maxmen & Ward, 2002). The chief side effects of ECT are cognitive. Treatment is most often associated with transient confusional state after single treatments, and with a longer period of antero-grade and retrograde memory interference (APA, 2000b).

Depressed clients with various medical conditions might be at risk, and, therefore, clients with cardiovascular disease, those with increased intracranial pressure, or those with cerebrovascular fragility might be poor candidates and would require careful medical work-up.

Essentially, ECT is the use of electrically induced repetitive firings of the neurons in the central nervous system. Electrodes are placed on the clients' temples (either bilaterally or unilaterally), and they are given a well-measured electric shock.

These electrical firings cause grand mal seizures in the brain. Therefore, clients are under a short-acting anesthesia, and they are also given a muscle-paralyzing agent to help prevent fractures. A course of ECT for depressed clients is approximately 6 to 12 treatments given two or three times per week. See Appendix F for a better understanding of the actual procedure and the nursing responsibilities involved in ECT.

## INTEGRATED APPROACHES (CAM)

Perhaps the best known of herbal remedies for depression is **St. John's wort**. St. John's wort has been reported in some studies to be effective for mild to moderate depressions. The herb should not be taken in certain situations (e.g., major depression, pregnancy, or children younger than 2 years old [Fuller & Sajatovic, 2000]). St. John's wort is not regulated as a drug by the FDA. St. John's wort has significant effects on liver metabolism and poses a danger of potentially harmful drug-drug interaction (Preston and associates, 2005). For example, the combined use of St. John's wort can have harmful effects with Digoxin, birth control pills, anesthesia, amphetamines, and other stimulants, and all other antidepressants.

SAM-e (s-adenosylmethionine), a synthetic form of a chemical produced naturally in the body, also proposed to be of a possible benefit in depression. To date, the possible benefits and long-term risks remain unclear (UC Berkeley Wellness Letter, 2005). One important problem with SAM-e is that it is converted into homocystine in the body and high levels of homoaptine appear to raise the risk of heart disease (UC Berkeley Wellness Letter, 2004). SAM-e should be used with caution in bipolar disorder as it may induce mania, and should not be taken with any other serotonin enhancing drugs since it may increase serotonin syndrome. Check out **consumerlab.com** for reputable brands of herbal and dietary supplements.

## NURSE, CLIENT, AND FAMILY RESOURCES

### ASSOCIATIONS

**National Alliance for the Mentally Ill (NAMI)**
Colonial Place Three
2107 Wilson Boulevard, Suite 300
Arlington, VA 22201-3042
(800) 950-NAMI

**Depressed Anonymous: Recovery from Depression**
http://www.nami.org
PO Box 17471
Louisville, KY 40217
(502) 569-1989
http://www.depressedanon.com

**National Foundation for Depressive Illness, Inc,**
PO Box 2257
New York, NY 10016
(800) 239-1265
http://www.depression.org

**National Organization for Seasonal Affective Disorders (NOSAD)**
PO Box 40190
Washington, DC 20016

**Depression and Bipolar Support Alliance**
730 N. Franklin, Suite 501
Chicago, IL 60610
(312) 642-0049
http://dbsalliance.org

## INTERNET SITES

**Depression Central**
www.psycom.net/depression.central.html

**Depression.com**
http://www.depression.com
Great general source

**Internet Mental Health**
http://www.mentalhealth.com
Great resource for everything

**NIMH: Depression**
www.nimh.nih.gov/publicat/depression.cfm

# CHAPTER 7

# Bipolar Disorders

## OVERVIEW

Bipolar disorders are mood disorders that include one or more manic or hypomanic episodes (elevated, expansive, or irritable mood) and usually one or more depressive episodes. Bipolar disorders are essentially related to biochemical imbalances in the brain, and the disease is thought to be genetically transferred. Medication adherence is key if nursing and counseling interventions are to be effective.

An acute or severe manic phase usually warrants hospitalization. A person experiencing hypomania, however, rarely needs hospitalization, unless there is a danger to self or others.

Bipolar disorders consist of three different categories of disorders: (1) **cyclothymia;** (2) **bipolar disorder (bipolar I and bipolar II)** and (3) **bipolar disorder not otherwise specified**. The symptoms seen in bipolar disorder (I and II) are more serious than those seen in cyclothymia. (American Psychiatric Association [APA], 2000)

### Cyclothymia

Cyclothymia is a chronic mood disturbance of at least 2 years duration. Cyclothymia is the recurrent experience of some of the symptoms of *hypomania* alternating with *dysthymic depression*. People with cyclothymia *do not* have severe impairment in their social or occupational functioning, nor do they experience psychotic symptoms such as delusions.

## Bipolar Disorder (Bipolar I and Bipolar II)

The manic episode in bipolar I might begin suddenly and last a few days to months. There can be impairments in reality testing, and, when severe, these impairments can take the form of grandiose or persecutory *delusions*. Considerable impairment in social, occupational, and interpersonal functioning exists. Hospitalization is often required to protect the person from the consequences of poor judgment and hyperactivity. **Bipolar disorder is classified as severe, biologically based mental illness by medical science**, in conjunction with the *Diagnostic and Statistical Manual of Mental Disorders* (4th edition, text revision) (DSM-IV-TR).

**Bipolar I** consists of one or more episodes of *major depression* plus one or more periods of clear-cut *mania*.

**Bipolar II** consists of one or more periods of *major depression* plus at least one *hypomanic episode*.

The distinction between hypomania and mania is made clear for diagnostic purposes in the DSM-IV-TR, and is presented in Box 7-1.

Bipolar disorder can be grouped into three phases:

1. **Acute Phase**—Hospitalization is usually indicated for a client in the acute manic or severe manic phase of bipolar disorder (particularly bipolar I). Hospitalization protects clients from harm (cardiac collapse, financial loss) and allows time for medication stabilization.
2. **Continuation Phase**—Usually lasts for 4 to 9 months, and the goal during this phase is to prevent relapse.
3. **Maintenance Treatment Phase**—Aimed at preventing the recurrence of an episode of bipolar illness.

Many of the interventions in this chapter address the client in the acute phase, because that is the phase that requires the most immediate and complex nursing care.

# ASSESSMENT

## Presenting Signs and Symptoms

- Periods of hyperactivity (pacing, restlessness, accelerated actions)
- Overconfident, exaggerated view of own abilities
- Decreased need for sleep; no acknowledgment of fatigue

Box
7-1

# DSM-IV-TR
## Criteria for Manic Episode and Hypomanic Episode

1. A distinct period of abnormality and persistently elevated, expansive, or irritable mood for at least:
   - 4 days for hypomania
   - 1 week for mania
2. During the period of mood disturbance, **at least three (or more)** of the following symptoms have persisted (four if the mood is only irritable) and have been present to a significant degree:
   - Inflated self-esteem or grandiosity
   - Decreased need for sleep (e.g., the person feels rested after only 3 hours of sleep)
   - Increased talkativeness or pressure to keep talking
   - Flight of ideas or subjective experience that thoughts are racing
   - Distractibility (i.e., the person's attention is too easily drawn to unimportant or irrelevant external stimuli)
   - Increase in goal-directed activity (either socially, at work or school, or sexually) or psychomotor agitation
   - Excessive involvement in pleasurable activities that have a high potential for painful consequences (e.g., the person engages in unrestrained buying sprees, sexual indiscretions, or foolish business investments)

### Hypomania
1. The episode is associated with an unequivocal change in functioning that is uncharacteristic of the person when not symptomatic.
2. Absence of marked impairment in social or occupational functioning.
3. Delusions are never present.
4. Hospitalization is not indicated.

### Mania
1. Severe enough to cause marked impairment in occupational activities, usual social activities, or relationships
   *or*
2. Hospitalization is needed to protect client and others from irresponsible or aggressive behavior
   *or*
3. There are psychotic features (e.g., grandiose and/or paranoid delusions)

Adapted from American Psychiatric Association. (2000). *Diagnostic and statistical manual of mental disorders* (4th ed., text revision). Washington, DC: American Psychiatric Association, pp. 362, 368; reprinted with permission.

- Poor social judgment, engaging in reckless and self-destructive activities (foolish business ventures, sexual indiscretions, buying sprees)
- Rapid-fire speech; pressured speech; loud, garrulous, rhyming or punning
- Brief attention span, easily distractible, flights of ideas, loosened associations, delusions
- Expansive, irritable, or paranoid behaviors
- Impatient, uncooperative, abusive, obscene, manipulative

## Assessment Tools

See Appendix D-4 for a questionnaire for mania. Clients might want to take this test frequently to monitor symptoms.

## Assessment Guidelines

Assessment will, of course, include identification of manic symptoms (Appendix D-4) and depressive symptoms (Appendix D-3). However, there are very important areas that need to be identified to secure safety, not just for the client, but perhaps others as well. Important overall assessment guidelines follow.

### Elated-Phase Bipolar

1. Assess if client is a danger to self or others:
   - Manic clients can exhaust themselves to the point of death.
   - Client might not eat or sleep for days at a time.
   - Poor impulse control might result in harm to others or self.
   - Uncontrolled spending.
2. Clients might give away all of their money or possessions, so might need controls to protect them from bankruptcy.
3. Assess for need for hospitalization to safeguard and stabilize client.
4. Assess medical status. A thorough medical examination helps to determine if mania is primary (a mood disorder—bipolar/cyclothymia) or secondary to another condition. Mania can be:
   - Secondary to a general medical condition
   - Substance induced (use or abuse of drug, medication, or toxin exposure)

5. Assess the client's and family's understanding of bipolar disorder, knowledge of medications, support groups, and organizations that provide information on bipolar disorder.

# NURSING DIAGNOSES WITH INTERVENTIONS

## Discussion of Potential Nursing Diagnoses

During an acutely or extremely manic episode, hospitalization is recommended to prevent physical exhaustion and to initiate and stabilize medication. The primary consideration is the prevention of exhaustion and death from cardiac collapse. Because of the client's poor judgment, excessive and constant motor activity, probably dehydration, and difficulty evaluating reality, the client is at risk for injury **(Risk for Injury)**.

Aggression is a common feature in mania. At times, intrusive and taunting behaviors can induce others to strike out against these clients. Conversely, when in a manic state, a client might evidence inability to control behavior, and destructive, hostile, and aggressive behaviors (range reaction) might occur and pose danger to the well-being of others and/or property **(Risk for Violence: Self-Directed or Other-Directed)**.

Grandiosity and poor judgment can result in the client giving away money and possessions indiscriminately, bankruptcy, and neglect of family. Clients might get involved in making foolish business deals or make impulsive major life changes (e.g., divorce, marriage, or career changes). Getting involved in impossible schemes, shady legal deals, and questionable business ventures can also be part of the picture. Because of the client's grandiose thinking and extremely poor judgment, **Disturbed Thought Processes** are present. The behaviors that stem from the client's faulty thinking usually result in **Ineffective Coping**.

Clients in the manic phase can be extremely manipulative, fault finding, and adept at exploiting other's vulnerabilities. They constantly push limits. Often the motivation for this manipulation is an attempt to gain a sense of control, when, in fact, the person is totally unable to control any aspect of his or her life: thoughts, feelings, and particularly behaviors. Therefore, **Defensive Coping** might be evidenced by the client's manipulative, angry, and hostile verbal behaviors.

The families of people with bipolar disorder often experience extreme disruptions in their lives, and might be in crises when their family member is in acute and severe mania. Infidelity and divorce is common; family savings might be wiped out and debt accumulated; relationships within the family unit might be strained beyond endurance; and friendships can be ruined. **Interrupted Family Processes** must always be assessed and information and referrals for support provided.

The client in the acute or extreme manic state might have numerous unmet physical needs. The manic client is too agitated and hyperactive to eat, sleep, or be appropriately groomed or dressed and can be constipated. Therefore, **Deficient Fluid Volume, Imbalanced Nutrition, Disturbed Sleep Pattern, Constipation, Dressing/Grooming Self-Care Deficit, and Bathing/Hygiene Self-Care Deficit** are all areas that need to be carefully assessed. When the client is severely manic, the nurse could target interventions for all of the above using **Total Self-Care Deficit** (eating, sleeping, dressing/grooming, bathing/hygiene, bowel functioning).

Table 7-1 provides a list of potential nursing diagnoses.

Table 7-1 **Potential Nursing Diagnoses for Bipolar Disorder**

| Signs and Symptoms | Nursing Diagnoses |
| --- | --- |
| Excessive and constant motor activity | **Risk for Injury** |
| Poor judgment | |
| Lack of rest and sleep | |
| Poor nutritional intake (Excessive/relentless mix of above behaviors can lead to cardiac collapse.) | |
| Loud, profane, hostile, combative, aggressive, demanding | **Risk for Violence: Self-Directed or Other-Directed** |
| Intrusive and taunting behaviors | **Ineffective Coping** |
| Inability to control behavior | |

*Continued*

Table 7-1 **Potential Nursing Diagnoses for Bipolar Disorder—cont'd**

| Signs and Symptoms | Nursing Diagnoses |
| --- | --- |
| Rage reaction | |
| Manipulative, angry, or hostile verbal and physical behaviors | **Defensive Coping** |
| Racing thoughts, grandiosity, poor judgment | **Disturbed Thought Processes Ineffective Coping** |
| Gives away valuables, neglects family, makes impulsive major life changes (divorce, career changes) | **Interrupted Family Processes Caregiver Role Strain** |
| Continuous, pressured speech jumping from topic to topic **(flights of ideas)** | **Impaired Verbal Communication** |
| Constant motor activity, going from one person or event to another; might annoy or taunt others; speech loud and crass; provocative behaviors | **Impaired Social Interaction** |
| Too distracted, agitated, and disorganized to eat, groom, bathe, dress self | **Imbalanced Nutrition: Less than Body Requirements** |
| Too frantic and hyperactive to sleep; sleep deprivation can lead to exhaustion and death | **Deficient Fluid Volume Self-Care Deficit (bathing/ hygiene, dressing/grooming) Disturbed Sleep Pattern** |

## Overall Guidelines for Nursing Interventions

Specific behaviors demonstrated by the manic client should be addressed separately, as follows in this text. However, there are overall guidelines that are effective with bipolar clients during periods of mania. Overall guidelines include:

### Elated-Phase Bipolar

1. Use a firm and calm approach.
2. Use short, concise explanations or statements.
3. Remain neutral, avoid power struggles.
4. Provide a consistent and structured environment.
5. Firmly redirect energy into appropriate and constructive channels.

6. Decrease environmental stimuli whenever possible.
7. Provide structured solitary activities; tasks that take minimal concentration are best. Avoid groups and stimulating activities until client can tolerate that level of activity.
8. Spend one-on-one time with the client if he/she is psychotic or anxious.
9. Provide frequent rest periods.
10. Provide high-calorie fluids and finger foods frequently throughout the day.
11. On a daily basis, monitor client's:
    • Sleep pattern
    • Food intake
    • Elimination (constipation often a problem)
12. Teach client and family about illness, and be sure client has written information regarding his or her medications.
13. Ascertain that client and family have information on supportive services in their community for further information and support.

## Selected Nursing Diagnoses and Nursing Care Plans

The following sections identify primary nursing diagnoses for use with a manic client, particularly in the acute and severely manic phases of the illness. Included are specific nursing interventions that are appropriate for meeting outcome criteria for each diagnosis.

### RISK FOR INJURY

A state in which the individual is at risk of injury as a result of environmental conditions interacting with the individual's adaptive and defensive resources

### Related To (Etiology)

▲ Cognitive, affective, and psychomotor factors
● Biochemical/neurologic imbalances
● Extreme hyperactivity/physical agitation
● Rage reaction
● Dehydration and exhaustion

---

▲ NANDA International accepted;  ● In addition to NANDA International

## As Evidenced By
## (Assessment Findings/Diagnostic Cues)

- Impaired judgment (reality testing, risk behavior)
- Excessive and constant motor activity—unable to rest for even short periods
- Lack of fluid ingestion
- Abrasions, bruises, cuts from running/falling into objects

## Outcome Criteria

- Response to medication will have expected therapeutic effects
- Maintenance of therapeutic blood levels
- Sustain optimum physical health through medication management and therapeutic regimen

## Long-Term Goals

Client will:
- Be free of injury within 2 to 3 weeks:
  - Cardiac status stable
  - Well hydrated
  - Skin free of abrasions and scrapes
- Be free of excessive physical agitation and purposeless motor activity within 2 weeks
- Take short voluntary rest periods during the day by (date)

## Short-Term Goals

- Client's cardiac status will remain stable while in the hospital
- While acutely manic, client will drink 8 oz of fluid every hour throughout the day
- Client will spend time with the nurse in a quiet environment three to four times a day between 7 AM and 11 PM with the aid of nursing guidance
- Client will remain free from falls and abrasions every day while in the hospital
- Client will be free of dangerous levels of hyperactive motor behavior with the aid of medications and nursing interventions within 24 hours

---

▲ NANDA International accepted; ● In addition to NANDA International

*Interventions and Rationales*

| Intervention | Rationale |
|---|---|
| 1. Maintain low level of stimuli in client's environment (e.g., away from bright lights, loud noises, and people). | 1. Helps decrease escalation of anxiety. |
| 2. Provide structured solitary activities with nurse or aide. | 2. Structure provides security and focus. |
| 3. Provide frequent high-calorie fluids. | 3. Prevents serious dehydration. |
| 4. Provide frequent rest periods. | 4. Prevents exhaustion. |
| 5. Redirect violent behavior. | 5. Physical exercise can decrease tension and provide focus. |
| 6. Acute mania might warrant the use of phenothiazines and seclusion to minimize physical harm. | 6. Exhaustion and death result from dehydration, lack of sleep, and constant physical activity. |
| 7. Observe for signs of lithium toxicity. | 7. There is a small margin of safety between therapeutic and toxic doses. |
| 8. Protect client from giving away money and possessions. Hold valuables in hospital safe until rational judgment returns. | 8. Client's "generosity" is a manic defense that is consistent with irrational, grandiose thinking. |

## RISK FOR VIOLENCE: SELF-DIRECTED OR OTHER DIRECTED

At risk for behaviors in which an individual demonstrates that he/she can be physically, emotionally, and/or sexually harmful to self or others

## Related To (Etiology)

- ▲ Psychotic symptomatology
- ▲ Rage reaction
- ▲ Impulsivity
- ▲ Manic excitement
- ● Biochemical/neurologic imbalances

## As Evidenced By
## (Assessment Findings/Diagnostic Cues)

- ▲ Verbal threats against others
- ▲ Verbal threats against self (suicidal threats/attempts, hitting or injuring self, banging head against wall)
- ▲ Provocative behaviors (e.g., argumentative)
- ● Loud, threatening, profane speech
- ● Poor impulse control
- ● Agitated behaviors (e.g., slamming doors, prowling hallways, increased muscle tension, knocking things over)

## Outcome Criteria

- • Displays nonviolent behaviors toward self and others
- • Verbalizes control of feelings
- • Interacts with others appropriately

## Long-Term Goals

Client will:
- • Refrain from verbal threats and loud, profane language toward others by (date)
- • Seek help when experiencing aggressive impulses by (date)

## Short-Term Goals

Client will:
- • Display nonviolent behavior toward others in the hospital, with the aid of medications and nursing interventions
- • Refrain from provoking others to physical harm, with the aid of seclusion or nursing interventions
- • Respond to external controls (medications, seclusion, nursing interventions) when potential or actual loss of control occurs

---

▲ NANDA International accepted; ● In addition to NANDA International

*Interventions and Rationales*

| Intervention | Rationale |
|---|---|
| 1. Use a calm and firm approach. | 1. Provides structure and and control for a client who is out of control. |
| 2. Use short and concise explanations or statements. | 2. Short attention span limits comprehension to small bits of information. |
| 3. Maintain a consistent approach, employ consistent expectations, and provide a structured environment. | 3. Clear and consistent limits and expectations minimize potential for client's manipulation of staff. |
| 4. Remain neutral: avoid power struggles and value judgments. | 4. Client can use inconsistencies and value judgments as justification for arguing and escalating mania. |
| 5. Decrease environmental stimuli (keep away from loud music/ noises, people, and bright lights). | 5. Helps decrease escalation of anxiety and manic symptoms. |
| 6. Assess client's behavior frequently (every 15 minutes) for signs of increased agitation and hyperactivity. | 6. Early detection and intervention of escalating mania might help prevent harm to self or others, and decrease need for seclusion. |
| 7. Redirect agitation and potentially violent behaviors with physical outlets in area of low stimulation (e.g., punching bag). | 7. Can help to relieve pent-up hostility and relieve muscle tension. |
| 8. Alert staff if potential for seclusion appears imminent. Usual priority of interventions would be: | 8. If nursing interventions (quiet environment and firm limit setting) and chemical restraints (tranquilizers—e.g., |

| Intervention | Rationale |
|---|---|
| a. Firmly setting limits<br>b. Chemical restraints (tranquilizers)<br>c. Seclusion | haloperidol [Haldol]) have not helped dampen escalating manic behaviors, then seclusion might be warranted. **See Chapter 17 for guidelines on secluding an individual**. |
| 9. Chart, in nurse's notes, behaviors; interventions; what seemed to escalate agitation; what helped to calm agitation; when as-needed (PRN) medications were given and their effect; and what proved most helpful. | 9. Staff will begin to recognize potential signals for escalating manic behaviors and have a guideline for what might work best for the individual client. |

## INEFFECTIVE COPING

Inability to form a valid appraisal of stressors, inadequate choice of practical responses, and/or inability to use available resources

### *Related To (Etiology)*

▲ Disturbance in tension release
▲ Inadequate level of perception of control
● Ineffective problem-solving strategies/skills
● Biochemical/neurologic changes in the brain

### *As Evidenced By*
*(Assessment Findings/Diagnostic Cues)*

▲ Inability to ask for help
▲ Inability to meet basic needs
▲ Inability to problem-solve
▲ Destructive behavior toward self or others
▲ Change in usual communication patterns

---

▲ NANDA International accepted; ● In addition to NANDA International

- Presence of delusions (grandeur, persecution)
- Using extremely poor judgment in business and financial negotiations
- Giving away valuables and financial savings indiscriminately, often to strangers

## Outcome Criteria

- Report an absence of delusions, racing thoughts, and irresponsible actions as a result of medication adherence and environmental structures
- Be protected from making any major life decisions (legal, business, marital) during an acute or severe manic phase
- Demonstrate an absence of destructive behavior toward self or others
- Cease use of manipulation to obtain needs and control others
- Return to pre-crisis level of functioning after acute/ severe manic phase is past

## Long-Term Goals

Client will:
- Demonstrate a decrease in manipulative behavior by (date)
- Demonstrate a decrease in demanding and provocative behavior by (date)
- Seek competent medical assistance and legal protection when signing any legal documents regarding personal or financial matters during manic phase of illness

## Short-Term Goals

Client will:
- Retain valuables or other possessions while in the hospital
- Respond to external controls (medication, seclusion, nursing interventions) when potential or actual loss of control occurs
- Respond to limit-setting techniques with aid of medication during acute and severe manic phase

---

▲ NANDA International accepted; ● In addition to NANDA International

*Interventions and Rationales*

**Intervention**

1. Administer an antimanic medication and PRN tranquilizers, as ordered, and evaluate for efficacy, and side and toxic effects.

2. Observe for destructive behavior toward self or others. Intervene in the early phases of escalation of manic behavior. Intervene using **Risk for Violence** in this Chapter and **Chapter 17 (Anger and Aggression)** as a guide for interventions.

3. Have valuables, credit cards, and large sums of money sent home with family or put in hospital safe until client is discharged.

4. Maintain a firm, calm, and neutral approach at all times.
   **Avoid:**
   a. Getting involved in power struggles
   b. Arguing with the client
   c. Joking or "clever" repartee in response and other clients. to client's "cheerful and humorous" mood

**Rationale**

1. Bipolar disorder is caused by biochemical/neurologic imbalances in the brain. Appropriate antimanic medications allow psychosocial and nursing interventions to be effective.

2. Hostile verbal behaviors, poor impulse control, provocative behaviors, and violent acting out against others or property are some of the symptoms of this disease and are seen in extreme and/or acute mania. Early detection and intervention can prevent harm to client or others int the environment.

3. During manic episodes, people give away valuables and money indiscriminately to strangers, often leaving themselves broke and in debt.

4. a-c. These behaviors by staff can escalate environmental stimulation and, consequently, manic activity. Once the manic client is out of control, seclusion might be required, which can be traumatic to the manic individual as well as the staff

| Intervention | Rationale |
|---|---|
| 5. Provide hospital legal service when and if client is involved in making or signing important legal documents during an acute manic phase. | 5. Judgment and reality testing are both impaired during acute mania. Clients might need legal advice and protection against making important decisions that are not in their best interest. |
| 6. Assess and recognize early signs of manipulative behavior, and intervene appropriately. For example:<br>a. Taunting staff by pointing out faults or oversights<br>b. Pitting one staff member against another ("You are much more understanding than Nurse X . . . do you know what he did?") or pitting one group against another (evening versus day shift)<br>c. Aggressively demanding behaviors that can trigger exasperation and frustration in staff | 6. Setting limits is an important step in the intervention of bipolar clients, especially when intervening in manipulative behaviors. Staff agreement on limits set and consistency is imperative if the limits are to be carried out effectively. **Refer to Chapter 19** for more on interviewing with manipulative behaviors. |

## IMPAIRED SOCIAL INTERACTION

The state in which an individual participates in an insufficient or excessive quantity or ineffective quality of social exchange

## Related To (Etiology)

- ▲ Disturbed thought processes
- ● Biochemical imbalances
- ● Excessive hyperactivity and agitation

## As Evidenced By
## (Assessment Findings/Diagnostic Cues)

- ▲ Observed use of unsuccessful social interaction behaviors
- ▲ Dysfunctional interaction with peers, family, and/or others
- ▲ Family reports change of style or patterns of interaction
- ● Intrusive and manipulative behaviors antagonizing others
- ● Loud, obscene, or threatening verbal behavior
- ● Poor attention span and difficulty focusing on one thing at a time
- ● Increase of manic behaviors when client is in a highly stimulating environment (e.g., with groups of people, loud music)

## Outcome Criteria

- Client initiates and maintains goal-directed and mutually satisfying activities/verbal exchanges with others
- Client and family state that there is an increase in stability and meaningfulness in social interactions

## Long-Term Goals

Client will:
- Put feelings into words instead of actions when experiencing anxiety or loss of control before discharge
- Participate in unit activities without disruption or demonstrating inappropriate behavior by discharge
- Demonstrate ability to remove self from stimulating environment in order to "cool down" by discharge

---

▲ NANDA International accepted; ● In addition to NANDA International

## Short-Term Goals

Client will:

- Focus on one activity requiring a short attention span for 5 minutes three times a day with nursing assistance by (date)
- Find one or two solitary activities that can help relieve tensions and minimize escalation of anxiety with aid of nurse or occupational/activity therapist by (date)
- Sit through a short, small group meeting free from disruptive outbursts by (date)

## Interventions and Rationales

| Intervention | Rationale |
|---|---|
| 1. When possible, provide an environment with minimum stimuli (e.g., quiet, soft music, dim lighting). | 1. Reduction in stimuli lessens distractibility. |
| 2. Solitary activities requiring short attention spans with mild physical exertion are best initially (e.g., writing, painting [finger painting, murals], woodworking, or walks with staff). | 2. Solitary activities minimize stimuli; mild physical activities release tension constructively. |
| 3. When less manic, client might join one or two other clients in quiet, nonstimulating activities (e.g., board games, drawing, cards). *Avoid competitive games.* | 3. As mania subsides, involvement in activities that provide a focus and social contact becomes more appropriate. Competitive games can stimulate aggression and can increase psychomotor activity. |

## TOTAL SELF-CARE DEFICIT

Impaired ability to perform or complete bathing/hygiene, dressing/grooming, feeding, or toileting activities for oneself

## Related To (Etiology)

▲ Perceptual or cognitive impairment
▲ Severe anxiety
● Manic excitement
● Racing thoughts and poor attention span
● Inability to concentrate on one thing at a time

## As Evidenced By
## (Assessment Findings/Diagnostic Cues)

▲ Observation or valid report of inability to eat, bathe, toilet, dress, and/or groom self independently

## Outcome Criteria

• Maintenance of pre-crisis level of self-care

## Long-Term Goals

• Client's weight will be within normal limits for age and height by (date)
• Client will sleep 6 to 8 hours per night by (date)
• Client will dress and groom self in appropriate manner consistent with pre-crisis level of dress and grooming by (date)
• Client's bowel habits will be within normal limits by (date)

## Short-Term Goals

Client will:
• Eat one half to one third of each meal plus one snack between meals with aid of nursing intervention by (date)
• Sleep 6 hours out of 24 with aid of medication and nursing measures within 3 days
• Wear appropriate attire each day while in hospital
• Bathe at least every other day while in hospital
• Have normal bowel movements within 2 days with the aid of high-fiber foods, fluids, and, if needed, medication

---

▲ NANDA International accepted; ● In addition to NANDA International

*Interventions and Rationales*

| Intervention | Rationale |
|---|---|

**Imbalanced Nutrition**

1. Monitor intake, output, and vital signs.

   1. Ensures adequate fluid and caloric intake; minimizes dehydration and cardiac collapse.

2. Encourage frequent high-calorie protein drinks and finger foods (e.g., sandwiches, fruit, milkshakes).

   2. Constant fluid and calorie replacement are needed. Client might be too active to sit at meals. Finger foods allow "eating on the run."

3. Frequently remind the client to eat (e.g., "Tom, finish your milkshake", "Sally, eat this banana.").

   3. The manic client is unaware of bodily needs and is easily distracted. Needs supervision to eat.

**Disturbed Sleep Pattern**

1. Encourage frequent rest periods during the day.

   1. Lack of sleep can lead to exhaustion and death.

2. Keep client in areas of low stimulation.

   2. Promotes relaxation and minimizes manic behavior.

3. At night, encourage warm baths, soothing music, and medication when indicated. Avoid giving the client caffeine.

   3. Promotes relaxation, rest, and sleep.

**Dressing/Grooming Self-Care Deficit**

1. If warranted, supervise choice of clothes; minimize flamboyant and bizarre dress, and sexually suggestive dress, such as bikini tops and bottoms.

   1. Lessens the potential for inappropriate attention, which can increase level of mania, or ridicule, which lowers self-esteem and increases the need for manic defense. Assists client in maintaining dignity.

**Intervention**

2. Give simple step-by-step reminders for hygiene and dress (e.g., "Here is your razor. Shave the left side . . . now the right side", "Here is your toothbrush. Put the toothpaste on the brush.").

**Rationale**

2. Distractibility and poor concentration are countered by simple, concrete instructions.

**Constipation**

1. Monitor bowel habits; offer fluids and food that is high in fiber. Evaluate the need for laxative. Encourage client to go to the bathroom.

1. Prevents fecal impaction resulting from dehydration and decreased peristalsis.

## INTERRUPTED FAMILY PROCESSES

Change in family relationships and/or functioning

### Related To (Etiology)

▲ Shift in health status of family member

▲ Situational crisis or transition (e.g., illness, manic episode of one member)

▲ Family role shift

● Erratic and out-of-control behavior of one family member with the potential for dangerous behavior affecting all family members (violence, leaving family in debt, risky behaviors in relationships and business, flagrant infidelities, unprotected and promiscuous sex)

● Nonadherence to antimanic and other medications

---

▲ NANDA International accepted; ● In addition to NANDA International

*As Evidenced By*
*(Assessment Findings/Diagnostic Cues)*

▲ Changes in effectiveness in completing assigned tasks
▲ Changes in participation in problem solving
▲ Changes in participation in decision making
▲ Changes in communication patterns
● Inability to deal with traumatic or crisis experiences constructively
● Deficient knowledge regarding disorder, need for medication adherence, and available support systems for both family members and client
● Family in crisis

*Outcome Criteria*

All members:
• Perform expected roles
• Adapt to unexpected crises
• Use stress reduction techniques

*Long-Term Goals*

Family members/significant others:
• State that they find needed support and information in a support group(s)
• Can identify the signs of increase manic behavior in their family member
• State what they will do (whom to call, where to go) when client's mood begins to escalate to dangerous levels
• Demonstrate an understanding of what a bipolar disorder is, the medications, the need for adherence to medication and treatment

*Short-Term Goals*

Family members/significant others will:
• Discuss with nurse/counselor three areas of family life that are most disruptive and seek alternative options with aid of nursing/counseling interventions by (date)
• State and have in writing the names and telephone numbers of at least two bipolar support groups by (date)

---

▲ NANDA International accepted; ● In addition to NANDA International

- State that they have gained support from at least one support group on how to work with family member when he or she is manic by (date)
- State their understanding for the need for medication adherence, and be able to identify three signs that indicate possible need for intervention when their family member's mood escalates by (date)
- Briefly discuss and have in writing the names and addresses of two bipolar organizations, two Internet site addresses, and medication information regarding bipolar disorder by (date)

*Interventions and Rationales*

| Intervention | Rationale |
|---|---|
| 1. During the first or second day of hospitalization, spend time with family identifying their needs during this time; for example:<br>  a. Need for information about the disease<br>  b. Need for information about lithium or other antimanic medications (e.g., need for adherence, side effects, toxic effects)<br>  c. Knowledge about bipolar support groups in the family's community and how they can help families going through crises | 1. This is a disease that can devastate and destroy some families. During an acute manic attack, families experience a great deal of disruption and confusion when their family member begins to act bizarre, out of control, and at times aggressive. Families need to understand about the disease, what can and cannot be done to help control the disease, and where to go for help for their individual issues. |

## MEDICAL TREATMENTS

The following discussion is for current treatment of bipolar clients. Please keep in mind that the treatment plan for a particular client needs to include other considerations as well. Is the client at risk for suicide, homicide, or violence? Is there evidence of psychotic or catatonic features? Does the client have a substance abuse disorder as well? Are there other psychiatric comorbidities, such as personality disorder or conduct disorder in a child or adolescent? Although there are clear-cut, acceptable primary treatments for bipolar disorder, the treatment plan might include a multimodal approach to a variety of client needs.

## Psychopharmacology

Pharmacologic treatment is a crucial component of treatment for people with bipolar disorders. Medications are effective in both the treatment of acute episodes and the prevention of future episodes. Lithium, valproate, carbamazepine, topiramate, and electroconvulsive therapy (ECT) are all used as primary agents in the treatment of people with bipolar disorders (APA, 2000b). A brief discussion of the mood stabilizers follows. Mood stabilizers are those medications with both antimanic and antidepressive action. Refer to Chapter 21 for specific information on these drugs, including side/toxic effects, nursing considerations, and client and family teaching.

### Lithium

Lithium or other mood stabilizers (particularly valproate [Depakote]) is an essential part of treatment. Lithium is particularly effective in reducing (Maxmen and Ward, 2002):
- Elation
- Flights of ideas
- Irritability and manipulativeness
- Anxiety

To a lesser extent, lithium controls:
- Insomnia
- Psychomotor agitation
- Threatening or assaultive behavior
- Distractibility
- Paranoia
- Hypersexuality

Lithium can calm manic clients, prevent or modify future manic episodes, and protect against future depressive episodes. Lithium must reach therapeutic levels in the client's blood to be effective. This usually takes from 7 to 14 days to be effective. Therefore, when a client is first brought to the hospital, he or she might be started on antipsychotic medications to help decrease psychomotor activity and aggressive behaviors, and prevent exhaustion, coronary collapse, and death.

As lithium reaches therapeutic levels, the antipsychotics are usually discontinued. A narrow range exists between the therapeutic dose and the toxic dose of lithium. Initially, blood levels can be checked weekly or biweekly until therapeutic levels are reached (0.8 to 1.4 mEq/L). Actual maintenance blood levels should reach between 0.4 and 1.0 mEq/L. To avoid serious toxicity, lithium levels should not exceed 1.5 mEq/L (Lehne, 2001).

Before the administration of lithium, a medical evaluation is performed to assess the client's ability to tolerate the drug. Lithium should not be given to people who are pregnant, have brain damage, or have cardiovascular, renal, or thyroid disease. Lithium is often the drug of choice for bipolar clients; however, some bipolar clients might not respond or might respond insufficiently to lithium, particularly in those who have four or more cycles per year, mixed manic/depressive features, or psychosis or neurologic disorders (Maxmen & Ward, 2002).

## Other Mood Stabilizers

Three anticonvulsants have demonstrated efficacy in the treatment of individuals with bipolar disease. These are carbamazepine (Tegretol), divalproex (Depakote), and lamotrigine (Lamictal) (Preston et al. 2005) Divalproex is particularly useful in mixed-state and rapid-cycling bipolar clients. Some clinicians find that divalproex is better tolerated than lithium, and as effective in preventing subsequent bipolar episodes.

Blood level monitoring is required for both carbamazepine and divalproex. The major worry with divalproex is the risk of severe, even fatal, hepatotoxicity. Carbamazepine (Tegretol) is used either alone or in combination with other mood stabilizers It is useful in clients with mixed states. Carbamazepine use is associated with potentially serious adverse reactions. Lamotrigine is a first line agent for bipolar depression and a second line agent for rapid cycling (Preston et al, 2005).

## Adjunctive and New or Atypical Medicines

Other antimanic drugs include some anticonvulsant drugs, such as, gabapentin (Neurotin), and topiramate (Topamax). Gabapentin (Neurotin) appears effective as an adjunct in the treatment of refractory bipolar clients as does topiramate (Topamax). Topiramate (Topamax) seems to be effective in acute mania as well as in adjunctive use in combination with other mood stabilizers. Some report success with rapid cycling as well.

Some benzodiazepines (e.g., clonazepam [Klonopin] and lorazepam [Ativan]) have been found to facilitate other antimanic treatments useful in treatment-resistant manic clients. Refer to Chapter 21 for a more thorough discussion of the mood stabilizers, along with adverse reactions, nursing measures, and client and family teaching.

## Other Medical Treatments

### Electroconvulsive Therapy

ECT is a primary consideration when a highly manic client is unable to wait until a medication starts to become effective; cannot tolerate one of the first-line medications listed earlier; or does not respond to the first-line medications. ECT has been found especially effective with rapid cycling clients (those who suffer four or more episodes of illness a year) as well as those with paranoid-destructive features that often respond poorly to lithium therapy (Abou-Saleh, 1992). ECT should also be considered for severe and dangerous manic clients and those in highly agitated states (Maxmen & Ward, 2002). ECT should also be considered for pregnant women. Refer to Appendix F for the nurse's responsibilities in ECT therapy.

### Psychotherapeutic Treatments

The primary goal of all therapies is to reduce the client's distress, to improve the client's ability to function between episodes, and to decrease the frequency of future episodes

(APA, 2000b). Because of the behaviors associated with the disorder, there are usually severe psychosocial consequences from past episodes. Bipolar disease appears to be a chronic, recurrent disease. Many clients do not fully recover between episodes. Some research suggests that between 30% and 60% of clients fail to regain full occupational and social functioning (Steinhauer, 2003). Therefore it becomes clear that adjuvant treatments are necessary along with medications.

No matter which therapy is chosen for a specific client, an approach that enforces clear limits in a firm and unprovacative manner is most recommended (APA 2000b). There are a number of psychotherapeutic approaches that can be helpful to some clients. Some of those therapies found helpful to some are (APA, 2000b):

- Inpatient family intervention
- Behavioral family management
- Family therapy and psychoeducation
- Cognitive behavioral treatment (Basco & Rush, 1996)

## NURSE, CLIENT, AND FAMILY RESOURCES

## ASSOCIATIONS

**National Alliance for the Mentally Ill (NAMI)**
Colonial Place Three
2107 Wilson Boulevard, Suite 300
Arlington, VA 22201-3042
(800) 950-NAMI

**Depressed Anonymous: Recovery from Depression**
PO Box 17471
Louisville, KY 40217
(502) 569-1989
http://www.depressedanon.com

**National Foundation for Depressive Illness, Inc.**
PO Box 2257
New York, NY 10116
(800) 239-1265
http://www.depression.org

**Depression and Bipolar Support Alliance**
730 N. Franklin, Suite 501
Chicago, IL 60610
(800) 82N-DMDA
http://www.dbsalliance.org

**Depression and Related Affective Disorders Association**
2330 West Joppa Road, Suite 100
Lutherville, MD 21093
(410) 583-2919
http://www.drada.org

## INTERNET SITES

**National Institute of Mental Health**
http://www.nimh.nih.gov/publicat/index.cfm
List of publications on bipolar disorder

**Bipolar Disorder Page**
http://mentalhelp.net/poc/center—index.php?id=4

**Med Help International**
http://www.medhelp.org
Many good links

**Bipolar Website**
http://www.bipolar.com
Good information and links

**Bipolar Disorder Guide at about.com**
http://bipolar.about.com

# CHAPTER 8

# Schizophrenia and Other Psychotic Disorders

## OVERVIEW

### Schizophrenia

The schizophrenias are severe and persistent neurologic diseases. These serious disorders affect a person's:
- Perceptions (hallucinations and delusions)
- Thinking (delusions, paranoia, disorganized thinking)
- Language (associative looseness, poverty of speech)
- Emotions (apathy, anhedonia, depression)
- Social behavior (aggressive, bizarre behaviors or extreme social withdrawal)

Schizophrenia affects approximately 1% of the population, and 95% of individuals who become schizophrenic have the condition throughout their lifetime. Schizophrenia is a relapsing psychotic disorder. A psychotic disorder is one in which people have difficulty with differentiating reality from fantasy (reality testing).

Major symptoms seen in psychotic disorders are hallucinations, delusions, and disorganized thinking. Hallucinations and delusions can be very frightening, often terrifying for individuals. They also can be very disconcerting initially and even frightening to nurses and other health care individuals. These are the **positive symptoms** of schizophrenia. Nurses can greatly benefit from individual or peer supervision when dealing with these challenging phenomena. Communicating with clients who are delusional and hallucinatory and have disorganized thinking is a skill that is learned with guidance and practice.

The **negative symptoms** of schizophrenia are more subtle and are the most damaging to the client's quality of life. **Negative symptoms** include feelings of emptiness, amotivational states, anhedonia, and apathy.

**Cognitive symptoms** (poor problem-solving, poor decision-making skills, illogical thinking) also need to be targeted when planning care.

The symptoms of schizophrenia usually become apparent during adolescence or early adulthood (15 to 25 for men, 25 to 35 for women). Paranoid schizophrenia has a later onset. The schizophrenias are severe, biologically based mental illnesses. Current theories of schizophrenia involve neuroanatomical and neurochemical abnormalities, which might be induced either genetically or environmentally (birth defects, viruses). Although the schizophrenias are not caused by psychological events, stressful life events can trigger an exacerbation of the illness. Therefore, psychoeducational and family treatment modalities can be crucial in helping clients in a number of ways. Psychoeducational, family, group, and behavioral approaches, for example, can help clients increase their social skills, maximize their ability in self-care and independent living, maintain medical adherence, and, most important, increase the quality of their lives. Client and family education greatly improves the management of schizophrenia.

Schizophrenia is not a single disease, but rather a syndrome that involves cerebral blood flow, neuroelectrophysiology, neuroanatomy, and neurobiochemistry. The *Diagnostic and Statistical Manual of Mental Disorders* (4th edition, text revision) (DSM-IV-TR) criteria for the diagnosis of schizophrenia are listed in Box 8–1.

Box 8–2 identifies five subtypes of schizophrenia.

## Other Psychotic Disorders

### Schizophreniform Disorder

The essential features of this disorder are exactly those of schizophrenia except that:

| Box 8-1 | DSM-IV-TR Criteria for Schizophrenia |

1. *Characteristic symptoms:* Two (or more) of the following, each present for a significant portion of the time during a 1-month period (or less if successfully treated):
   * Delusions
   * Hallucinations
   * Disorganized speech (e.g., frequent derailment or incoherence)
   * Grossly disorganized or catatonic behavior
   * Negative symptoms, (i.e., affective flattening, alogia, or avolition)

Note: Only one Criterion 1 symptom is required if delusions are bizarre or hallucinations consist of a voice keeping up a running commentary on the person's behavior or thoughts, or two or more voices conversing with each other.

2. *Social/occupational dysfunction:* For a significant portion of the time since the onset of the disturbance, one or more major areas of functioning, such as work, interpersonal relations, or self-care, are markedly below the level achieved prior to the onset (or when the onset is in childhood or adolescence, failure to achieve expected level of interpersonal, academic, or occupational achievement).

3. *Duration:* Continuous signs of the disturbance persist for at least 6 months. This 6-month period must include at least 1 month of symptoms (or less if successfully treated) that meet Criterion 1 (i.e., active-phase symptoms) and might include periods of prodromal or residual symptoms.

4. Symptoms are not caused by (a) another psychotic disorder; (b) a substance or general medical disorder; or (c) a pervasive developmental disorder, unless prominent delusions or hallucinations are also present for at least 1 month.

Adapted from American Psychiatric Association (2000). *Diagnostic and statistical manual of mental disorders* (4th ed., text revision). Washington, DC: American Psychiatric Association, p. 312; reprinted with permission.

* The total duration of the illness is at least 1 month, but less than 6 months.
* Impaired social or occupational functioning during some part of the illness is not apparent (although it might occur).

This disorder might or might not have a good prognosis.

---

## Box 8-2 Subtypes of Schizophrenia

### Paranoid

Onset usually in the late 20s to 30s. People who develop this disorder usually function well before the onset of the disorder (good premorbid functioning). *Paranoia* (any intense and strongly defended irrational suspicion) is the main characteristic; the main defense is projection. *Hallucinations, delusions, and ideas of reference* are dominant.

### Disorganized

The most *regressed and socially impaired* of all the schizophrenias. The person has highly disorganized speech and behavior and inappropriate affect. Bizarre mannerisms include grimacing, along with other oddities of behavior.

### Catatonia

The essential feature is abnormal motor behavior. Two extreme motor behaviors are seen in catatonia. One extreme is psychomotor agitation, which can lead to exhaustion. The other extreme is psychomotor retardation and *withdrawal* to the point of stupor. The onset is usually acute, and the prognosis is good with medications and swift interventions. Other behaviors might include autism, waxy flexibility, and negativism.

### Undifferentiated (Mixed Type)

Clients experience active hallucinations and delusions, but no one clinical picture dominates (e.g., not paranoid, catatonic, or disorganized; rather the clinical picture is one of a *mixture* of symptoms).

### Residual

A person who is referred to as having residual schizophrenia no longer has active symptoms of the disease, such as delusions, hallucinations, or disorganized speech and behaviors. However, there is a persistence of some symptoms—for example, marked social withdrawal; impairment in role function (wage earner, student, or homemaker); eccentric behavior or odd beliefs; poor personal hygiene; lack of interest, energy, initiative; and inappropriate affect.

## Brief Psychotic Disorder

This is a disorder in which there is a sudden onset of psychotic symptoms (delusions, hallucinations, disorganized speech) or grossly disorganized or catatonic behavior. The episode lasts at least 1 day, but less than 1 month, and then the individual returns to his or her premorbid level of functioning. Brief psychotic disorders often follow extremely stressful life events.

## Schizoaffective Disorder

This disorder is characterized by an uninterrupted period of illness during which there is a major depressive, manic, or mixed episode, concurrent with symptoms that meet the criteria for schizophrenia. The symptoms must not be due to any substance use or abuse or general medical condition.

## Delusional Disorder

This disorder involves nonbizarre delusions (situations that occur in real life, such as being followed, infected, loved at a distance, deceived by a spouse, or having a disease) of at least 1 month's duration. The person's ability to function is not markedly impaired, nor is the person's behavior obviously odd or bizarre. Common types of delusions seen in this disorder are delusions of grandeur, persecution, or jealousy, or somatic or mixed delusions.

## Shared Psychotic Disorder (Folie à Deux)

A shared psychotic disorder is an occurrence in which one individual, who is in a close relationship with another who has a psychotic disorder with a delusion, eventually comes to share the delusional beliefs either in total or in part. Apart from the shared delusion, the person who takes on the other's delusional behavior is not otherwise odd or unusual. Impairment of the person who shares the delusion is usually much less than the person who has the psychotic disorder with the delusion. The cult phenomenon is an example, as was demonstrated at Waco and Jonestown.

## *Induced or Secondary Psychosis*

Psychosis can be induced by substances (drugs of abuse, alcohol, medications, or toxin exposure) or caused by the physiologic consequences of a general medical condition (delirium, neurologic conditions, metabolic conditions, hepatic or renal diseases, and many more). **Medical conditions and substances of abuse must always be ruled out before a primary diagnosis of a schizophrenia or other psychotic disorder can be made.**

## *Phases of Schizophrenia*

Schizophrenia has been divided into three phases:

**Phase I—Onset.** This phase (acute phase) includes the prodromal symptoms (e.g., acute or chronic anxiety, phobias, obsessions, compulsions, dissociative features) as well as the acute psychotic symptoms of hallucinations, delusions, and/or disorganized thinking.

**Phase II—Years following onset.** Patterns that characterize this phase are the ebb and flow of the intensity and disruption caused by symptoms, which might, in some cases, be followed by complete or relatively complete recovery.

**Phase III—Long-term course and outcome.** This is the course that the severely and persistently mentally ill client follows when the disease becomes chronic. For some clients, the intensity of the psychosis might diminish with age; however, the long-term dysfunctional effects of the disorder are not as amenable to change.

# ASSESSMENT

## Presenting Signs and Symptoms

1. Positive symptoms
   - Delusions
   - Hallucinations
   - Disorganized thinking/speech
   - Disorganized or catatonic behavior
2. Negative symptoms
   - Flat emotional affect
   - Sparse productivity of thought (Alogia)
   - Lack of goal directed activity (Avolition)

3. Cognitive symptoms
   • Memory and attention deficits
   • Language difficulties
   • Monitor personal behavior, ability to establish goals, maintain tasks, and so on.

## Assessment Tool

The Brief Psychiatric Rating Scale (BPRS) (Appendix D-5) is a useful tool for evaluating overall psychiatric functioning. It is particularly helpful in evaluating the degree to which psychotic symptoms affect a person's ability to function.

## Assessment Guidelines
### Schizophrenias
**Assessing Positive Symptoms**
1. Assess for command hallucinations (e.g., voices telling the person to harm self or another). **If yes:**
   • Do you plan to follow the command?
   • Do you believe the voices are real?
2. Assess if the client has fragmented, poorly organized, well-organized, systematized, or extensive system of beliefs that are not supported by reality (delusions). **If yes:**
   • Assess if delusions have to do with someone trying to harm the client and if the client is planning to retaliate against a person or organization.
   • Assess if precautions need to be taken.
3. Assess for pervasive suspiciousness about everyone and their actions, for example:
   • Is on guard, hyperalert, vigilant
   • Blames others for consequences of own behavior
   • Is hostile, argumentative, or often threatening, in verbalization or behavior

**Assessing Negative Symptoms**
4. Assess for negative symptoms of schizophrenia (see Table 8-1 for definitions and suggested interventions).
5. Assess if client is on medications, what the medications are, and if treatment is adherent with medications.
6. How does the family respond to increased symptoms? Overprotective? Hostile? Suspicious?
7. How do family members and client relate?

8. Assess support system. Is family well informed about the disease (e.g., schizophrenia)? Does family understand the need for medication adherence? Is family familiar with family support groups in the community, or where to go for respite and family support?

# NURSING DIAGNOSES WITH INTERVENTIONS

People with schizophrenia often have multiple needs. Basic to these is safety. Refer to Chapters 16 and 17 for nursing care plans identifying nursing interventions for **suicide intent and violence toward others.** Suicide and threat of violence to others are basic to nursing interventions for all clients in all settings, not just for people with schizophrenia or the hospitalized person.

Relating to people with schizophrenia can be a challenge, especially in the acute phase; therefore guidelines for

Table 8-1 **Negative (Deficit) Symptoms of Schizophrenia**

| Symptoms | Clinical Findings | Treatment |
|---|---|---|
| Apathy<br>Poverty of speech or content of speech<br>Poor social functioning<br>Anhedonia<br>Social withdrawal | Slow onset<br>Interferes with a person's life<br>Positive premorbid history<br>Chronic deterioration<br>Family history of schizophrenia<br>Cerebellar atrophy and lateral and third ventricular enlargement on computed tomography scan<br>Abnormalities on neuropsychologic testing<br>Poor response to antipsychotics | The newer atypical (novel) antipsychotics might target some of the negative symptoms. The most used interventions include:<br>1. Skill training interventions:<br>• Identify areas of skill deficit person is willing to work on.<br>• Prioritize skills important to the person.<br>2. Working with person to identify stressors:<br>• Identify which stressors contribute to maladaptive behaviors.<br>3. Work with person on increasing appropriate coping skills. |

**Impaired Verbal Communication** are included. Again, during the acute phase, relating to others is difficult. Guidelines for interacting and gradually adding social skills are included in **Impaired Social Interaction.** Working with clients who are hallucinating **(Disturbed Sensory Perception),** delusional **(Disturbed Thought Processes),** and paranoid **(Defensive Coping)** can be a great challenge. Therefore, these are included.

Also, importantly, often the families are left to cope with the exhaustive needs of their family member. **Interrupted Family Processes** should always be assessed, and referrals and teaching should be readily available.

Nonadherence to medications or treatment is a huge challenge for mental health professionals. Nursing care plans for **Nonadherence/Noncompliance** are found in Chapter 20. Table 8-2 provides a list of potential nursing diagnoses.

Table 8-2 **Potential Nursing Diagnoses for Schizophrenia**

| Symptoms | Nursing Diagnoses |
| --- | --- |
| **Positive Symptoms** | |
| **Hallucinations:** | Disturbed Sensory Perception: Auditory/Visual |
| • Hears voices (loud noises) that others do not hear. | Risk for Violence: Self-Directed and Other-Directed |
| • Hears voices telling them to hurt self or others (*command hallucinations*). | |
| **Distorted thinking not based in reality,** for example: | Disturbed Thought Processes Defensive Coping |
| • **Persecution:** thinking others are trying to harm them. | |
| • **Jealousy:** thinking spouse or lover is being unfaithful, or thinks others are jealous when they are not. | |
| • **Grandeur:** thinking they have powers they do not possess, or they are someone powerful or famous. | |
| • **Reference:** believing all events within the environment are directed at or hold special meaning for them. | |

Table 8-2 **Potential Nursing Diagnoses for Schizophrenia—cont'd**

| Symptoms | Nursing Diagnoses |
| --- | --- |
| • Loose association of ideas **(looseness of association)**. | **Impaired Verbal Communication** |
| • Uses words in a meaningless, disconnected manner **(word salad)**. | **Disturbed Thought Processes** |
| • Uses words that rhyme in a nonsensical fashion **(clang association)**. | |
| • Repeats words that are heard (*echolalia*). | |
| • Does not speak **(mutism)**. | |
| • The person delays getting to the point of communication because of unnecessary and tedious details **(circumstantiality)**. | |
| • Concrete thinking: The inability to abstract; uses literal translations concerning aspects of the environment. | |
| Negative Symptoms | |
| Uncommunicative, withdrawn, no eye contact. | **Social Isolation** |
| Preoccupation with own thoughts. | **Impaired Social Interaction** |
| Expression of feelings of rejection or of aloneness (lies in bed all day; positions back to door). | **Risk for Loneliness** |
| Talks about self as "bad" or "no good." | **Chronic Low Self-Esteem** |
| Feels guilty because of "bad thoughts"; extremely sensitive to real or perceived slights. | **Risk for Self-Directed Violence** |
| Lack of energy **(anergia)**. | **Ineffective Coping** |
| Lack of motivation **(avolition)**; unable to initiate tasks (social contact, grooming, and other aspects of daily living). | **Self-Care Deficit (bathing/hygiene, dressing/grooming) Constipation** |

*Continued*

Table 8-2 **Potential Nursing Diagnoses for Schizophrenia—cont'd**

| Symptoms | Nursing Diagnoses |
| --- | --- |
| **Other** | |
| Families and significant others become confused, overwhelmed, lack knowledge of disease or treatment, feel powerless in coping with client at home | **Compromised Family Coping** <br> **Disabled Family Coping** <br> **Impaired Parenting** <br> **Caregiver Role Strain** |
| **Nonadherence to medications and treatment:** Client stops taking medication (often because of side effects), stops going to therapy groups. | **Deficient Knowledge** <br> **Nonadherence (Noncompliance)** |

## Selected Nursing Diagnoses and Nursing Care Plans

### IMPAIRED VERBAL COMMUNICATION

Decreased, delayed, or absent ability to receive, process, transmit, or use a system of symbols

*Related To (Etiology)*

- ▲ Psychologic barriers (e.g., psychosis, lack of stimuli)
- ▲ Side effects of medication
- ▲ Altered perceptions
- ● Biochemical alterations in the brain of certain neurotransmitters

*As Evidenced By*
*(Assessment Findings/Diagnostic Cues)*

- ▲ Inappropriate verbalization
- ▲ Difficulty expressing thoughts verbally
- ▲ Difficulty in comprehending and maintaining the usual communication pattern
- ● Poverty of speech
- ● Disturbances in cognitive associations (e.g., looseness of association, perseveration, neologisms)

---

▲ NANDA International accepted; ● In addition to NANDA International

- Inability to distinguish internally stimulated thoughts from actual environmental events or commonly shared knowledge

## Outcome Criteria

- Communicates thoughts and feelings in a coherent, goal-directed manner (to client's best ability)
- Demonstrates reality-based thought processes in verbal communication (to client's best ability)

## Long-Term Goals

Client will:
- Be able to speak in a manner that can be understood by others with the aid of medication and attentive listening by discharge
- Learn two diversionary tactics that work for him/her to lower anxiety, thus enhancing ability to think clearly and speak more logically by (date)

## Short-Term Goals

Client will:
- Spend three 5-minute periods with nurse sharing observations in the environment within 4 days
- Spend time with one or two other people in structured activity involving neutral topics by (date)

## Interventions and Rationales

| Intervention | Rationale |
|---|---|
| 1. Assess if incoherence in speech is chronic or if it is more sudden, as in an exacerbation of symptoms. | 1. Establishing a baseline facilitates the establishment of realistic goals, the cornerstone for planning effective care. |
| 2. Identify how long client has been on antipsychotic medication. | 2. Therapeutic levels of an antipsychotic helps clear thinking and diminishes looseness of association (LOA). |
| 3. Plan short, frequent periods with client throughout the day. | 3. Short periods are less stressful, and periodic meetings give client a chance to develop familiarity and safety. |

●In addition to NANDA International

| Intervention | Rationale |
|---|---|
| 4. Use simple words, and keep directions simple. | 4. Client might have difficulty processing even simple sentences. |
| 5. Keep voice low and speak slowly. | 5. High pitched/loud tone of voice can raise anxiety levels; slow speaking aids understanding. |
| 6. Look for themes in what is said, even though spoken words appear incoherent (e.g., anxiety, fear, sadness). | 6. Often client's choice of words is symbolic of feelings. |
| 7. When you do not understand a client, let him/her know you are having difficulty understanding (e.g., "I want to understand what you are saying, but I am having difficulty.") | 7. Pretending to understand (when you do not) limits your credibility in the eyes of your client and lessens the potential for trust. |
| 8. Use therapeutic techniques to try to understand client's concerns (e.g., "Are you saying . . .?" "You mentioned demons many times. Are you feeling frightened?"). | 8. Even if the words are hard to understand, try getting to the feelings behind them. |
| 9. Focus on and direct client's attention to concrete things in the environment. | 9. Helps draw focus away from delusions and focus on reality-based things. |
| 10. Keep environment quiet and as free of stimuli as possible. | 10. Keeps anxiety from escalating and increasing confusion and hallucinations/delusions. |
| 11. Use simple, concrete, and literal explanations. | 11. Minimizes misunderstanding and/or incorporating those misunderstandings into delusional systems. |

| Intervention | Rationale |
|---|---|
| 12. When client is ready, introduce tactics that can lower anxiety and minimize voices and "worrying" thoughts. Teach client to do the following:<br>• Take time out.<br>• Read aloud to self.<br>• Seek out staff, family, or other supportive person.<br>• Listen to music.<br>• Learn to replace irrational thoughts with rational statements.<br>• Learn to replace "bad" thoughts with constructive thoughts.<br>• Perform deep breathing exercises. | 12. Helping client to use tactics to lower anxiety can help enhance functional speech. |

## IMPAIRED SOCIAL INTERACTION

The state in which an individual participates in an insufficient or excessive quantity or ineffective quality of social exchange

### Related To (Etiology)

▲ Impaired thought processes (hallucinations or delusions)
▲ Self-concept disturbance (might feel "bad" about self or "no-good")
▲ Difficulty with communication (e.g., associative looseness)
● Inappropriate or inadequate emotional responses
● Feeling threatened in social situations
● Exaggerated response to stimuli
● Difficulty with concentration

---

▲ NANDA International accepted; ● In addition to NANDA International

## As Evidenced By
## (Assessment Findings/Diagnostic Cues)

- ▲ Verbalized or observed discomfort in social situations
- ▲ Observed use of unsuccessful social interactions behaviors
- ▲ Dysfunctional interaction with peers
- ● Spends time alone by self
- ● Inappropriate or inadequate emotional response
- ● Does not make eye contact, or initiate or respond to social advances of others
- ● Appears agitated or anxious when others come too close or try to engage him in an activity

## Outcome Criteria

- Improves social interaction with family, friends, and neighbors
- Engages in social interactions in goal directed manner
- Uses appropriate social skills in interactions
- ■ Seeks out supportive social contacts

## Long-Term Goals

Client will:
- Engage in one or two activities with minimal encouragement from nurse or family members by (date)
- Use appropriate skills to initiate and maintain an interaction by (date)
- State that he or she is comfortable in at least three structured activities that are goal directed by (date)
- Demonstrate interest to start coping skills training when ready for learning

## Short-Term Goals

Client will:
- Engage in one activity with nurse by the end of the day
- Attend one structured group activity within 1 week
- Maintain an interaction with another client while doing an activity (drawing, playing cards, cooking a meal)

---

▲ NANDA International accepted; ● In addition to NANDA International; ■ Adapted from NOC Outcome Social Supports

## Interventions and Rationales

| Intervention | Rationale |
|---|---|
| 1. Assess if medication has reached therapeutic levels. | 1. Many of the positive symptoms (paranoia, delusions, and hallucinations) will subside with medications, which will facilitate interactions. |
| 2. Ensure that the goals set are realistic, whether in the hospital or community. | 2. Avoids pressure on client, and sense of failure on part of nurse/family. This sense of failure can lead to mutual withdrawal. |
| 3. Keep client in an environment as free of stimuli (loud noises, high traffic areas) as possible. | 3. Client might respond to noises and crowding with agitation, anxiety, and increased inability to concentrate on outside events. |
| 4. Avoid touching the client. | 4. Touch by a "stranger" can be misinterpreted as a sexual or threatening gesture. This is particularly true for a **paranoid** client. |
| 5. If client is unable to respond verbally or in a coherent manner, spend frequent, short periods with client. | 5. An interested presence can provide a sense of being worthwhile. |
| 6. Structure times each day to include planned times for brief interactions and activities with the client on a one-on-one basis. | 6. Helps client to develop a sense of safety in a nonthreatening environment. |

| Intervention | Rationale |
|---|---|
| 7. If client is delusional/ hallucinating or is having trouble concentrating at this time, provide very simple concrete activities with client (e.g., looking at a picture book with nurse, drawing, painting). | 7. Even simple activities help draw client away from delusional thinking onto reality in the environment. |
| 8. Structure activities that work at the client's pace and ability. | 8. Client can lose interest in activities that are too ambitious, which can increase a sense of failure. |
| 9. Try to incorporate the strengths and interests the client had when not as impaired into the activities planned. | 9. Increases likelihood of client's participation and enjoyment. |
| 10. If client is very **paranoid,** solitary or one-on-one activities that require concentration are appropriate. | 10. Client is free to choose his level of interaction; however, the concentration can help minimize distressing paranoid thoughts or voice (e.g., chess). |
| 11. If client is very **withdrawn,** one-on-one activities with a "safe" person initially should be planned. | 11. Learns to feel safe with one person, then gradually might participate in a structured group activity. |
| 12. As client progresses, provide the client with graded activities according to level of tolerance e.g., (1) simple games with one "safe" person; (2) slowly add a third person into "safe" | 12. Gradually the client learns to feel safe and competent with increased social demands. |

| Intervention | Rationale |
|---|---|
| activities; (3) introduce simple group activities; and then (4) groups in which clients participate more. | |
| 13. Eventually engage other clients and significant others in social interactions and activities with the client (card games, ping-pong, sing-a-longs, group outings, etc) at client's level. | 13. Client continues to feel safe and competent in a graduated hierarchy of interactions. |
| 14. Identify with client symptoms he experiences when he/she begins to feel anxious around others. | 14. Increased anxiety can intensify agitation, aggressiveness, and suspiciousness. |
| 15. Teach client to remove himself briefly when feeling agitated and work on some anxiety-relief exercises (e.g., deep breathing, thought stopping). | 15. Teaches client skills in dealing with anxiety and increasing a sense of control. |
| 16. Provide opportunities for the client to learn adaptive social skills in a nonthreatening environment. Initial social skills training could include basic social behaviors (e.g., maintain good eye contact, appropriate distance, calm demeanor, moderate voice tone). | 16. Social skills training helps client adapt and function at a higher level in society, and increases clients quality of life. These simple skills might take time for a client with schizophrenia, but can increase self confidence as well as more positive responses from others. |

| Intervention | Rationale |
|---|---|
| 17. As client progresses, Coping Skills Training should be available to him/her (nurse, staff, or others). Basically the process is:<br>  a. Define the skill to be learned.<br>  b. Model the skill.<br>  c. Rehearse skills in a safe environment, then in the community.<br>  d. Give corrective feedback on the implementation of skills. | 17. Increases client's ability to derive social support and decrease loneliness. Clients will not give up substances of abuse unless they have alternative means to facilitate socialization and feel they belong. |
| 18. Useful coping skills that client will need include conversational and assertiveness skills. | 18. These are fundamental skills for dealing with the world, which everyone uses daily with more or less skill. |
| 19. Remember to give acknowledgment and recognition for positive steps client takes in increasing social skills and appropriate interactions with others. | 19. Recognition and appreciation go a long way to sustaining and increasing a specific behavior. |

## Hallucinations

### Presenting Signs and Symptoms

- Clients state they hear voices.
- Client denies hearing voices, but observer notes client('s):
  - Eyes following something in motion that observer cannot see
  - Staring at one place in room
  - Head turning to side as if listening

- ○ Mumbling to self or conversing when no one else is present
- ○ Inappropriate facial expressions, eye blinking
- If hallucinations are from other causes (e.g., drugs, alcohol, delirium), the underlying cause needs to be treated as soon as possible using accepted medical and nursing protocols.

## Assessment Guidelines
### Hallucinations

1. Assess for command hallucinations (e.g., voices telling the person to harm self or another).
2. Assess when hallucinations seem to occur the most (e.g., times of stress, at night).

## Selected Nursing Diagnoses and Nursing Care Plans

### DISTURBED SENSORY PERCEPTION: AUDITORY/VISUAL

Change in the amount or patterning of incoming stimuli accompanied by a diminished, exaggerated, distorted, or impaired response to such stimuli

### Related To (Etiology)

- ▲ Altered sensory reception: transmission or integration
- ▲ Biochemical imbalance
- ▲ Chemical alterations (e.g., drugs, electrolyte imbalances)
- ▲ Altered sensory perception
- ▲ Psychologic stress
- ● Neurologic/biochemical changes

---

▲NANDA International accepted; ●In addition to NANDA International

## As Evidenced By
## (Assessment Findings/Diagnostic Cues)

- ▲ Disorientation to time/place/person
- ▲ Auditory distortions
- ▲ Hallucinations
- ● Tilting the head as if listening to someone
- ● Frequent blinking of the eyes and grimacing
- ● Mumbling to self, talking or laughing to self
- ▲ Altered communication pattern
- ▲ Change in problem-solving pattern
- ▲ Reported or measured change in sensory acuity
- ▲ Inappropriate responses

## Outcome Criteria

- • Maintains social relationships
- • Maintains role performance
- • States that the voices are no longer threatening, nor do they interfere with his or her life
- ■ Learns ways to refrain from responding to hallucinations

## Long-Term Goals

Client will:
- • Demonstrate techniques that help distract him or her from the voices by (date)
- • Monitor intensity of anxiety

## Short-Term Goals

Client will:
- • State, using a scale from 1 to 10, that "the voices" are less frequent and threatening when aided by medication and nursing intervention by (date)
- • State three symptoms they recognize when their stress levels are high by (date)

---

▲ NANDA International accepted; ● In addition to NANDA International; ■ Adapted from NOC Objective Distortive Thought Self-Control

- Identify two stressful events that trigger hallucinations by (date)
- Demonstrate one stress reduction technique by (date)
- Identify two personal interventions that decrease or lower the intensity or frequency of hallucinations (e.g., listening to music, wearing headphones, reading out loud, jogging, socializing) by (date)

## *Interventions and Rationales*

| Intervention | Rationale |
|---|---|
| 1. If voices are telling the client to harm self or others, take necessary environmental precautions.<br>  a. Notify others and police, physician, and administration according to unit protocol.<br>  b. If in the hospital, use unit protocols for **suicidal** or **threats of violence** if client plans to act on commands.<br>  c. If in the community, evaluate need for hospitalization. Clearly document what client says and, if he/she is a threat to others, document who was contacted and notified (use agency protocol as a guide). | 1. People often obey hallucinatory commands to kill self or others. Early assessment and intervention might save lives. |
| 2. Decrease environmental stimuli when possible (low noise, minimal activity). | 2. Decrease potential for anxiety that might trigger hallucinations. Helps calm client. |

| Intervention | Rationale |
|---|---|
| 3. Accept the fact that the voices are real to the client, but explain that you do not hear the voices. Refer to the voices as "your voices" or "voices that you hear." | 3. Validating that your reality does not include voices can help client cast "doubt" on the validity of his or her voices. |
| 4. Stay with clients when they are starting to hallucinate, and direct them to tell the "voices they hear" to go away. Repeat often in a matter-of-fact manner. | 4. Clients can sometimes learn to push voices aside when given repeated instruction, especially within the framework of a trusting relationship. |
| 5. Keep to simple, basic, reality-based topics of conversation. Help client to focus on one idea at a time. | 5. Client's thinking might be confused and disorganized; this intervention helps client focus and comprehend reality-based issues. |
| 6. Explore how the hallucinations are experienced by the client. | 6. Exploring the hallucination and sharing the experience can help give the person a sense of power that he or she might be able to manage the hallucinatory voices. |
| 7. Help the client to identify the needs that might underlie the hallucination. What other ways can these needs be met? | 7. Hallucinations might reflect needs for:<br>a. Power<br>b. Self-esteem<br>c. Anger<br>d. Sexuality |

| Intervention | Rationale |
|---|---|
| 8. Help client to identify times that the hallucinations are most prevalent and frightening. | 8. Helps both nurse and client identify situations and times that might be most anxiety producing and threatening to client. |
| 9. Engage client in simple physical activities or tasks that channel energy (writing, drawing, crafts, noncompetitive sports, treadmill, walking on track, exercise bike). | 9. Redirecting client's energies to acceptable activities can decrease the possibility of acting on hallucinations and help distract from voices. |
| 10. Work with the client to find which activities help reduce anxiety and distract the client from hallucinatory material. Practice new skills with client. | 10. If clients' stress triggers hallucinatory activity, they might be more motivated to find ways to remove themselves from a stressful environment or try distraction techniques. |
| 11. Be alert for signs of increasing fear, anxiety, or agitation. | 11. Might herald hallucinatory activity, which can be very frightening to client, and client might act upon command hallucinations (harm self or others). |
| 12. Intervene with one-on-one, seclusion, or PRN medication (as ordered) when appropriate. | 12. Intervene before anxiety begins to escalate. If client is already out of control, use chemical or physical restraints following unit protocols. |

# Delusions

## Presenting Signs and Symptoms

- The client has fragmented, poorly organized, well-organized, systematized, or extensive system of beliefs that are not supported by reality.
- The content of the delusions can be grandiose, persecutory, jealous, somatic, or based on guilt.

## Assessment Guidelines

*Delusions*

1. Assess if delusions have to do with someone trying to harm the client, or if the client is planning to retaliate against a person or organization.
   a. If client is a threat to self or others, notify person and authorities.
   b. Confer with physician and administration if precautions need to be taken.
2. Assess when delusional thinking is the most prominent (e.g., when under stress, in the presence of certain situations or people, at night).

## Selected Nursing Diagnoses and Nursing Care Plans

### DISTURBED THOUGHT PROCESSES

Disruption in cognitive operations and activities

*Related To (Etiology)*

- Biochemical/neurologic imbalances
- Panic levels of anxiety
- Overwhelming stressful life events
- Chemical alterations (e.g., drugs, electrolyte imbalances)

*As Evidenced By*
*(Assessment Findings/Diagnostic Cues)*

- ▲ Inaccurate interpretation of environment
- ▲ Memory deficit/problems
- ▲ Egocentricity
- ▲ Inappropriate non-reality-based thinking
- Delusions

---

▲ NANDA International accepted; ● In addition to NANDA International

## Outcome Criteria

- Refrains from acting on delusional thinking
- Demonstrates satisfying relationships with real people.
- Delusions no longer threaten or interfere with his or her ability to function in family, social, and work situations.
- Perceives environment correctly

## Long-Term Goals

Client will:
- Demonstrate two effective coping skills that minimize delusional thoughts by (date)

## Short-Term Goals

Client will:
- State that the "thoughts" are less intense and less frequent with aid of medications and nursing interventions by (date)
- Talk about concrete happenings in the environment without talking about delusions for 5 minutes by (date)
- Begin to recognize that his or her frightening (suspicious) "thinking" occurs most often at times of stress and when he or she is anxious

## Interventions and Rationales

| Intervention | Rationale |
|---|---|
| 1. Utilize safety measures to protect clients or others, if clients believe they need to protect themselves against a specific person. Precautions are needed. | 1. During acute phase, client's delusional thinking might dictate to them that they might have to hurt others or self in order to be safe. External controls might be needed. |
| 2. Attempt to understand the significance of these beliefs to the client at the time of their presentation. | 2. Important clues to underlying fears and issues can be found in the client's seemingly illogical fantasies. |

---

- NOC objective Disturbed Thought Self-Control

| Intervention | Rationale |
|---|---|
| 3. Be aware that client's delusions represent the way that he or she experiences reality. | 3. Identifying the client's experience allows the nurse to understand the client's feelings. |
| 4. Identify feelings related to delusions. For example:<br>a. If client believes someone is going to harm him/her, client is experiencing fear.<br>b. If client believes someone or something is controlling his/her thoughts, client is experiencing helplessness. | 4. When people believe that they are understood, anxiety might lessen. |
| 5. Do not argue with the client's beliefs or try to correct false beliefs using facts. | 5. Arguing will only increase client's defensive position, thereby reinforcing false beliefs. This will result in the client feeling even more isolated and misunderstood. |
| 6. Do not touch the client; use gestures carefully. | 6. A psychotic person might misinterpret touch as either aggressive or sexual in nature and might interpret gestures as aggressive moves. People who are psychotic need a lot of personal space. |
| 7. Interact with clients on the basis of things in the environment. Try to distract client from their delusions by engaging in reality-based activities (cards, simple board games, simple arts and crafts projects, cooking with another person, etc.). | 7. When thinking is focused on reality-based activities, the client is free of delusional thinking during that time. Helps focus attention externally. |

| Intervention | Rationale |
|---|---|
| 8. Teach client coping skills that minimize "worrying" thoughts. Coping skills include:<br>• Talking to a trusted friend<br>• Phoning a helpline<br>• Singing<br>• Going to a gym<br>• Thought-stopping techniques | 8. When client is ready, teach strategies client can do alone. |
| 9. Encourage healthy habits to optimize functioning:<br>• Maintain regular sleep pattern.<br>• Reduce alcohol and drug intake.<br>• Maintain self-care.<br>• Maintain medication regimen. | 9. All are vital to help keep client in remission. |

## Paranoia

### Presenting Signs and Symptoms

- Pervasive suspiciousness about one or more persons and their actions
- On guard, hyperalert, vigilant
- Blames others for consequences of own behavior
- Hostile, argumentative, often threatening verbalizations or behavior
- Poor interpersonal relationships
- Has delusions of influence, persecution, and grandiosity
- Often refuses medications because "nothing is wrong with me"
- Might refuse food if believes it is poisoned

### Assessment Guidelines

*Paranoia*

1. Assess for suicidal or homicidal behaviors.
2. Assess for potential for violence.
3. Assess need for hospitalization.

## Selected Nursing Diagnoses and Nursing Care Plans

### DEFENSIVE COPING

Repeated projection of falsely positive self-evaluation based on a self-protective pattern that defends against underlying perceived threats to positive self-regard

### *Related To (Etiology)*

- ● Perceived threat to self
- ● Suspicions of the motives of others
- ● Perceived lack of self-efficacy/vulnerability

### *As Evidenced By (Assessment Findings/Diagnostic Cues)*

- ▲ Projection of blame/responsibility
- ▲ Grandiosity
- ▲ Denial of obvious problems
- ▲ Rationalization of failures
- ▲ Superior attitude toward others
- ▲ Hostile laughter or ridicule of others
- ▲ Difficulty in reality testing of perceptions
- ▲ Difficulty establishing/maintaining relationships
- ● Hostility, aggression, or homicidal ideation
- ● Fearful
- ● False beliefs about the intentions of others

### *Outcome Criteria*

- • Interacts with others appropriately
- • Maintains medical compliance
- • Demonstrates decreased suspicious behaviors interacting with others
- ■ Avoids high-risk environments and situations

---

▲ NANDA International accepted; ● In addition to NANDA International; ■ NOC Outcome for Impulse Self-Control

## Long-Term Goals

Client will:

- Acknowledge that medications help lower suspiciousness
- State that he/she feels safe and more in control in interactions with environment/family/work/social gatherings by (date)
- Be able to apply a variety of stress/anxiety-reducing techniques on own by (date)

## Short-Term Goals

Client will:

- Remain safe with the aid of medication and nursing interventions (either interpersonal, chemical, or seclusion), as will others in the client's environment
- Focus on reality-based activity with the aid of medication/nursing intervention by (date)
- Demonstrate two newly learned constructive ways to deal with stress and feelings of powerlessness by (date)
- Demonstrate the ability to remove himself or herself from situations when anxiety begins to increase with the aid of medications and nursing interventions by (date)
- Identify one action that helps client feel more in control of his or her life

## Interventions and Rationales

| Intervention | Rationale |
|---|---|
| 1. Use a nonjudgmental, respectful, and neutral approach with the client. | 1. There is less chance for a suspicious client to misconstrue intent or meaning if content is neutral and approach is respectful and nonjudgmental. |
| 2. Be honest and consistent with client regarding expectations and enforcing rules. | 2. Suspicious people are quick to discern dishonesty. Honesty and consistency provide an atmosphere in which trust can grow. |

| Intervention | Rationale |
|---|---|
| 3. Use clear and simple language when communicating with a suspicious client. | 3. Minimize the opportunity for miscommunication and misconstruing the meaning of the message. |
| 4. Explain to client what you are going to do before you do it. | 4. Prepares the client beforehand and minimizes misinterpreting your intent as hostile or aggressive. |
| 5. Be aware of client's tendency to have ideas of reference; do not do things in front of client that can be misinterpreted:<br>a. Laughing<br>b. Whispering<br>c. Talking quietly when client can see but not hear what is being said | 5. Suspicious clients will automatically think that they are the target of the interaction and interpret it in a negative manner (e.g., you are laughing at them, whispering about them, etc.). |
| 6. Diffuse angry and hostile verbal attacks with a nondefensive stand. | 6. When staff become defensive, anger escalates for both client and staff. A nondefensive and nonjudgmental attitude provides an atmosphere in which feelings can be explored more easily. |
| 7. Assess and observe client regularly for signs of increasing anxiety and hostility. | 7. Intervene before client loses control. |
| 8. Provide verbal/physical limits when client's hostile behavior escalates: *We won't allow you to hurt anyone here. If you can't control yourself, we will help you.* | 8. Often verbal limits are effective in helping a client gain self-control. |

| Intervention | Rationale |
|---|---|
| 9. Set limits in a clear, matter-of-fact way, using a calm tone. *Threatening John is not acceptable. Let's talk about appropriate ways to deal with your feelings.* | 9. Calm and neutral approach may diffuse escalation of anger. Offer an alternative to verbal abuse by finding appropriate ways to deal with feelings. |
| 10. Maintain low level of stimuli and enhance a nonthreatening environment (avoid groups). | 10. Noisy environments might be perceived as threatening. |
| 11. Initially, provide solitary, noncompetitive activities that take some concentration. Later a game with one or more clients that takes concentration (e.g., chess, checkers, thoughtful card games such as bridge or rummy). | 11. If a client is suspicious of others, solitary activities are the best. Concentrating on environmental stimuli minimizes paranoid rumination. |

# Providing Support to Family/Others

## INTERRUPTED FAMILY PROCESSES

Change in family relationships and/or functioning

### Related To (Etiology)

▲ Shift in health status of a family member
▲ Situational crisis or transition
▲ Family role shift
▲ Developmental crisis or transition
● Mental or physical disorder of family member

---

▲ NANDA International accepted; ● In addition to NANDA International

## As Evidenced By
### (Assessment Findings/Diagnostic Cues)

- ▲ Changes in participation in decision making
- ▲ Changes in mutual support
- ▲ Changes in stress reduction behavior
- ▲ Changes in communication patterns
- ▲ Changes in participation in problem solving
- ▲ Changes in expression of conflict in family
- ● Inability to meet needs of family and significant others (physical, emotional, spiritual)
- ● Knowledge deficit regarding the disease and what is happening with ill family member (might believe client is more capable than they are)
- ● Knowledge deficit regarding community and health-care support

## Outcome Criteria

Family members/significant others will:
- State they have received needed support from community and agency resources that offer support, education, coping skills training, and/or social network development (psychoeducational approach)
- Demonstrate problem-solving skills for handling tensions and misunderstanding within the family environment
- Recount in some detail the early signs and symptoms of relapse in their ill family member, and know whom to contact

## Long-Term Goals

Family members/significant others will:
- Know of at least two contact people when they suspect potential relapse by (date)
- Discuss the disease (schizophrenia) knowledgeably by (date):
  - ○ Understand the need for medical adherence
  - ○ Support the ill family member in maintaining optimum health

---

▲ NANDA International accepted; ● In addition to NANDA International

    ○ Know about community resources (e.g., help with self-
      care activities, private respite)
- Have access to family/multiple family support groups
  and psychoeducational training by (date)

## Short-Term Goals

Family members/significant others will:
- Meet with nurse/physician/social worker the first day
  of hospitalization and begin to learn about this neuro-
  logic/biochemical disease, treatment, and community
  resources
- Attend at least one family support group (single family,
  multiple family) within 4 days from onset of acute
  episode
- Problem-solve, with the nurse, two concrete situations
  within the family that all would like to change
- State what the medications can do for their ill member,
  the side effects and toxic effects of the drugs, and the
  need for adherence to medication at least 2 to 3 days
  before discharge
- Be included in the discharge planning along with client
- State and have written information identifying the signs
  of potential relapse and whom to contact before discharge
- Name and have complete list of community supports for
  ill family member and supports for all members of the
  family at least 2 days before discharge

## Interventions and Rationales

| Intervention | Rationale |
|---|---|
| 1. Identify family's ability to cope (e.g., experience of loss, caregiver burden, needed supports). | 1. Family's needs must be addressed to stabilize family unit. |
| 2. Provide opportunity for family to discuss feelings related to ill family member and identify their immediate concerns. | 2. Nurses and staff can best intervene when they understand the family's experience and needs. |

| Intervention | Rationale |
|---|---|
| 3. Assess the family members' current level of knowledge about the disease and medications used to treat the disease. | 3. Family might have misconceptions and misinformation about schizophrenia and treatment, or no knowledge at all. Teach at client's and family's level of understanding and readiness to learn. |
| 4. Provide information on disease and treatment strategies at family's level of knowledge. | 4. Meet family members' needs for information. |
| 5. Inform the client and family in clear, simple terms about psycho-pharmacologic therapy: dosage, the need to take medication as prescribed, side effects, and toxic effect. Written information should be given to client and family members as well. **Refer to the client and family teaching guidelines in Chapter 21 under Antipsychotic Medication.** | 5. Understanding of the disease and the treatment of the disease encourages greater family support and client adherence. |
| 6. Provide information on family and client community resources for client and family after discharge: support groups, organizations, day hospitals, psycho-educational programs, respite centers, etc. **See list of associations and Internet sites at end of chapter.** | 6. Schizophrenia is an over-whelming disease for both the client and the family. Groups, support groups, and psychoeducational centers can help:<br>a. Develop family skills<br>b. Access resources<br>c. Access support<br>d. Access caring |

| Intervention | Rationale |
|---|---|
| | e. Minimize isolation |
| | f. Improve quality of life for all family members |
| 7. Teach family and client the warning symptoms of potential relapse. | 7. Rapid recognition of early warning symptoms can help ward off potential relapse when immediate medical attention is sought. |

## MEDICAL TREATMENT

### Psychopharmacology

Antipsychotic medications are indicated for nearly all psychotic episodes of schizophrenia. To delay medication therapy too long can put the client at risk for suicide or other dangerous behaviors.

Medications used to treat schizophrenia are called antipsychotic medications. Two groups of antipsychotic drugs exist: *standard* (traditional/conventional) and the newer *atypical* (or novel) medications. **Many physicians urge the use of the *atypical* medications initially because of their better side effect profile and the fact that the atypical medications target the negative symptoms (apathy, lack of motivation) and anhedonia (lack of pleasure in life), thereby increasing the quality of life for clients.**

### *Atypical (Novel) Antipsychotic Medications*

During the early 1990s, new types of antipsychotics began appearing on the market, and they are currently used as first-line medications. (Clozapine [Clozaril] is the exception because of its tendency to cause agranulocytosis and its high incidence for seizures.) These drugs not only target the acute and disturbing symptoms seen in acute active episodes of schizophrenia (hallucinations, delusions, associative looseness, paranoia), called positive symptoms, but also target the negative symptoms, which allows improvement in the quality of life for clients (increased motivation, improved judgment, increased energy, ability to experience pleasure and increased cognitive function). These drugs also have a very low extrapyramidal symptom (EPS) profile and, in general, have a more favorable side-effect profile.

**Pros**

- Target negative and positive symptoms
- Lower risk of EPS
- Lowers incidence of adverse reactions, increased compliance
- May improve symptoms of:
  - Anxiety
  - Depression
  - Decreased suicidal behavior

**Cons**

- Increased weight gain
- Metabolic abnormalities (glucose dysregulation, hypercholesterolemia)
- Are more expensive

Table 8-3 provides a list of atypical antipsychotics, their dosages, and the side effects.

## Standard Medications

The standard antipsychotic drugs target the more flagrant symptoms of schizophrenia (hallucinations, delusions, suspiciousness, associative looseness). These drugs can:

- Reduce disruptive and violent behavior
- Increase activity, speech, and sociability in withdrawn clients
- Improve self-care
- Improve sleep patterns
- Reduce the disturbing quality of hallucinations and delusions
- Improve thought processes
- Decrease resistance to supportive therapy
- Reduce rate of relapse
- Decrease intensity of paranoid reactions

Antipsychotic agents are usually effective 3 to 6 weeks after the regimen is started.

**Adverse Reactions** There are some troubling side effects of these drugs that can at times limit medical adherence.

Table 8-3 **Antipsychotic Medications**

| Drug | Dose Range (mg/day) | Atypical Antipsychotic Agents | | | | | Special Considerations |
|------|---------------------|------|-----|----|-----|-----|------------------------|
| | | EPS | ACH | OH | SED | | |
| Clozapine (Clozaril) P.O. ODT: FazaClo | 300–900 | No | High | High | High | | Used in treatment-refractory clients—**non–first-line** 0.8%–0.1% incidence of agranulocytosis—weekly WBC High seizure rate |
| Risperidone (Risperdal) P.O. (Consta: LAI) ODT: M-Tabs | 2–16 | Low | Very low | Mod | Low | | Weight gain significant Doses >6 mg might see TD |
| Olanzapine (Zyprexa) Zydis: ODT | 2.5–20 | Low | Low | Mod | Low | | Weight gain significant Once-daily dose (long half-life) Interaction with SSRIs might occur |

Drug dosages from Fuller and Sajatovic, 2000, Lieberman and Tasman, 2000, and Kennedy 2000; adapted from Varcarolis et al: *Foundations of psychiatric mental health nursing* (5th ed.). Philadelphia: WB Saunders, 2005.

*Dosages vary with individual responses to antipsychotic agent used.

*ACH,* Anticholinergic side effects (e.g., dry mouth, blurred vision, urinary retention, constipation, agitation); *ECG,* electrocardiograph; *EPS,* extrapyramidal side effects; *HDL,* high-density lipoprotein; *IM,* intramuscular; *IV,* intravenous; *LDL,* low-density lipoprotein; *OH,* orthostatic hypotension; *NMS,* neuroleptic malignant syndrome; *PO,* oral; *R,* rectal; *SC,* subcutaneous; *L.A.I.-*Long acting injection, *O.D.T.-*Orally disintegrating tablets. *SED,* sedation; *SSRI,* selective serotonin reuptake inhibitor; *TD,* tardive dyskinesia; *WBC,* white blood cell count.

*Continued*

Table 8-3 **Antipsychotic Medications—cont'd**

| | Dose Range (mg/day) | EPS | ACH | OH | SED | Special Considerations |
|---|---|---|---|---|---|---|
| | | | Atypical Antipsychotic Agents | | | |
| **Drug** | | | | | | |
| Quetiapine (Seroquel) | 150–750 | Low | Low-None | Mod | Low | Risk of TD and NMS very low |
| Ziprasidone (Geodon) PO/IM | 40–160 | Low-None | Mild-Mod | Mild | Low | ECG changes-QT prolongation; not to be used with other drugs known to prolong QT interval<br>Effective with the depressive symptoms of schizophrenia<br>Low propensity for weight gain |
| Aripiprazole (Abilify) PO/IM | 10–30 | Low | Low-None | Low-Mild | Low- | Teach about and check for akathisia; reported in some children<br>TD and sedation dose related NMS rare<br>Little or no weight gain or increase in glucose, HDL, LDL, or triglycerides<br>First of a new class of atypical antipsychotics |

| | Standard (Traditional) Antipsychotic Medications | | | |
|---|---|---|---|---|
| Drug | Routes of Administration | Acute (mg/day)* | Maintenance (mg/day)* | Special Considerations |
| Haloperidol (Haldol) | PO, IM | 5–50 | 2–20 | Has low sedative properties; is used in large doses for assaultive patients, thus avoiding the severe side effect of hypotension<br>Appropriate for the elderly for the same reason as above; lessens the chance of falls from dizziness or hypotension<br>High incidence of extrapyramidal side effects |
| Trifluoperazine (Stelazine) | PO, IM | 10–60 | 5–30 | Low sedation—good for withdrawn or paranoid symptoms<br>High incidence of EPS<br>NMS might occur |

Drug dosages from Fuller and Sajatovic, 2000, Lieberman and Tasman, 2000, and Kennedy 2000; adapted from Varcarolis, et al: *Foundations of psychiatric mental health nursing* (5th ed.). Philadelphia: WB Saunders, 2005.

*Dosages vary with individual responses to antipsychotic agent used.

*ACH,* Anticholinergic side effects (e.g., dry mouth, blurred vision, urinary retention, constipation, agitation); *ECG,* electrocardiograph; *EPS,* extrapyramidal side effects; *HDL,* high-density lipoprotein; *IM,* intramuscular; *IV,* intravenous; *LDL,* low-density lipoprotein; *OH,* orthostatic hypotension; *NMS,* neuroleptic malignant syndrome; *PO,* oral; *R,* rectal; *SC,* subcutaneous; *L.A.I.*-Long acting injection, *O.D.T.*-Orally disintegrating tablets. *SED,* sedation; *SSRI,* selective serotonin reuptake inhibitor; *TD,* tardive dyskinesia; *WBC,* white blood cell count.

*Continued*

Table 8-3 **Antipsychotic Medications—cont'd**

| | Standard (Traditional) Antipsychotic Medications | | |
| Drug | Routes of Administration | Acute (mg/day)* | Maintenance (mg/day)* | Special Considerations |
|---|---|---|---|---|
| Fluphenazine (Prolixin) | PO, IM, SC | 2.5–20 | 2–20 | Among the least sedative |
| Thiothixene (Navane) | PO, IM | 6–30 | 5–40 | High incidence of akathisia |
| Loxapine (Loxitane) | PO, IM | 60–100 | 20–200 | Possibly associated with weight reduction |
| Molindone (Moban) | PO | 50–100 | 20–200 | Possibly associated with weight reduction |
| Perphenazine (Trilafon) | PO, IM, IV | 12–32 | 8–64 | Can help control severe vomiting |
| Chlorpromazine (Thorazine) | PO, IM, R | 200–1600 | 200–1000 | Increases sensitivity to sun (as with other phenothiazines) Highest sedation and hypotension effects; least potent Can cause irreversible retinitis pigmentosis at 800 mg/day |
| Chlorprothixene (Taractan) | PO, IM | 50–600 | 75–600 | Weight gain common |

| | | | | |
|---|---|---|---|---|
| Thioridazine (Mellaril) | PO | 200-600 | 200-600 | **Not recommended as first-line antipsychotic** Dose-related severe ECG changes; might cause sudden death |
| Mesoridazine (Serentil) | PO, IM | 75-300 | 100-400 | Among the most sedative; severe nausea and vomiting might occur in adults |
| Decanoate: Long-Acting | | | | |
| Haloperidol (Haldol) LAI, IM | | 0 | 50-300 | Given deep muscle z-track IM **Give every 3-4 weeks** |
| Fluphenazine (Prolixin) IM, LAI | | 0 | 12.5-50 | Given deep muscle z-track IM **Give every 2-4 weeks** |

Drug dosages from Fuller and Sajatovic, 2000, Lieberman and Tasman, 2000, and Kennedy 2000; adapted from Varcarolis, et al: *Foundations of psychiatric mental health nursing* (5th ed.). Philadelphia: WB Saunders, 2005.

*Dosages vary with individual responses to antipsychotic agent used.

*ACH,* Anticholinergic side effects (e.g., dry mouth, blurred vision, urinary retention, constipation, agitation); *ECG,* electrocardiograph; *EPS,* extrapyramidal side effects; *HDL,* high-density lipoprotein; *IM,* intramuscular; *IV,* intravenous; *LDL,* low-density lipoprotein; *OH,* orthostatic hypotension; *NMS,* neuroleptic malignant syndrome; *PO,* oral; *R,* rectal; *SC,* subcutaneous; *L.A.I.*-Long acting injection, *O.D.T.*-Orally disintegrating tablets. *SED,* sedation; *SSRI,* selective serotonin reuptake inhibitor; *TD,* tardive dyskinesia; *WBC,* white blood cell count.

Some of these side effects can be managed with other medications. EPS, cardiac side effects, and toxic effects of these drugs are discussed further in Chapter 21.

One of the most disturbing side effects to clients are the EPS; medication is used to treat the EPS caused by these standard antipsychotics. Refer to Chapter 21 for a client and family medication teaching plan.

# PSYCHOSOCIAL APPROACHES

## Treatment of Comorbid Conditions

There are many treatment approaches that can help clients with schizophrenia better adjust to their environment and increase their quality of life when used in conjunction with medications. Some of the psychotherapeutic approaches that seem to be useful for many people with these disorders are discussed here. However, treatment should not only be aimed at the symptoms of schizophrenia but also need to target some of the comorbid conditions that a client might exhibit. Some of the more common comorbid conditions in people with schizophrenia include:

• Substance use problems
• Depressive symptoms or disorders
• Risk for suicide
• Violent behaviors

If a comorbid condition is identified, it must be treated, if overall adherence to a second treatment approach is followed and/or successful.

## Specific Psychosocial Treatments

### Individual Therapy

There is evidence that *supportive therapy* that includes problem-solving techniques and social skills training helps reduce relapse and enhance social and occupational functioning when added to medication treatment for schizophrenic individuals who are treated in an outpatient environment. Cognitive behavioral therapy (CBT), cognitive rehabilitation, and social skills training (SST) are particularly helpful in people with chronic schizophrenia who have cognitive impairments.

## Family Intervention

Families with a schizophrenic member endure considerable hardships while coping with the psychotic and residual symptoms of schizophrenia. Often families are the sole caretakers of their schizophrenic member and need education, guidance, and support as well as training to help them manage (APA, 2000b). A **Psychoeducational family approach** provides support, education, coping skills training, and social network expansion and has been proven very successful with both decreasing family stress and increasing client adherence to treatment. Families can be helped by:

- Understanding the disease and the role of medications
- Setting realistic goals for their schizophrenic member
- Developing problem-solving skills for handling tensions and misunderstanding within the family environment
- Identifying early signs of relapse
- Having knowledge of where they can go for guidance and support within the community and nationally

## Group Therapy

The goals of group therapy for individual members are to increase problem-solving ability, to enable realistic goal planning, to facilitate social interactions, and to manage medication side effects (Kanas, 1996). Groups can help clients develop interpersonal skills, resolution of family problems, utilization of community supports as well as increase medication compliance by learning to deal with troubling side effects.

# NURSE, CLIENT, AND FAMILY RESOURCES

## ASSOCIATIONS

**National Alliance for the Mentally III (NAMI)**
Colonial Place Three
2107 Wilson Boulevard, Suite 300
Arlington, VA 22201-3042
(800) 950-NAMI (check this one out!)
http://www.nami.org

**Schizophrenics Anonymous**
403 Seymour Avenue, Suite 202
Lansing, MI 48933
(517) 485-7168;(800) 482-9534 (consumer line) (check this
    one out!)

**Recovery, Inc.**
802 North Dearborn Street
Chicago, II, 60610
(312) 337-5661

## INTERNET SITES

**Doctors Guide to the Internet**
http://www.pslgroup.com/schizophr.htm
Many articles; good site for schizophrenia information

**Internet Mental Health**
http://www.mentalhealth.com
Vast amount of information/booklets/articles and general
    information

**National Alliance for Research on Schizophrenia and
    Depression**
http://www.narsad.org

**Schizophrenia.com**
http://www.schizophrenia.com

# CHAPTER 9

# Personality Disorders

## OVERVIEW

Clients diagnosed as having personality disorders (PDs) have multiple needs that pose many challenges to nurses and other health care providers. PDs occur in approximately 10% of the population; however, they are often overdiagnosed in clients who are ethnically and culturally different from the health care practitioner (Sadock & Sadock, 2000). Therefore, it is important that assessment be performed in the context of the client's national, cultural, spiritual, and ethnic background.

Personality disorders are a major source of long-term disability and frequently occur in conjunction with other psychiatric disorders, or with general medical conditions. For example, both major depression and panic disorder have a high rate of comorbidity (co-occurrence) with PDs, estimated to occur in approximately 25% to 50% of clients. Comorbid PDs are likely to be found in clients with somatization, eating disorder, chronic pain, recurrent suicide attempts, and posttraumatic stress disorder (Goldberg, 1998). People with a substance abuse problem might also have a comorbid PD, which can complicate the therapeutic working relationship and interfere with treatment.

Personality disorders comprise personality traits that are maladaptive, persistent, and inflexible. The intensity and manifestation of presenting problems can vary widely among clients with PDs depending on diagnoses and individual characteristics. Some clients with PDs have milder forms of disability, whereas other clients' symptoms present

as extreme, even psychotic. However, all of the PDs have four common characteristics:
1. Inflexible and maladaptive responses to stress
2. Disability in working and loving
3. Ability to evoke interpersonal conflict in health care providers as well as family and friends
4. Capacity to have an intense effect on others (this process is often unconscious and generally produces undesirable results)

Box 9-1 identifies the *Diagnostic and Statistical Manual of Mental Disorders* (4th edition, text revision) (DSM-IV-TR) criteria for a person with a PD.

The DSM-IV-TR organizes the 10 PDs into three clusters (Box 9-2).

| Box 9-1 | **DSM-IV-TR** <br> **Criteria for a Personality Disorder** |
|---|---|

1. An enduring pattern of inner experience and behavior that deviates markedly from the expectations of the individual's culture. This pattern is manifested in two (or more) of the following areas:
   - Cognition (i.e., ways of perceiving and interpreting self, other people, and events)
   - Affect (i.e., the range, intensity, liability, and appropriateness of emotional response)
   - Interpersonal functioning
   - Impulse control
2. The enduring pattern is inflexible and pervasive across a broad range of personal and social situations.
3. The enduring pattern leads to clinically significant distress or impairment in social, occupational, or other important areas of functioning.
4. The pattern is stable and of long duration, and its onset can be traced back at least to adolescence or early adulthood.
5. The enduring pattern is not better accounted for as manifestation or consequence of another mental disorder.
6. The enduring pattern is not due to the direct physiological effects of a substance (e.g., a drug of abuse, a medication) or a general medical condition (e.g., head trauma).

Adapted from American Psychiatric Association. (2000). *Diagnostic and statistical manual of mental disorders* (4th ed., text revision). Washington, DC: American Psychiatric Association, p. 689; reprinted with permission.

| Box 9-2 | DSM-IV-TR Personality Disorder Clusters |
| --- | --- |

**Cluster A Disorders—Odd or Eccentric**
Paranoid Personality Disorder
Schizoid Personality Disorder
Schizotypal Personality Disorder

**Cluster B Disorders—Dramatic, Emotional, or Erratic**
Antisocial Personality Disorder
Borderline Personality Disorder
Histrionic Personality Disorder
Narcissistic Personality Disorder

**Cluster C Disorders—Anxious or Fearful**
Dependent Personality Disorder
Obsessive-Compulsive Personality Disorder
Avoidant Personality Disorder

Because each of the PDs has its own characteristics, personality traits, and effects on self and others, it is best to deal with them individually. The following sections (1) describe the defining characteristics, (2) identify some intervention guidelines, and (3) offer the most recent treatment modalities for each PD.

Some of the most problematic behaviors that nurses are confronted with in the health care setting are similar for many of the PDs. These behaviors in part include manipulation (see Chapter 19), self-mutilation, suicide (see Chapter 16), anger and hostility (see Chapter 17), low self-esteem, ineffective coping and/or impaired social interaction, and nonadherence to medication or treatment (see Chapter 20). **Self-mutilation, low self-esteem, impaired social interaction, and ineffective coping** are covered in this chapter. The other common nursing diagnoses of clients with PD are covered in separate chapters. All of these behaviors are commonly seen in a host of disorders, and the guidelines for intervention are similar for all clients.

Although people with PDs might be hospitalized briefly during a crisis, generally long-term treatment takes place in clinics and community settings.

## DSM-IV-TR Cluster A Disorders— Odd or Eccentric

Cluster A disorders, often referred to as "odd" or "eccentric", comprise PDs that have been established to have some relationship to schizophrenia. Of the Cluster A disorders, schizotypal PD is most strongly related to schizophrenia. The following discussion gives defining characteristics, guidelines for care, and treatments for the Cluster A disorders.

## Paranoid Personality Disorder (PPD)

### Presenting Signs and Symptoms

- Vigilant and suspicious of others' motives—believe people mean to exploit, harm, or deceive them in some manner
- Bear grudges; are unforgiving of insults, injuries, or slights
- Read hidden, demeaning, or threatening meanings into benign remarks or events
- Have difficulty establishing close relationships; usually work alone
- Perceived as cold and unemotional, and do not share their thoughts with others; lack a sense of humor
- Very critical of others but have a great deal of difficulty accepting criticism
- Are prone to file suit

### Nursing Guidelines

1. Avoid being too "nice" or "friendly."
2. Give clear and straightforward explanations of tests and procedures beforehand.
3. Use simple, clear language; avoid ambiguity.
4. Project a neutral but kind affect.
5. Warn about any changes, side effects of medications, and reasons for delay. Such interventions might help allay anxiety and minimize suspiciousness.
6. A written plan of treatment might help encourage cooperation.

### Treatment

Paranoid clients will initially mistrust their therapist's motives and find it difficult to share personal information.

For that reason, therapy is often not sought or sustained among these clients. However, when a person with PPD does enter therapy, initially supportive therapy might help the client experience trust and even begin to feel some amount of safety in an interpersonal relationship. If a therapeutic alliance can be achieved, cognitive and behavioral techniques might be useful to the client. The focus is on enhancing coping strategies and relieving stress and worry that are expressed as hypervigilance and social withdrawal (Zale et al., 1997). Severe symptoms of paranoia can be attenuated with careful use of antipsychotic medication.

## Schizoid Personality Disorder

*Presenting Signs and Symptoms*

- Neither desire nor enjoy close relationships, even within their own family
- Prefer to live apart from others, choose solitary activities, have little interest in sexual activity with others, and might describe themselves as "loners"
- Show emotional coldness, detachment, or flattened affect
- Occupation often involves little interpersonal contact

*Nursing Guidelines*

1. Avoid being too "nice" or "friendly."
2. Do not try to re-socialize these clients (Goldberg, 1998).
3. A thorough diagnostic assessment might be needed to identify symptoms or disorders that the client is reluctant to discuss.

*Treatment*

A schizoid individual is apt to seek treatment only in a crisis situation, and only then to seek relief from acute symptoms. In some cases, supportive psychotherapy with cognitive-behavioral techniques can help reinforce socially outgoing behaviors. Group therapy might be appropriate if the individual needs of each client are addressed. In some cases, social skills training groups might be an effective intervention (Zale et al., 1997). Short-term use of psychopharmacology might be appropriate for treating anxiety or depression.

Low-dose antipsychotic medication can target symptoms such as anger, hostility, paranoia, and ideas of reference if such symptoms are part of the clinical picture.

# Schizotypal Personality Disorders

*Presenting Signs and Symptoms*

- Share many of the withdrawn, aloof, and socially distant characteristics listed for the schizoid PD client described earlier
- Ideas of reference, odd beliefs, magical thinking, or unusual perceptual experiences, including bodily illusions, might be present
- Excessive and unrelieved social anxiety frequently associated with paranoid fears
- Lack of close friends and confidants
- Inappropriate or constricted affect
- Behavior or appearance that is odd, eccentric, or peculiar
- Some individuals diagnosed with schizotypal PD will go on to present with a full-blown schizophrenic illness

*Nursing Guidelines*

1. Respect the client's need for social isolation.
2. Be aware of client's suspiciousness and employ appropriate interventions (see Chapter 8).
3. As with the schizoid client, careful diagnostic assessment might be needed to uncover any other medical or psychological symptoms that might need intervention (e.g., suicidal thoughts).

*Treatment*

As with the schizoid client, allowing distance and providing supportive measures might encourage the gradual development of a therapeutic alliance. Cognitive and behavioral measures might help clients gain basic social skills. Low-dose therapy with the newer atypical antipsychotics (risperidone [Risperdal], olanzapine [Zyprexa]) can be effective in allowing the schizotypal client to be more comfortable, less anxious, less prone to suspiciousness, and more organized in his or her thinking (Zale et al., 1997).

## DSM-IV-TR Cluster B Disorders— Dramatic, Emotional, or Erratic

These four disorders appear to share dramatic, erratic, or flamboyant behavior as part of their presenting symptoms. As yet, no empirical evidence for this manner of clustering exists (Zale et al., 1997), but there does seem to be a high degree of overlap among these disorders. There is also a great deal of comorbidity with Axis I disorders such as substance abuse, mood, and anxiety disorders as well as other PDs (cluster A, B, or C) that are found on Axis II. It is often difficult for the clinician to know which disorder is primary and which should take precedence in treatment (Zale et al., 1997).

## Antisocial Personality Disorder (ASPD)

### Presenting Signs and Symptoms

- An extended history of antisocial behaviors (stealing, persistent lying, cruelty to animals or people, vandalism, substance abuse) usually beginning before the age of 15 and continuing into adulthood
- Deceitfulness (use of aliases, conning others for personal profit or pleasure, repeated lying)
- Consistent irresponsibility (failure to honor financial obligations, work responsibilities, family/parenting obligations)
- Impassivity and repeated aggressiveness toward others
- Total lack of remorse for physically or emotionally hurting or mistreating others or swindling or stealing from others
- At times presents as charming, self-assured, and adept
- Interaction with others through **manipulation, aggressiveness**, and **exploitation**, totally lacking in empathy or concern for others
- Substance abuse is the most frequent comorbid Axis I disorder.
- There is a significant familial pattern to criminality in general and ASPD in particular (McGee & Linehan, 1997).

### Nursing Guidelines

1. Try to prevent or reduce untoward effects of manipulation (flattery, seductiveness, instilling guilt).
   - Set clear and realistic limits on specific behavior.

- All limits should be adhered to by all staff involved.
- Carefully document objective physical signs of manipulation or aggression when managing clinical problems.
- Document behaviors objectively (give times, dates, circumstances).
- Provide clear boundaries and consequences.
2. Be aware that antisocial clients can instill guilt when they are not getting what they want. Guard against being manipulated through feeling guilty.
3. Treatment of substance abuse is best handled through a well-organized treatment *before* counseling and other forms of therapy are started.

## Treatment

Unfortunately, there is no treatment of choice for ASPD. The most useful approach is to target specific problem behaviors that have been shown to be amenable to modification, combined with other therapies such as psychopharmacology and family therapy. Lithium carbonate, divalproex sodium (Depakote), and carbamazepine have effectively decreased violent behaviors in some individuals. The selective serotonin reuptake inhibitors (SSRIs) (e.g., fluoxetine) have been effective in decreasing the occurrence of aggressive behaviors in others (McGee & Linehan, 1997). Some positive results have been obtained through milieu programs (e.g., token economy systems and therapeutic communities).

# Borderline Personality Disorder (BPD)

## Presenting Signs and Symptoms

- Relationships with others are intense and unstable, and alternate between intense dependence and rejection.
- Behaviors are often impulsive and self-damaging (e.g., spending, unsafe sex, substance abuse, reckless driving, binge eating).
- Recurrent suicidal and/or self-mutilating behaviors are common, often in response to perceived threats of rejection, separation.
- Chronic feelings of emptiness or boredom, and an absence of self-satisfaction.

- Frantic efforts to avoid real or imagined abandonment.
- Intense affect is manifested in outbursts of anger, hostility, depression, and/or anxiety.
- Intense and primitive rage often complicates therapy and takes the form of extreme sarcasm, enduring bitterness, and angry outbursts at others.
- Major defense is **splitting**, which often manifests in pitting one person or group against another (good guy versus bad guy).
- Splitting is only one form of **manipulation** that individuals with BPD use.
- Rapid idealization-devaluation is a classic signal behavior suggestive of borderline psychopathology or some other primitive personality.
- Transient quasipsychotic symptoms might develop in the form of paranoid or dissociative symptoms during times of stress.

*Nursing Guidelines*

1. Set realistic goals, use clear action words.
2. Be aware of manipulative behaviors (flattery, seductiveness, guilt instilling).
3. Provide clear and consistent boundaries and limits.
4. Use clear and straightforward communication.
5. When behavioral problems emerge, calmly review the therapeutic goals and boundaries of treatment.
6. Avoid rejecting or rescuing.
7. Assess for suicidal and self-mutilating behaviors, especially during times of stress.

*Treatment*

There is no one treatment that has emerged as a guaranteed treatment for BPD. Although psychodynamically oriented therapy is commonly recommended for BPD, there are no randomized, controlled trials demonstrating the efficacy of any psychodynamic approach. Linehan has developed a behaviorally based treatment that targets the highly dysfunctional behaviors seen in clients with BPD. Her treatment approach is called dialectical behavioral therapy, and has proved promising in a randomized, controlled study (McGee & Linehan, 1997). Therapy is often marked by a period of improvement with alternating periods of worsening. Short-term hospitalization is not uncommon during periods of suicidal or self-mutilating behaviors or severe depression. Long-term outpatient therapy, and at times carefully chosen group therapy if appropriate for the client, has provided improvement for many clients.

A combination of psychotherapy and medication seems to provide the best results for treatment of clients diagnosed with BPD. Medications can reduce anxiety, depression, and disruptive impulses. Approximately 50% of people with BPD experience serious episodes of depression. Low-dose antipsychotics might prove useful for severely cognitively disturbed individuals. The newer antidepressants (SSRIs) have helped some BPD clients in dealing with their anger. The anticonvulsant carbamazepine has demonstrated some efficacy in decreasing the frequency and severity of behavioral dyscontrol episodes, suicidality, and temper outbursts (McGee & Linehan, 1997).

Clients with BPD pose great challenges for nurse clinicians, and supervision is advised to help with the inevitable strong countertransference issues.

## Histrionic Personality Disorder (HPD)

*Presenting Signs and Symptoms*

- Consistently draw attention to themselves; very concerned about being attractive and use physical appearance to gain center stage
- Show excessive emotionality and attention-getting behavior (e.g., display sexually seductive, provocative, or self-dramatizing behaviors)
- Intense emotional expressions are shallow, with rapid shifts from person to person or idea to idea
- Prone to describe more intimacy in a relationship than is there (e.g., show intense attention to a casual acquaintance)
- Are suggestible (easily influenced by others or circumstances)
- Others experience them as smothering, destructive; unable to understand/insensitive to anyone else's experience
- Without instant gratification or admiration from others, clients can experience depression and become suicidal

## Nursing Guidelines

1. Understand seductive behavior as a response to distress.
2. Keep communication and interactions professional, despite temptation to collude with the client in a flirtatious and misleading manner.
3. Encourage and model the use of concrete and descriptive rather than vague and impressionistic language.
4. Teach and role model assertiveness.

### Treatment

People with HPD use indirect means to get others to take care of them (physical attractiveness, charm, temper outbursts), and this can greatly complicate the therapeutic process. Therapeutic approaches used are psychoanalytic and cognitive-behavioral methods; however, research on the treatment of HPD is lacking. Most of the literature consists of case reports using various approaches (McGee & Linehan, 1997).

# Narcissistic Personality Disorder (NPD)

## Presenting Signs and Symptoms

- Exploit others to meet their own needs and desires
- Come across as arrogant and demonstrate a demeanor of "persistent entitlement"
- Portray a demeanor of grandiosity, a need for admiration, and a lack of empathy for others (American Psychiatric Association [APA], 2000)
- May begrudge others their success or possessions, feeling that they deserve the admiration and privileges more (APA, 2000)
- Relationships are characterized by disruption (frequently provoke arguments) or control (consistently in power struggles)

## Nursing Guidelines

1. Remain neutral and avoid power struggles or becoming defensive in response to the client's disparaging remarks, no matter how provocative the situation might be.
2. Convey unassuming self-confidence.

*Treatment*

There have been no controlled trials of efficacy for any one therapeutic approach. The main approaches are supportive or insight-oriented psychotherapy. Milieu therapy might be useful for some NPD clients. Treatment difficulties are based in preserving the client's self-esteem in the face of psychiatric interventions (Kaplan & Sadock, 2002). Most of these clients do not seek treatment unless they seek treatment for an Axis I disorder and have comorbid NPD.

## DSM-IV-TR Cluster C Disorders— Anxious or Fearful

These disorders have been clustered together because their common property is the experience of high levels of anxiety and the outward signs of fear. These personality types also show social inhibitions, mostly in the sexual sphere (e.g., shyness or awkwardness with potential sexual partners; impotence; or frigidity). Many people with a Cluster C disorder have a fearful reluctance to express irritation or anger, even in an interpersonal encounter that justifies these feelings (Stone, 1997).

Inhibited clients tend to *internalize* blame for the frustrations in their lives even when they are not to blame for these frustrations. This willingness to accept responsibility for contributing to their own unhappiness can foster a good working relationship between clinician and client. Therefore, this can be a useful trait. Those who blame others for their problems (*externalize* blame outward), such as antisocial, paranoid, and sadistic people, pose great challenges in therapy and have a guarded prognosis (Stone, 1997).

## Dependent Personality Disorder (DPD)

*Presenting Signs and Symptoms*

- Might manifest an unusual degree of agreeableness or friendliness
- These qualities are meant to enhance the dependent person's ability to attach to another who can act as protector; urgently seeks another relationship as a source of care and support when a close relationship ends

- Clinging is a common manifestation, but unfortunately this trait eventually alienates people and threatens to drive them away
- Often perfecting the technique of clinging to others takes the place of outside interests, reading, cultivation of friends, or other sustaining activities
- Have difficulty making everyday decisions without excessive advice and support from others
- Go to excessive lengths to obtain nurture and support from others, even to the point of being mistreated or abused, or suffering extreme self-sacrifice
- Need others to assume responsibility for most major areas of life. When others do not take initiative or take responsibility for them, their needs go unmet
- Have difficulty expressing disagreements with others for fear of loss of support or approval
- Is at risk for anxiety and mood disorders. DPD can occur in conjunction with BPD, avoidant personality disorder, and HPD
- Fear not getting enough care, and often insist on having everything done for them

## Nursing Guidelines

1. Identify and help address current stresses.
2. Try to satisfy client's needs, but set limits in such a manner that the client does not feel punished, which might lead to withdrawal.
3. Strong countertransference often develops in clinicians because of the client's excessive clinging (demands of extra time, nighttime calls, crisis before vacations); therefore, supervision is well advised.
4. Teach and role model assertiveness.

## Treatment

A variety of therapies are useful, and might all be appropriate during different phases while working on specific issues. Therapies include psychoanalytic psychotherapy, supportive therapy, cognitive-behavioral therapy, group therapy, and family therapy. Therapy is usually long-term and is dependent on the motivation of the client and how realistic the goals are (Stone, 1997).

# Obsessive-Compulsive Personality Disorder (OCPD)

## Presenting Signs and Symptoms

- Inflexible, rigid, and need to be in control
- Perfectionists to a degree that it interferes with completion of work; cannot delegate
- Overemphasis on work to the exclusion of friendships and pleasurable leisure activities
- Preoccupied with details to the extent that decision-making is impaired
- Intimacy in relationships is superficial and rigidly controlled, even though clients with OCPD might feel deep and genuine affection for friends and family
- Highly critical of self and others in matters of morality, ethics, or values
- The term *compulsive* refers to the behavioral aspects: preoccupation with lists, rules, schedules, and more. Other traits include indecisiveness, hoarding, and stinginess with money or time
- Clients with OCPD are often overwhelmed with a concern about loss of control (being too messy, sexy, or naughty); hence, their need to overcontrol and dominate people and situations in their lives (Stone, 1997)

## Nursing Guidelines

1. Guard against engaging in power struggles with an OCPD client. Need for control is very high for these clients.
2. Intellectualization, rationalization, and reaction formation are the most common defense mechanisms that clients with OCPD use.

## Treatment

Individual psychotherapy, supportive or insight-oriented therapy, and cognitive-behavioral therapy might all be useful depending on goals and the ego strengths of the client. Therapeutic issues usually include those of control, submission, and intellectualization. Some medications found to be useful for the obsessional component are clomipramine (tricyclic antidepressant [TCA]), fluoxetine (SSRI), and clonazepam (anxiolytic). Group therapy can also be a useful adjunct to therapy.

# Avoidant Personality Disorder (APD)

## Presenting Signs and Symptoms

- Pervasive pattern of social inhibition; virtually all people with APD have social phobias
- Strong feelings of inadequacy; APD clients experience fear of rejection and/or criticism; These individuals are very reticent in social situations because of this fear
- Avoid occupational activities that involve significant interpersonal contact because of fears of criticism, disapproval, or rejection
- View themselves as socially inept, personally unappealing, or inferior to others
- Might be inhibited and reluctant to involve themselves in new interpersonal situations or new activities
- Not uncommon for some clients with APD to have comorbid agoraphobia and obsessive-compulsive disorder as well as social phobia

## Nursing Guidelines

1. A friendly, gentle, reassuring approach is the best way to treat clients with APD.
2. Being pushed into social situations can cause extreme and severe anxiety for APD clients.

## Treatment

Each client needs to be assessed individually. For example, if the client has been taught fearfulness and withdrawal by avoidant parents, treatment would differ from that for the client whose behavioral and cognitive traits stem from parental brutalization, incest, or sexual molestation in childhood (Stone, 1997). Because of the inherent social phobia, various forms of treatment can prove useful, such as cognitive therapy, desensitization, social skills training, and other cognitive-behavioral techniques. Group therapy has not proven advantageous over one-on-one supportive or exploratory psychotherapies. However, in the case of incest or other interpersonal trauma, special groups that include people with similar backgrounds are considered quite beneficial (Stone, 1997). Social anxiety might respond to a monoamine oxidase inhibitor (MAOI). Benzodiazepine anxiolytics might help to contain brief panic episodes. The lowering of the frightening anxiety can help clients engage more readily into therapy and can aid compliance when clients are very fearful and anxious.

# ASSESSMENT

## Presenting Signs and Symptoms

In assessing for a PD, the client's history might reveal persistent traits held for long periods of time causing distress or impairment in functioning. Refer to the sections on individual PDs for specific signs and symptoms earlier. What follows are assessment guidelines for identifying if a client fits into a specific Cluster A, B, or C. Does the client:

**Cluster A**

1. Suspect others of exploiting or deceiving him or her? Bear grudges and not forget insults?
2. Detach self from social relationships? Not desire close relationships or being part of a family? Take pleasure in few, if any, activities?
3. Have a history of social and interpersonal deficits marked by acute discomfort? Have any cognitive or perceptual distortions?

**Cluster B**

4. Have a pervasive pattern of disregard for and violation of the rights of others? Act deceitfully (repeated lying, use others for own needs)? Act consistently irresponsible toward others?
5. Have a pattern of unstable and chaotic personal relationships? Have a history of suicide attempts or self-mutilation? Have chronic feelings of emptiness, or show intense anger, intense anxiety, and dysphoria?
6. Have a pattern of excessive emotionality and attention-seeking behaviors (e.g., sexually seductive or provocative)? Have very self-dramatic, theatrical, and exaggerated expressions of emotion?
7. Act grandiose, need admiration, lack empathy for others? Have unreasonable expectations of favored treatment? Act interpersonally exploitive?

**Cluster C**

8. Persistently avoid social situations because of feelings of inadequacy and hypersensitivity to negative evaluation? View self as socially inept or inferior to others?

9. Have an excessive need to be taken care of, show cling-ing behaviors within relationships, have intense fear of separation? Have difficulty making everyday decisions without excessive amount of advice and reassurance from others?

10. Have a preoccupation with neatness, perfectionism, and mental and interpersonal control? Show rigidity and stubbornness?

Clients with PDs rarely seek treatment unless:

1. Client usually comes to the attention of the health care system through a crisis situation.

2. Antisocial clients most often come into the health care system through the courts by means of a court order.

3. Suicide attempts, self-mutilation, or substance abuse are common crises that bring people with PD into treat-ment.

## Assessment Tools

Refer to Appendix D-6 for a sample questionnaire helpful in identifying personality traits.

## Assessment Guidelines
### Personality Disorders

1. Assessment about personality functioning needs to be viewed within the person's ethnic, cultural, and social background.

2. PDs are often exacerbated following the loss of signifi-cant supporting people or in a disruptive social situation.

3. A change in personality in middle adulthood or later signals the need for a thorough medical workup or assessment for unrecognized substance abuse disorder.

4. Be cognizant that social stereotypes can muddy a clini-cian's judgment in that a particular diagnosis can be over- or underdiagnosed (e.g., for males or females because of sexual bias; because of social class or immigrant status).

# NURSING DIAGNOSES WITH INTERVENTIONS

## Discussion of Potential Nursing Diagnoses

The data the nurse clinician collects provide information about the client's presenting problem or behaviors, emotional state, precipitating situations, and maladaptive coping behaviors. Clients with PDs present with any number of problematic behaviors. These behaviors can be pathological or maladaptive. Behaviors that are repetitive or rigid, or those that present an obstacle to meaningful relationships or functioning, are considered behaviors that will be focused on during management of care. Many of the dysfunctional thought processes and behaviors are described in the individual presentations of these disorders earlier.

**Short-term goals** usually center on the client's safety and comfort, and are pertinent to the client's physical and mental well-being. Often, the first goals for the management of an *acute crisis* are to evaluate the need for medication and to identify appropriate verbal interventions to decrease the client's immediate emotional stress (Profiri, 1998). **Keep in mind that clients have varied degrees of cognitive functioning and disabilities. What might be a short-term goal for one is likely a long-term goal for another**. The goals cited here and in other chapters are helpful guidelines, but often the clinician is the one to best estimate client strengths, capabilities, supports, and current level of functioning when setting specific time limits on goals. (For more on this topic, see Chapter 1.)

**Long-term goals** are targeted for the long term, and center on skill attainment. It is important to keep goals realistic. Changing lifelong patterns of behaviors that are inflexible and persistent takes a great deal of time, as well as engagement by the client. Outcome criteria usually include the following areas (Profiri, 1998):

- Linking consequences to both functional and dysfunctional behaviors
- Learning and mastering skills that facilitate functional behaviors
- Practicing the substitution of functional alternatives during crisis
- Ongoing management of anger, anxiety, shame, and happiness

- Creating a lifestyle that prevents regressing (e.g., **HALT:** never getting too Hungry, too Angry, too Lonely, or too Tired)
- Nursing crisis intervention strategies

These clients often act very impulsively. The nurse will be called upon to intervene in many acting-out behaviors, often marked by impulsivity, such as self-mutilation and/or suicide attempts, anger and hostility toward the nurse clinician, extreme paranoia and blaming others for problems, manipulation and splitting, and intense anxiety for example. Acting-out behaviors are often most intense during the initial phases of therapy. Dealing with clients when they are acting out, especially during crises, takes persistence, patience, and learned skill on the part of the clinician. Some of the more common behavioral defenses PD clients employ require rigorous interventions. Because it is impossible to deal with all the problem areas of the 10 PDs, we will identify common behaviors for which all nurses are encouraged to develop skills. Common phenomena related to PD clients are (1) manipulation, (2) self-mutilation/suicide attempts, (3) intense low self-esteem, (4) intense anxiety, (5) anger and physical fighting, (6) projecting identification and blame to others, and (7) impulsivity. PD clients are often very demanding of health care personnel and others.

Four common phenomena and nursing diagnoses are presented here: **Risk for Self-Mutilation** (scratching, burning, cutting), **Chronic Low Self-Esteem, Impaired Social Interaction,** and **Ineffective Coping**. Nursing interventions for minimizing and preventing **manipulation** are presented in Chapter 19. **Suicide** is covered in Chapter 16. Intense **anger and hostility** are addressed in Chapter 17.

People with PDs have great difficulty getting along with others and often elicit intense negative feelings from others. The following behaviors are found in a variety of combinations: demanding, angry, fault finding, suspicious, insensitive to the needs of others, manipulative, clinging, at times withdrawn, and often intensely lonely. Therefore, the interpersonal relationships of those with PDs are often chaotic and unsatisfying for all concerned. **Impaired Social Interaction (Defensive Coping/Avoidance, Ineffective Coping)** are key nursing diagnoses for people with PD; these problems are always present, most often in response to intense feelings of powerlessness. Table 9-1 identifies other possible nursing diagnoses.

Table 9-1 **Potential Nursing Diagnoses for Personality Disorders**

| Symptoms | Nursing Diagnosis |
| --- | --- |
| Crisis, high levels of anxiety | **Ineffective Coping** |
| | **Anxiety** |
| Anger and aggression; child, elder, or spouse abuse | **Risk for Other-Directed Violence** |
| | **Ineffective Coping** |
| | **Impaired Parenting** |
| | **Disabled Family Coping** |
| Withdrawal | **Social Isolation** |
| Paranoia | **Fear** |
| | **Disturbed Sensory Perception** |
| | **Disturbed Thought Processes** |
| | **Defensive Coping** |
| Depression | **Hopelessness** |
| | **Helplessness** |
| | **Risk for Self-Directed Violence** |
| | **Self-Mutilation** |
| | **Chronic Low Self-Esteem** |
| | **Spiritual Distress** |
| Difficulty in relationships, manipulation | **Ineffective Coping** |
| | **Impaired Social Interaction** |
| | **Defensive Coping** |
| | **Interrupted Family Processes** |
| | **Risk for Loneliness** |
| Not keeping medical appointments, late for appointments, not following prescribed medical procedure/medication | **Ineffective Therapeutic Regimen Management** |
| | **Nonadherence (Non-compliance) to Medications or Treatments (specify)** |

Many people with PDs leave therapy after a crisis is over and things have settled down somewhat. Therefore, nonadherence to therapy or medication is common. **Nonadherence to medications or treatment** is addressed in Chapter 20.

The nurse should remember, however, that each client is uniquely individual, and although many of the phenomena are shared among several of the PDs, the manifestations of these behaviors can take many forms. The difficulty PD clients have in their interpersonal relationships is carried over to the health care setting, and poses challenges for nurses, physicians, and other health care personnel.

Supervision and case discussion are usually extremely useful in guarding against getting caught up in counter-transferential power struggles and nontherapeutic encounters that threaten any therapeutic alliance.

Whatever nursing diagnoses you choose, keep in mind that nursing diagnoses must be uniquely crafted to the specific individual, the presenting symptoms, the individual circumstances, and the personal manifestation of these symptoms. This is especially true for people with PDs.

## Overall Guidelines for Nursing Interventions
### Personality Disorders

1. Understand that creating a therapeutic alliance with clients with PD is going to be difficult. A history of interrupted therapeutic alliances, in addition to the client's suspiciousness, aloofness, secretive style, and hostility, can be a setup for failure.
2. Giving PD clients some choices (e.g., time they wish to set up appointments) might enhance compliance, because these clients often require a sense of control.
3. A feeling of being threatened and vulnerable might lead to blaming or verbally attacking others.
4. Clients with PD are hypersensitive to criticism, and, therefore, one of the most effective methods of teaching new behaviors is to build on the client's existing skills.
5. Setting limits is an important part of the work with PD clients. It is important for nurses to take time setting clear boundaries (nurse's responsibilities and client's responsibility) and repeat the limits frequently when working with PD clients.

## Selected Nursing Diagnoses and Nursing Care Plans

### RISK FOR SELF-MULTILATION

At risk for deliberate self-injurious behavior causing tissue damage with the intent of causing nonfatal injury to attain relief of tension

## *Related To (Etiology)*

▲ High-risk populations (BPD, psychotic states)
▲ History of self-injury
▲ History of physical, emotional, or sexual abuse
▲ Feelings of depression, rejection, self-hatred, separation anxiety, guilt, and depersonalization
▲ Emotionally disturbed or battered children
▲ Mentally retarded and autistic children
● Ineffective coping skills
● Desperate need for attention
● Inability to verbally express feelings
● Impulsive behavior

## *As Evidenced By*
## *(Assessment Findings/Diagnostic Cues)*

● Signs of old scars on wrists and other parts of the body (cigarette burns, superficial knife/razor marks)
● Fresh superficial slashes on wrists or other parts of the body
● Statements as to self-mutilation behaviors
● Intense rage focused inward

## *Outcome Criteria*

• Be free of self-inflicted injury
• Participate in impulse control training
• Participate in coping skills training
■ Seeks help when experiencing self-destructive impulses

## *Long-Term Goals*

Client will:
• Demonstrate a decrease in frequency and intensity of self-inflicted injury by (date)
• Participate in therapeutic regimen
• Demonstrate two new coping skills that work for client for when tension mounts and impulse returns by (date)

---

▲ NANDA International accepted; ● In addition to NANDA International; ■ NOC Outcome for Impulse Self-Control

## Short-Term Goals

Client will:
- Respond to external limits
- Sign a "no-harm" contract that identifies steps he or she will take when urges return (date)
- Express feelings related to stress and tension instead of acting-out behaviors (date)
- Discuss alternative ways client can meet demands of current situation (date)

## Interventions and Rationales

| Intervention | Rationale |
|---|---|
| 1. Assess client's history of self-mutilation:<br>  a. Types of mutilating behaviors<br>  b. Frequency of behaviors<br>  c. Stressors preceding behavior | 1. Identifying patterns and circumstances surrounding self-injury helps nurse plan interventions and teaching strategies to fit the individual. |
| 2. Identify feelings experienced before and around the act of self-mutilation. | 2. Feelings are a guideline for future intervention (e.g., rage at feeling left out or abandoned). |
| 3. Explore with client what these feelings might mean. | 3. Self-mutilation might also be:<br>  a. A way to gain control over others<br>  b. A way to feel alive through pain<br>  c. An expression of guilt or self-hate |
| 4. Secure a written or verbal no-harm contract with the client. Identify specific steps (e.g., persons to call upon when prompted to self-mutilate). | 4. Client is encouraged to take responsibility for healthier behavior. Talking to others and learning alternative coping skills can reduce frequency and severity until such behavior ceases. |

| Intervention | Rationale |
|---|---|
| 5. Use a matter-of-fact approach when self-mutilation occurs. Avoid criticizing or giving sympathy. | 5. A neutral approach prevents blaming, which increases anxiety, giving special attention that encourages acting out. |
| 6. After treatment of the wound, discuss what happened right before, and the thoughts and feelings that the client had immediately before self-mutilating. | 6. Identify dynamics for both client and clinician. Allows the identification of less harmful responses to help relieve intense tensions. |
| 7. Work out a plan identifying alternatives to self-mutilating behaviors.<br>  a. Anticipate certain situations that might lead to increased stress (e.g., tension or rage).<br>  b. Identify actions that might modify the intensity of such situations.<br>  c. Identify two or three people whom the client can contact to discuss and examine intense feelings (rage, self-hate) when they arise. | 7. Plan is periodically reviewed and evaluated. Offers a chance to deal with feelings and struggles that arise. |
| 8. Set and maintain limits on acceptable behavior and make clear client's responsibilities. If client is hospitalized at the time, be clear regarding the unit rules. | 8. Clear and nonpunitive limit setting is essential for decreasing negative behaviors. |
| 9. Be consistent in maintaining and enforcing the limits, using a nonpunitive approach. | 9. Consistency can establish a sense of security. |

## CHRONIC LOW SELF-ESTEEM

Longstanding negative self-evaluation/feelings about self or self-capabilities

*Related To (Etiology)*

- Childhood physical/sexual/psychologic abuse and/or neglect
- Avoidant and dependent patterns
- Persistent lack of integrated self-view, with splitting as a defense
- Shame and guilt
- Substance abuse
- Lack of realistic ego boundaries
- Dysfunctional family of origin

*As Evidenced By*
*(Assessment Findings/Diagnostic Cues)*

- ▲ Longstanding or chronic self-negating verbalizations; expressions of shame/guilt
- ▲ Evaluates self as unable to deal with events
- ▲ Rationalizes away/rejects positive feedback and exaggerates negative feedback about self
- ▲ Hesitant to try new things/situations
- ▲ Overly conforming, dependent on others' opinions, indecisive
- ▲ Excessively seeks reassurance
- ▲ Expresses longstanding shame/guilt

*Outcome Criteria*

- Demonstrate ability to reframe negative self-thoughts into more realistic appraisals
- Behavioral manifestations of depression greatly reduced and controlled with medication
- ■ Uses effective coping strategies

---

▲ NANDA International accepted; ● In addition to NANDA International; ■ NOC Objective Psychosocial Adjustment: Life Change

## Long-Term Goals

Client will:

- Demonstrate ability to reframe and dispute cognitive distortions with assistance of nurse/clinician by (date)
- State a willingness to work on two realistic future goals by (date)
- Identify one new skill he or she has learned to help meet personal goals by (date)

## Short-Term Goals

Client will:

- Identify three strengths in work/school life by (date)
- Identify two cognitive distortions that affect self-image
- Reframe and dispute one cognitive distortion with nurse
- Set one realistic goal with nurse that he or she wishes to pursue
- Identify one skill he or she will work on to meet future goals by (date)

## Interventions and Rationales

| Intervention | Rationale |
|---|---|
| 1. Maintain a neutral, calm, and respectful manner, although with some clients this is easier said than done. | 1. Helps client see himself or herself as respected as a person even when behavior might not be appropriate. |
| 2. Keep in mind PD clients might defend against feeling of low-self esteem through blaming, projection, anger, passivity, and demanding behaviors. | 2. Many behaviors seen in PD clients cover a fragile sense of self. Often these behaviors are the crux of clients' interpersonal difficulties in all their relationships. |
| 3. Assess with clients their self-perception. Target different areas of the client's life: | 3. Identify with client **realistic** areas of strength and weakness. Client and nurse can |

| Intervention | Rationale |
|---|---|
| a. Strengths and weaknesses in performance at work/school/daily-life tasks<br>b. Strengths and weaknesses as to physical appearance, sexuality, personality | then work on the realities of the self-appraisal, and target those areas of assessment that do not not appear accurate. |
| 4. Review with the client the types of cognitive distortions that affect self-esteem (e.g., self-blame, mind reading, overgeneralization, selective inattention, all-or-none thinking). | 4. These are the most common cognitive distortions people use. Identifying them is the first step to correcting distortions that form one's self-view. |
| 5. Work with client to recognize cognitive distortions. Encourage client to keep a log. | 5. Cognitive distortions are automatic. Keeping a log helps make automatic, unconscious thinking clear. |
| 6. Teach client to reframe and dispute cognitive distortions. Disputes need to be strong, specific, and nonjudgmental. | 6. Practice and belief in the disputes over time help clients gain a more realistic appraisal of events, the world, and themselves. |
| 7. Discourage client from dwelling on and "reliving" past mistakes. | 7. **The past cannot be changed**. Dwelling on past mistakes prevents the client from appraising the present and planning for the future. |
| 8. Discourage client from making repetitive self-blaming and negative remarks. | 8. Unacceptable behavior does not make the client a bad person, it means that the client made some poor choices in the past. |

| Intervention | Rationale |
|---|---|
| 9. Focus questions in a positive and active light; helps client refocus on the present and look to the future. For example: **"What could you do differently now?"** *or* **"What have you learned from that experience?"** | 9. Allows client to look at past behaviors differently, and gives the client a sense that he or she has choices in the future. |
| 10. Give the client honest and genuine feedback regarding your observations as to his or her strengths, and areas that could use additional skills. | 10. Feedback helps give clients a more accurate view of self, strengths, areas to work on, as well as a sense that someone is trying to understand them. |
| 11. Do not flatter or be dishonest in your appraisals. | 11. Dishonesty and insincerity undermine trust and negatively affect any therapeutic alliance. |
| 12. Set goals realistically, and renegotiate goals frequently. Remember that client's negative self-view and distrust of the world took years to develop. | 12. Unrealistic goals can set up hopelessness in clients and frustration in nurse clinicians. Clients might blame the nurse for not "helping them," and nurses might blame the client for not "getting better." |
| 13. Discuss with client his or her plans for the future. Work with client to set realistic short-term goals. Identify skills to be learned to help client reach his or her goals. | 13. Looking toward the future minimizes dwelling on the past and negative self-rumination. When realistic short-term goals are met, client can gain a sense of accomplishment, direction, and purpose in life. Accomplishing goals can bolster a sense of control and enhance self-perception. |

## IMPAIRED SOCIAL INTERACTION

Insufficient or excessive quantity or ineffective quality of social exchange

---

### *Related To (Etiology)*

- ▲ Unacceptable social behavior or values
- ▲ Immature interests
- ● Biochemical changes in the brain
- ● Genetic factors
- ● Disruptive or abusive early family background

### *As Evidenced By*
### *(Assessment Findings/Diagnostic Cues)*

- ▲ Observed use of unsuccessful social interaction behaviors
- ▲ Dysfunctional interaction with peers, family, and/or others
- ● Alienating others through angry, clinging, demeaning, and/or manipulative behavior or ridicule toward others
- ● Destructive behavior toward self or others

### *Outcome Criteria*

- Demonstrates an ability to use constructive criticism
- Demonstrates newly acquired social skills in social situations
- Identifies and problem solves with counselor factors that interfere with social interaction
- Demonstrates a willingness to participate in follow-up therapy
- Demonstrates a reduction in clinging, splitting, manipulation, and other distancing behaviors

---

▲ NANDA International accepted; ● In addition to NANDA International

## Long-Term Goals

Client will:
- Demonstrate, with the aid of the nurse/clinician, the ability to identify at least two unacceptable social behavior (manipulation, splitting, demeaning attitudes, angry acting out) that client is willing to change by (date)
- Work with nurse/clinician on substituting positive behaviors for those unacceptable behaviors identified earlier on an ongoing basis by (date)

## Short-Term Goals

Client will:
- Begin to demonstrate a reduction in manipulative behaviors as evidenced by nurse/staff
- Begin to demonstrate an increase in nonviolent behaviors as evidenced by a reduction in reported outbursts
- Identify two personal behaviors that are responsible for relationship difficulties within 2 weeks
- Verbalize decreased suspicion and increased security
- Identify one specific area that requires change
- Identify and express feelings as they occur with nurse
- State he or she is willing to continue in follow-up therapy
- Keep follow-up appointments

## Interventions and Rationales

| Intervention | Rationale |
|---|---|
| 1. In a respectful, neutral manner, explain expected client behaviors, limits, and responsibilities during sessions with nurse clinician. Clearly state the rules and regulations of the institution, and the consequences when these rules are not adhered to. | 1. From the beginning, clients need to have explicit guidelines and boundaries for expected behaviors on their part, as well as what client can expect from the nurse. Clients need to be fully aware that they will be held responsible for their behaviors. |

| Intervention | Rationale |
|---|---|
| 2. Set limits on any manipulative behaviors:<br>a. Arguing or begging<br>b. Flattery or seductiveness<br>c. Instilling guilt, clinging<br>d. Constantly seeking attention<br>e. Pitting one person, staff, group against another<br>f. Frequently disregarding the rules<br>g. Constant engagement in power struggles<br>h. Angry, demanding behaviors | 2. From the beginning, limits need to be clear. It will be necessary to refer to these limits frequently, because it is to be expected that the client will test these limits repeatedly. |
| 3. Intervene in manipulative behavior.<br>a. **All limits should be adhered to by all staff involved.**<br>b. **Objective physical signs in managing clinical problems should be carefully documented.**<br>c. **Behaviors should be documented objectively (give times, dates, circumstances).**<br>d. **Provide clear boundaries and consequences.**<br>e. **Enforce the consequences.** | 3. Clients will test limits, and, once they understand that the limits are solid, this understanding can motivate them to work on other ways to get their needs met. Hopefully, this will be done with the nurse clinician through problem-solving alternative behaviors and learning new effective communication skills. |

| Intervention | Rationale |
|---|---|
| 4. Expand limits by clarifying expectations for clients in a number of settings. | 4. When time is taken in initial meetings to clarify expectations, confrontations and power struggles with clients can be minimized and even avoided. |
| 5. Collaborate with the client, as well as the multidisciplinary team, to establish a reward system for compliance with clearly defined expectations (Krupnick & Wade, 1993). | 5. Tangible reinforcement for meeting expectations can strengthen the client's positive behaviors (Krupnick & Wade, 1993). |
| 6. Monitor own thoughts and feelings constantly regarding your response to the PD client. Supervision is strongly recommended for new and seasoned clinicians alike when working with PD clients. | 6. Strong and intense countertransference reactions to PD clients are bound to occur. When the nurse is enmeshed in his or her own strong reactions toward the client (either positive or negative), nurse effectiveness suffers, and the therapeutic alliance might be threatened. |
| 7. Problem solve and role play with client acceptable social skills that will help obtain needs effectively and appropriately. | 7. Over time, alternative ways of experiencing interpersonal relationships might emerge. Take one small skill that client is willing to work on, break it down into small parts, and work on it with client. |

| Intervention | Rationale |
|---|---|
| 8. Assess need for and encourage skills training workshop. | 8. Skills training workshops offer the client ways to increase social skills through role play and interactions with others who are learning similar skills. This often acts as a motivating factor where positive feedback and helpful suggestions are readily available. |
| 9. Understand that PD clients in particular will be resistant to change and that this is symptomatic of PDs. This is particularly true in the beginning phases of therapy. | 9. Responding to client's resistance and seeming lack of change in a neutral manner is part of the foundation for trust. In other words, the nurse does not have a vested interest in the client "getting better." The nurse remains focused on the client's needs and issues in any event. |

## INEFFECTIVE COPING

Inability to form a valid appraisal of stressors, inadequate choice of practiced responses, and/or ability to use available resources

### Related To (Etiology)

- ▲ Intense emotional state
- ▲ Failure to intend to change behavior
- ▲ Lack of motivation to change behaviors
- ▲ Negative attitudes toward health behavior
- ● Neurobiologic factors
- ● Trauma early in life (sexual, physical, or emotional abuse)

---

▲ NANDA International accepted; ● In addition to NANDA International

## As Evidenced By
## (Assessment Findings/Diagnostic Cues)

- ▲ Failure to achieve optimal sense of control
- ▲ Failure to take actions that would prevent further health problems
- ▲ Demonstration of nonacceptance of health status
- ● Anger or hostility
- ● Dishonesty
- ● Superficial relationships with others
- ● Manipulations of others
- ● Dependency
- ● Intense emotional dysregulation
- ● Extreme distrust of others

## Outcome Criteria

- Increase in frequency of expressing needs directly without ulterior motives
- Demonstrates decreased manipulative, attention-seeking behaviors
- Learn and master skills that facilitate functional behavior
- Ongoing management of anger, anxiety, shame, and loneliness
- Identifies behaviors leading to hospitalization
- Demonstrates use of a newly learned coping skill to modify anxiety and frustration
- Demonstrates increase in impulse control

## Long-Term Goals

Client will:
- State that he/she will continue treatment on an outpatient basis by (date)
- Focus on one problem and work through the problem-solving process with nurse by (date)
- Talk about feelings and perceptions and not act on them at least twice by (date)
- Practice the substitution of functional skills for times of increased anxiety with nurse by (date)

---

▲ NANDA International accepted; ● In addition to NANDA International

## *Short-Term Goals*

Client will:
- Remain safe while hospitalized
- Not act out anger toward others while hospitalized
- Spend time with nurse and focus on one thing he/she would like to change

## General Interventions for All Personality Disorders

| Intervention | Rationale |
|---|---|
| 1. Review intervention guidelines for each PD in this chapter. | 1. All clients are individuals, even within the same diagnostic category. However, guidelines for specific categories are helpful for planning. |
| 2. Ascertain from family/ friends how the person interacts with significant people. Is the client always withdrawn, hostile, distrustful, have continuous physical complaints? | 2. Identifying baseline behaviors helps with setting goals. |
| 3. Identify what the client sees as the behaviors and circumstances that lead to hospitalization. | 3. Ascertain client's understanding of behaviors and responsibility for own action. |
| 4. Identify behavioral limits and behaviors that are expected. Do not argue, debate, rationalize, or bargain. | 4. Client needs clear structure. Expect frequent testing of limits initially. Maintaining limits can enhance feelings of safety in the client. |
| 5. Be clear with the client as to the unit/ hospital/clinic policies. Give brief concrete reasons for the rules, if asked, and then move on. | 5. Institutional policies provide structure and safety. |

| Intervention | Rationale |
|---|---|
| 6. Be very clear about the consequences if policies/limits are not adhered to. | 6. Client needs to understand the consequences of breaking the rules. |
| 7. When limits or policies are not followed, enforce the consequences in a matter-of-fact, nonjudgmental manner. | 7. Enforces that the client is responsible for his/her own actions. |
| 8. Approach client in a consistent manner in all interactions. | 8. Enhances feelings of security and provides stucture. Exceptions encourage manipulative behaviors. |
| 9. Make a clear and concrete written plan of care so other staff can follow. | 9. Helps minimize manipulations and might help encourage cooperation. |
| 10. If feasible, devise a care plan with the client. | 10. If goals and interventions are agreed upon, cooperation with plan is optimized. |
| 11. Refrain from sharing **personal information** with client. | 11. Opens up areas for manipulation and undermines professional boundaries. |
| 12. Do not take **gifts** from the client (any client). | 12. Again, clouds the boundaries and can give client the idea that he is due special consideration. |
| 13. Be aware of **flattery** as an attempt to feed into your needs to feel special. | 13. Giving into client's thinking that you are "the best" or "the only one" can pit you against other staff and undermine client's needs for limits. |
| 14. If client becomes **seductive**, reiterate the therapeutic goals and boundaries of treatment. | 14. The client is in the hospital/clinic for a reason. Being taken in by by seductive behavior undermines effectiveness of treatment. |

| Intervention | Rationale |
|---|---|
| 15. Some clients might attempt to **instill guilt** when they do not get what they want. Remain neutral but firm. | 15. Nurses often want to be seen as "nice." However, being professional and maintaining limits is the better therapeutic approach. |
| 16. If client becomes **hostile** or **projects blame** onto you or staff, project a neutral, calm demeanor, and avoid power struggles. Focus on the client's underlying feelings. | 16. Defuses tension and opens up productive interaction. |
| 17. When appropriate, attempt to understand underlying feelings prompting inappropriate behaviors. (Those with ASPD might not be good candidates for this.) | 17. Often acting out behaviors stem from underlying feelings of shame, fear, anger, loneliness, insecurity, etc. Talking about feelings can lead to problem solving and growth for client. |
| 18. Work with client on problem-solving skills using a situation that is bothering the client. Go step by step:<br>• Define the problem<br>• Explore alternatives<br>• Make decisions | 18. Client might not know how to articulate the problem. Helping identify alternatives gives the client a sense of control. Evaluating the pros and cons of the alternatives facilitates choosing potential solutions. |
| 19. When client is ready and interested, teach client coping skills to help defuse tension and troubling feelings (e.g., anxiety reduction, assertiveness skills). | 19. Increasing skills helps client use healthier ways to defuse tensions and get needs met. |

| Intervention | Rationale |
|---|---|
| 20. Keep goals very realistic and go in small steps. There are no overnight successes with people with PDs. | 20. It can take a long time to positively change ingrained, life-long, maladaptive habits; however, change is always possible. |
| 21. Give client positive attention when behaviors are appropriate and productive. Avoid giving any attention (when possible and not dangerous to self or others) when client's behaviors are inappropriate. | 21. Reinforcing positive behaviors might increase likelihood of repetition. Ignoring negative behaviors (when feasible) robs client of even negative attention. |
| 22. Guard against personal feelings of frustration and lack of progress. | 22. Change is often very slow and may seem to take longer than it actually is. Nurture yourself outside the job. Keep your "bucket" full with laughter and high regard from friends and family. |
| 23. Understand that many people with PDs do not stay in treatment and often come to facilities because of crisis or court order. | 23. Even short encounters with therapeutic persons can make a difference when a client is ready to learn more adaptive ways of living his or her life. |

Three diagnostic categories are the most likely to come into contact with the mental health system. These include people with the diagnoses of **Borderline Personality Disorder (BPD), Antisocial Personality Disorder (ASPD),** and **Paranoid Personality Disorder (PPD)**.

All of the above would apply to all clients with PD. However, some additional interventions are suggested below for clients with these traits.

## *Borderline Personality Disorder (BPD)*

| Intervention | Rationale |
|---|---|
| 1. Assess for self-mutilating or suicide thoughts or behaviors (see Chapter 16 for nursing care plans related to suicide behaviors). | 1. Self-mutilating and suicide threats are common behaviors for clients with BPD. |
| 2. Interventions often call for responses to client's intense and labile mood swings, anxiety, depression, and irritability. | 2. Many of the dysfunctional behaviors of BPD clients (e.g., parasuicidal, anger, manipulation, substance abuse) are used as "behavioral solutions" to intense pain. |
| a. Anxiety: Teach stress-reduction techniques such as deep breathing, relaxation, mediation, and exercise. | a. Clients experience intense anxiety and fear of abandonment. Stress reduction techniques help client focus more clearly. |
| b. Depression: Client might need medications to help curb depression. Observe for side effects and mood level. | b. Most clients with BPD suffer profound depression. |
| c. Irritability, anger: Use interventions early before anxiety and anger escalate. See Chapter 17 for nursing care plans related to angry and aggressive behaviors. | c. Clients with BPD are extremely uncomfortableand want immediate relief from painful feelings. Anger is a response to this pain. Intervening early can help avoid escalation. |

| Intervention | Rationale |
|---|---|
| 3. Clients with BPD can be manipulative (see Chapter 19 for nursing care plans). Be consistent: Set and maintain limits regarding behavior, responsibilities, and unit/community rules. | 3. Consistent limit setting helps provide structure and decrease negative behaviors. |
| 4. Use assertiveness when setting limits on client's unreasonable demands for time and attention. | 4. Firm, clear, nonjudgmental limits give client structure. |
| 5. Be nonjudgmental and respectful when listening to client's thoughts, feelings, or complaints. | 5. Clients have an intense fear of rejection. |
| 6. Encourage client to explore feelings and concerns (e.g., identify fears, loneliness, self-hate). | 6. Client is used to acting out feelings. |
| 7. Clients with BPD benefit from coping skills training (e.g., interpersonal skills, anger management skills, emotional regulation skills). Provide referrals and/or involve professional experts. | 7. Client learns to refine skills in changing behaviors, emotions, and thinking patterns associated with problems in living that are causing misery and distress (Linehan, 1993). |
| 8. Treatment of substance abuse is best handled by well-organized treatment systems, not by an individual nurse/clinician. | 8. Keeping detailed records and having a team involved with each client can minimize manipulation. |

| Intervention | Rationale |
|---|---|
| 9. Provide and encourage the client to use professionals in other disciplines such as social services, vocational rehabilitation, social work, or the law. | 9. Clients with BPD often have multiple social problems. Often they do not know how to obtain these services. |
| 10. Clients with BPD often drop out of treatment prematurely. However, when they return, they can still draw upon what they have learned from previous encounters with health care personnel. | 10. Clients might become impatient and leave, then return in a crisis situation. It is a good thing when they are able to tolerate longer periods of learning. |

## *Antisocial Behaviors*

People with antisocial traits are usually hospitalized against their will and often involve some law violations, marital discord (battering), or other. They rarely want to change their behaviors, and have no motivation to do so.

These clients relate through manipulation and do not have the ability to care for others physical or emotional well being; however, they may be "friendly" with others if there is something in it for them. Often these clients resort to **manipulation or violence** to get what they want. **Refer to Chapter 19 for nursing care plans dealing with manipulative behaviors, and Chapter 17 on anger and aggression.**

## *Paranoid Behaviors*

Often these clients function on the outside, even though they have a deep abiding distrust of the motives of others. Under stress, they might seek crisis help or act out in such a way to require hospitalization. The biggest challenge to nurses and other health care providers is working with the client's suspiciousness of others. **See Chapter 8 under Defensive Coping for a nursing care plan for a suspicious person.**

# MEDICAL TREATMENTS

## Psychopharmacology

There are no medications for treating PDs per se. There are, however, medications that can target some of the symptoms clients' experience, and, prescribed on an individual basis, can be very helpful for many clients as an adjunct in their therapy. Counseling/psychotherapy is probably the best primary approach to care, but psychopharmacology can be an important part of the therapeutic regimen in decreasing a client's anxiety, paranoia, aggressiveness, or other symptoms. Specific medications that are often used for a particular PD are mentioned in the earlier discussions of each of the PDs. Medications can facilitate a client's comfort, and make people with PDs more amenable to therapy. Refer to the discussion of the individual PDs for those medications that have been helpful for some individuals.

## Other Treatments

Because people with PDs rarely seek treatment or adhere to treatment unless they are under undue stress, depressed, exhibiting suicidal behaviors, remanded by the courts, and so on, therapeutic approaches are sometimes difficult. Refer to the individual discussion of PDs to identify which therapeutic modalities have proven to alleviate pain and/or helps modify behavior for some individuals.

Inherent in the diagnosis of PDs are longstanding traits that interfere with a person's social, occupational, and/or intimate relationships and functioning, and usually the person's sense of well-being as well. Therefore, as mentioned earlier, changing or modifying dysfunctional traits might take a long time.

**NURSE, CLIENT, AND FAMILY RESOURCES**

## ASSOCIATIONS

**National Alliance for the Mentally III (NAMI)**
Colonial Place Three
2107 Wilson Boulevard, Suite 300
Arlington, VA 22201-3042
(800) 950-NAMI
http://www.nami.org

# INTERNET SITES

**Borderline Personality Disorder Sanctuary**
http://www.navicom.com/~patty
Recovery information for people with BPD

**Self-Injury Page**
http://www.mhsanctuary.com/borderline
Self-mutilation

**BPD Central**
http://www.bpdcentral.com
Borderline personality disorder website

**Internet Mental Health**
http://www.mentalhealth.com
A good overview of all the personality disorders

**Personality Disorders**
www.focusas.com/Personality Disorder

# CHAPTER 10

# Chemical Dependencies

## OVERVIEW

Alcohol and drug dependencies are among the most prevalent illnesses. Although there has been a decrease in the use of marijuana, cocaine, and heroin in the United States over the last decade, there has been a dramatic increase in substances often referred to as "club drugs." These substances include MDMA (Ecstasy), gamma-hydroxybutyrate (GHB) (G, liquid ecstasy), flunitrazepam (Rohypnol), and methamphetamines (Gahlinger, 2004). Crystal methamphetamine is exceedingly addictive, cheap to produce, causes severe brain damage, and is becoming a public health crisis of epidemic proportions (NACO, 2006).

Treatment for individuals with substance use disorders includes an assessment phase, the treatment of the intoxication and withdrawal when necessary, and the development and implementation of an overall treatment strategy (APA, 2000b). Parent and child/adolescent teaching and recognition of potential harm various drugs can cause is a vital part of prevention.

**Substance-related disorders** refer to those disorders that are related to the taking of a drug of abuse (i.e., alcohol, cocaine, heroin, amphetamines), to the side effects of a prescribed medication (including over-the-counter medications), and to toxin exposure (e.g., heavy metals—lead or aluminum; rat poisons; pesticides; nerve gases). Knowledge of "club drugs" is increasingly important for health care workers to include in their teaching (*Diagnostic and Statistical Manual of Mental Disorders* [4th edition, text revision] [DSM-IV-TR]; APA, 2000). The DSM-IV-TR divides substance-related disorders into two groups.

1. *Substance Use Disorders* (**substance dependence and substance abuse).** Refer to Box 10-1 for the DSM-IV-TR definitions of substance dependence and substance abuse.
2. *Substance-Induced Disorders* **include substance intoxication, substance withdrawal, and substance-induced disorders (delirium, substance-induced psychotic disorders, etc.).** Refer to Box 10-2 for the DSM-IV-TR definition and criteria for substance intoxication and substance withdrawal.

---

| Box 10-1 | DSM-IV-TR Criteria for Substance Abuse and Dependence |

**Substance Abuse**
Maladaptive pattern of substance use leading to clinically significant impairment or distress, manifested by one or more of the following occurring within a 12-month period:
1. Inability to fulfill major role obligations at work, school, and home
2. Recurrent legal or interpersonal problems
3. Continued use despite recurrent social or interpersonal problems
4. Participation in physically hazardous situations while impaired (driving a car, operating a machine, exacerbation of symptoms—e.g., ulcers)

**Substance Dependence**
Maladaptive pattern of substance use leading to clinically significant impairment or distress, manifested by three or more of the following within a 12-month period:
1. Presence of tolerance to the drug
   *or*
2. Presence of withdrawal syndrome
3. Substance taken in larger amounts or for longer period than intended
4. Reduction or absence of important social, occupational, or recreational activities
5. Unsuccessful or persistent desire to cut down or control use
6. Increased time spent in getting, taking, and recovering from the substance; possibly withdrawn from family or friends
7. Substance use continual despite knowledge of recurrent physical or psychologic problems or that problems were caused or exacerbated by one substance

Adapted from American Psychiatric Association. (2000). *Diagnostic and statistical manual of mental disorders* (4th edition, text revision). Washington, DC, American Psychiatric Association, pp. 197-199; reprinted with permission.

| Box 10-2 | **DSDSM-IV-TR Criteria for Substance Intoxication and Withdrawal** |
| --- | --- |

**Substance Intoxication**

A. The development of a reversible substance-specific syndrome due to recent ingestion of (or exposure to) a substance. **Note:** Different substances might produce similar or identical syndromes.

B. Clinically significant maladaptive behavioral or psychological changes that are caused by the effect of the substance on the central nervous system (e.g., belligerence, mood lability, cognitive impairment, impaired judgment, impaired social or occupational functioning), and develop during or shortly after use of the substance.

C. The symptoms are not due to a general medical condition and are not better accounted for by another mental disorder.

**Substance Withdrawal**

A. The development of a substance-specific syndrome due to the cessation of (or reduction in) substance use that has been heavy and prolonged.

B. The substance-specific syndrome causes clinically significant distress or impairment in social, occupational, or other important areas of functioning.

C. The symptoms are not due to a general medical condition and are not better accounted for by another medical disorder.

Adapted from American Psychiatric Association. (2000). *Diagnostic and statistical manual of mental disorders* (4th edition, text revision). Washington, DC, American Psychiatric Association, pp. 201-202; reprinted with permission.

Substance use disorders (dependence and abuse), substance intoxication, and substance withdrawal are presented here with the more common substances of use (alcohol, amphetamines, cannabis, cocaine, hallucinogens, opioids, phencyclidine [PCP], sedatives, hypnotics, or anxiolytics). Some of these classes of drugs share similar features; for example:

• Alcohol shares features with the sedatives, hypnotics, and anxiolytics.
• Cocaine shares features with amphetamines and similarly acting sympathomimetics.

Table 10-1 identifies common drugs of abuse, therapeutic uses they might have, the properties of these drugs, and the symptoms of intoxication and overdose.

Table 10-1 **Common Drugs of Abuse**

| Class | Therapeutic Use | Symptoms of Use | Intoxication | Dependence (Physical/Psychologic) | |
|---|---|---|---|---|---|
| **CNS Depressants** Alcohol (ETOH) Barbiturates Benzodiazepines Chloral hydrate Other sedative-hypnotics | Antidote for methanol consumption | Relaxation, euphoria, decreased inhibitions, lack of concentration, poor judgment, slurred speech, decreased coordination | Slurred speech, nausea, vomiting, incoordination, sedation, drowsiness, emotional instability | Yes | Yes |
| **CNS Stimulants** Cocaine (short-acting) Amphetamines | Topical anesthetic Management of narcolepsy, hyperkinesia, and questionable at present, weight control | Euphoria, initial CNS stimulation, then depression, wakefulness, hypersexuality, impaired judgment, irritability, anxiety, panic attacks, paranoia, agitation, loss of appetite | Psychomotor activation, sweating, ↑ blood pressure, ↑ heart and respirations, tremors, dilated pupils, insomnia, assaultive, grandiose, impaired judgment and social and occupational functioning | Yes | Yes |

*Continued*

Table 10-1 **Common Drugs of Abuse—cont'd**

| Class | Therapeutic Use | Symptoms of Use | Intoxication | Dependence (Physical/ Psychologic) |
|-------|-----------------|-----------------|--------------|-------------------------------------|
| **Opioids** Opium (paregoric) Heroin Meperidine (Demerol) Morphine Codeine Methadone (Dolophine) Hydromorphine (Dilaudid) Fentanyl | Analgesic Methadone use in treatment of heroin dependency • Heroin has NO therapeutic use | Euphoria, sedation, reduced libido, emotional lability, impaired judgment, lack of motivation | Euphoria followed by dysphoria and impairment in attention, judgment, and memory. Pupils constrict, ↓ respiration, ↓ blood pressure, slurred speech, psychomotor retardation | Yes Yes |
| **Hallucinogens** Lysergic Acid (LSD) | LSD has no recognized therapeutic application | Euphoria, altered body image, altered perceptual alterations, alteration in judgment and memory, | Fear of going crazy, marked anxiety/ depression, depersonalization, grandiosity, | No No |

*Continued*

| | | |
|---|---|---|
| Phencyclidine (PCP) Mescaline Dimethyltryptamine (DMT) | detachment from surroundings, distortions in thinking (delusions), paranoia, confusion), hallucinations, disorientation, anxiety, panic, increased pulse Experiences range from sublime to terrifying | hallucinations, synesthesia, ↑ blood pressure, ↑ pulse, ↑ temperature, ↑ respiration, incoordination |
| | | Ataxia, muscle rigidity, seizures, regressive behaviors, belligerence, assaultiveness, vertical or horizontal nystagmus, bizarre, violent, labile behavior, ↑ blood pressure, ↑ pulse, ↑ temperature, blank stare |

Table 10-1 **Common Drugs of Abuse—cont'd**

| Class | Therapeutic Use | Symptoms of Use | Intoxication | Dependence (Physical/Psychologic) |
|---|---|---|---|---|
| **Cannabis** Marijuana Hashish, THC | Marijuana has been known to: • Reduce eye pressure in glaucoma patients • Relieve nausea and vomiting associated with chemotherapy in treatment of cancer patients • Stimulate appetite in AIDS patients | Relaxation, sexual arousal, talkativeness, increased appetite, altered state of awareness, mild euphoria or dysphoria, increased pulse, red eyes, dry mouth | Anxiety, suspiciousness, in high doses sensation of slowed time, social withdrawal, impaired judgment, possible hallucinations, ↑ pulse, conjunctival redness | Yes Yes in high doses |
| **Inhalants** Glue, lighter fluid, spray paint, paint thinner | None | Euphoria, giddiness, excitation | Excitation, followed by drowsiness, staggering, lightheadedness, agitation, disinhibition | Yes Yes |

**Club Drugs**

| Drug | Therapeutic Uses | Effects Sought | Adverse Effects | | |
|---|---|---|---|---|---|
| Ecstasy (MDMA) | None | Agitation followed by euphoria, sense of profound insight, intimacy, and well-being; Increased thirst | Sympathetic overload, some of which includes tachycardia, hypertension, arrhythmias, parkinsonism; Toxic and potentially fatal outcomes are extreme; hyperthermia, and the associated "serotonin syndrome," which can result in acute renal and hepatic failure, adult respiratory distress, and end organ damage as examples | Yes | Yes |
| Gamma-hydroxybutyrate (GHB) | Narcolepsy | ↓ Social inhibation ↑ Libido Euphoria | Hypersalivation, hypotonia, amnesia, ↑ BP, mood swings, seizures | Yes | Yes |
| Flunitrazepam (Rohypnol) Date Rape Drug | Anesthesia, sedation | Reduced anxiety, muscular tension; drowsiness, headaches; nightmares, confusion | Anterograde amnesia, lack of muscle control, loss of consciousness | Yes | Yes |

## Other Disorders Associated with Substance Use Disorders

The DSM-IV-TR identifies a number of other disorders for each of the substances besides dependence, abuse, intoxication, and withdrawal; for example:

Substance-induced:
Intoxication delirium
Withdrawal delirium
Persisting dementia
Persisting amnesic disorder
Psychotic disorder
Psychotic disorder with hallucinations/delusions
Mood disorder
Anxiety disorder
Sexual dysfunction
Sleep disorder
Disorder not otherwise specified (NOS)

In this chapter, common drugs of abuse are introduced, and symptoms of use, intoxication, overdose, and withdrawal are discussed. This chapter is focused on assessment data, identifying nursing diagnoses, goals, and interventions the nurse can implement.

### Nurses Need to Know

Before planning nursing care, the nurse needs to be aware of four phenomena that are inherent in the planning of treatment. These four phenomena are:

1. Tolerance
2. Polydrug use
3. Dual diagnoses
4. Medical comorbidity

Without through considerations of these four phenomena, safe and effective nursing or medical care cannot be implemented.

### *Tolerance*

Tolerance and withdrawal are two characteristics of physiologic addiction to a drug. When the body requires larger and larger amounts of a drug to achieve the same effect, the body builds up a **tolerance** to the drug. When the dose of the drug is reduced or the drug is no longer available, the lack of a certain level of the drug in the body produces **withdrawal symptoms.** Each drug has its own specific withdrawal syndrome. Some drugs, if stopped abruptly, can cause a medical emergency (Table 10-2).

## Polydrug Abuse

Use of two or more substances of abuse (polydrug abuse) is quite common. Alcohol dependence in conjunction with other drug dependence is prevalent, especially but not exclusively, for people younger than 30 years of age. This is especially true with drugs taken at nightclubs, raves, or music festivals (club drugs).

## Dual Diagnosis

The co-occurrence of a substance use disorder with another psychiatric disorder is called dual diagnosis. The Epidemiologic Catchment Area Study reported that more than 50% of substance-abusing individuals also were diagnosed with another psychiatric disorder (Beeder & Mellman, 1992). Common comorbid psychiatric disorders include personality disorders (borderline and antisocial), major depression, bipolar disorder, and schizophrenia. Dual diagnoses must always be identified and the comorbid disorder treated simultaneously if any change in drug-related behavior is to occur.

## Medical Comorbidity

Many serious and life-threatening medical problems are associated with the consequences of illicit injection drug use and its associated lifestyle. For example, systemic and organ-specific bacterial infections, viral hepatitis, tuberculosis, sexually transmitted disease, complications of pregnancy, pulmonary edema, and trauma are all found in injection drug users.

Another important consideration when working with substance-dependent individuals is that approximately 40% to 50% of clients with substance abuse problems have mild to moderate cognitive problems while actively using. These problems usually get better with long-term abstinence. However, it is best in the beginning to keep their treatment plan simple, because these clients are not

Table 10-2 **Drug Overdose and Withdrawal**

| Drug | Overdose | | Withdrawal | |
| | Effects | Possible Treatments | Effects | Possible Treatments |
| --- | --- | --- | --- | --- |
| **CNS Depressants**<br>Barbiturates<br>Benzodiazepines<br>Chloral hydrate<br>Glutethimide<br>Meprobamate<br>Alcohol (ETOH) | Cardiovascular or respiratory depression or arrest (mostly with barbiturates)<br>Coma<br>Shock<br>Convulsions<br>Death | *If awake:*<br>Keep awake.<br>Induce vomiting.<br>Give activated charcoal to aid absorption of drug.<br>Every 15 min, check vital signs (VS).<br>*Coma:*<br>Clear airway—endotracheal tube<br>Intravenous (IV) fluids<br>Gastric lavage with activated charcoal<br>Frequent VS checks for shock and cardiac arrest after client is stable<br>Seizure precautions | *Cessation of prolonged, heavy use:*<br>Nausea-vomiting<br>Tachycardia<br>Diaphoresis<br>Anxiety or irritability<br>Tremors in hands, fingers, eyelids<br>Marked insomnia<br>Grand mal seizures<br>*After 5-15 years of heavy use:*<br>Delirium | Carefully titrated detoxification with similar drug<br>*Note:* Abrupt withdrawal can lead to death. |

| | Overdose | Treatment | Withdrawal | Treatment |
|---|---|---|---|---|
| **Stimulants** | | Possible hemodialysis or peritoneal dialysis Flumazenil (Romazicon) IV | | |
| **Cocaine—crack** (short-acting) *Note:* High obtained: snorted for 3 min; injected for 30 sec; smoked for 4–6 sec (crack) Average high lasts: cocaine 15–30 min; crack 5–7 min | Respiratory distress Ataxia Hyperpyrexia Convulsions Coma Stroke Myocardial infarction Death | Antipsychotics medical and nursing management for: Hyperpyrexia (ambient cooling) Convulsions (diazepam) Respiratory distress Cardiovascular shock Acidify urine (ammonium chloride for amphetamine) | Fatigue Depression Agitation Apathy Anxiety Sleepiness Disorientation Lethargy Craving | Antidepressants (desipramine) Dopamine agonist |
| **Amphetamines** (long-acting) Dextroamphetamine Methamphetamine Ice (synthesized for street use) | Same as above | Same as above | Same as above | Same as above |

*Continued*

Table 10-2 **Drug Overdose and Withdrawal—cont'd**

| Drug | Overdose | | Withdrawal | |
|------|----------|--------------------|-----------|---------------------|
| | Effects | Possible Treatments | Effects | Possible Treatments |
| **Opioids** | | | | |
| **Opium** (paregoric) | Pupils might be dilated due to anoxia | Narcotic antagonist, e.g., naloxone (Narcan), quickly reverses central nervous system depression | Yawning | Methadone/ LAAM tapering |
| **Heroin** | Respiratory depression/arrest | | Insomnia | Clonidine-naltrexone detoxification |
| **Meperidine** (Demerol) | Coma | | Irritability | Buprenorphine substitution |
| **Codeine** | Shock | | Runny nose (rhinorrhea) | |
| **Methadone** (Dolophine) | Convulsions | | Panic | |
| **Hydromorphine** (Dilaudid) | Death | | Cramps | |
| **Fentanyl** (Sublimaze) | | | Diaphoresis | |
| **Fentanyl analogs** | | | Nausea-vomiting | |
| | | | Muscle aches ("bone pain") | |
| | | | Chills | |
| | | | Fever | |
| | | | Lacrimation | |
| | | | Diarrhea | |

*Continued*

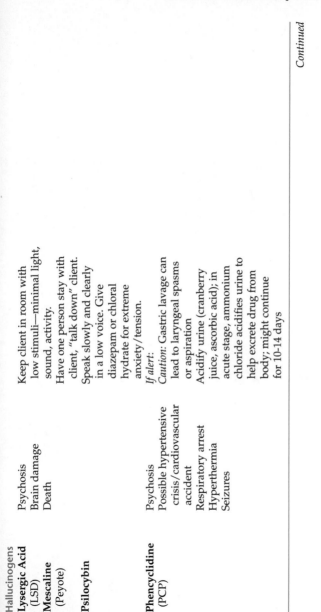

| | | |
|---|---|---|
| **Hallucinogens** | | |
| **Lysergic Acid** (LSD) **Mescaline** (Peyote) **Psilocybin** | Psychosis Brain damage Death | Keep client in room with low stimuli—minimal light, sound, activity. Have one person stay with client, "talk down" client. Speak slowly and clearly in a low voice. Give diazepam or chloral hydrate for extreme anxiety/tension. |
| **Phencyclidine** (PCP) | Psychosis Possible hypertensive crisis/cardiovascular accident Respiratory arrest Hyperthermia Seizures | *If alert:* *Caution:* Gastric lavage can lead to laryngeal spasms or aspiration Acidify urine (cranberry juice, ascorbic acid); in acute stage, ammonium chloride acidifies urine to help excrete drug from body; might continue for 10-14 days |

Table 10-2 **Drug Overdose and Withdrawal—cont'd**

| Drug | Overdose | | Withdrawal | |
|---|---|---|---|---|
| | Effects | Possible Treatments | Effects | Possible Treatments |
| | | Room with minimal stimuli **Do not attempt to talk down!** Speak slowly, clearly, and in a low voice. Diazepam Haloperidol can be used for severe behavioral disturbance (not a phenothiazine). *Medical intervention for:* Hyperthermia High blood pressure Respiratory distress Hypertension | | |
| **Club Drugs** Ecstasy (MDMA) | • Hyperthermia • Serotonin Syndrome Acute hepatic/renal failure. Elevated body temperature. ↑Water intake leads to hyponatremia | **No Antidote:** • Treat symptoms • Cardiac monitoring • Comprehensive chemistry panel identifies complications | Profound Depression secondary to Serotonin depletion Repeated use associated with cognitive impairment (potentially permanent memory loss) | |

| | Neurologic effects (confusion, delirium, paranoia) | (e.g. hepatic or renal damage) | Withdrawal symptoms include: |
|---|---|---|---|
| **Gamma-hydroxy-butyrate (GBA)**<br>*Street Names*<br>Fantasy<br>GBH<br>Liquid Ecstasy<br>Cherry Meth<br>(Date Rape Drug) | • Cheyne-Stokes respirations<br>• Seizures<br>• Coma<br>• Death | **No Antidote**<br>• Treat symptoms<br>• Monitor cardiac Status<br>• Comprehensive chemistry panel (to check renal, hepatic, or other complications) | • Anxiety<br>• Insomnia<br>• Tremors |
| **Flunitrazepam** (Rohypnol)<br>(Date Rape Drug) | • Hypotension<br>• Confusion<br>• Visual disturbances<br>• Urinary retention<br>• Aggressive behavior | **Antidote**<br>Flumazenil | Like other benzodiazepines<br>• ↑ Seizure potential<br>• Anxiety<br>• Muscle pain<br>• Photosensitivity<br>• Headache |

Data from American Psychiatric Association (2000). *Diagnostic and statistical manual of disorders* (4th ed., text revision). Washington, DC: American Psychiatric Association; Bohn, M.J. (2000). Alcoholism. *Psychiatric Clinics of North America, 16(4),* 679; O'Connor, P.G., Samet J.H., & Stein, M.D. (1994). Management of hospitalized drug users: Role of the internist. *American Journal of Medicine, 96,* 551; Bell K. (1992). Identifying the substance abuser in clinical practice. *Orthopedic Nursing,* 11(2):29.

Gahlinger, P.M. (2004). Club Drugs: MDMA, Gamma-hydroxybutyrate (GHB), Rohypnol, and ketamine, *American Family Physician,* (69) 11 (June 2004). http://www.aafp.org/afp/20040601/2619.html. Retrieved 2/22/05.

thinking or functioning at their optimum level (Zerbe, 1999).

Recovering is a lifetime process, and it comes about in steps. Because each client has different strengths, backgrounds, and supports, goals of treatment should be tailored to the individual's immediate needs and abilities. Initially, however, a 12-step program based on Alcoholics Anonymous **(AA)** is the most effective treatment modality for all addictions. The 12 steps ("working the steps") are designed to help a person refrain from addictive behaviors as well as to foster individual change and growth.

Such support groups include **PA** (Pills Anonymous), **NA** (Narcotics Anonymous), **WFS** (Women for Sobriety), and **CA** (Cocaine Anonymous), among others. These groups help break down denial in an atmosphere of support, understanding, and acceptance. It is strongly advised that individuals find a reliable sponsor within the support group, especially for the early period of sobriety. A relationship has been established between a person's feelings of "belonging" and treatment outcome. The more the client feels socially involved with peers, the greater the likelihood of successful treatment outcome, continuation of treatment, and lower relapse rates.

There are self-help groups for families and friends of an addicted person. They are also based on the 12 steps. These groups help clients, family, and friends work through accepting the disease model of addiction. This acceptance can remove the burdens of guilt, hostility, and shame from family members. They also offer pragmatic methods for identifying and avoiding enabling behaviors. Such support groups include **Al-Anon** (for friends and family members of an alcoholic), **Narc-Anon** (for friends and family members of a narcotic addict), and **ACOA** (for Adult Children of Alcoholics). **NOTE: Be aware that several sessions over weeks or months might be necessary for the client to reach the point of accepting the reality of the problem and the need for treatment** (Dunner, 1997).

## ASSESSMENT

### Presenting Signs and Symptoms

- The client might exhibit any of the signs and symptoms of **intoxication or withdrawal** (see Table 10-2).

- The client might have needle tracts in the antecubital fossa, wrist, or feet, or behind the knees.
- The client might have suicidal thoughts. If yes, assess for lethality of ideations. **(See Chapter 16 for discussion on assessment and interventions for suicidal individuals.)**
- The client might have a history of blackouts, delirium, or seizures.
- The client might have a coexisting medical condition related to the substance of abuse—for example: AIDS, central nervous system (CNS) disease or deterioration.

## Assessment Tools

It is often less threatening to people when assessing their drug history to start with "safe" questions first, such as:
1. "What prescription drugs do you currently take?"
2. "What over-the-counter drugs do you currently take?"
3. "What social drugs do you currently take?"
   a. Start with nicotine and caffeine.
   b. Ask about alcohol.
   c. Ask about other social drugs (marijuana, cocaine, and heroin).

There are many helpful assessment tools that nurses can use to assess if the individual has an alcohol or drug problem. Three that can be very useful are:
1. Nurse's assessment tool in emergencies (see Appendix D-7C).
2. **Alcohol problems**—The Brief Version of the Michigan Alcohol Screening Test (MAST) (see Appendix D-7A).
3. **Other drug-related problems**—The Drug Abuse Screening Test (DAST) (see Appendix D-7B).

## Assessment Guidelines

### Substance Abuse

1. Is immediate medical attention warranted for a severe or major withdrawal syndrome? For example, alcohol and sedative use can be life threatening during a major withdrawal.
2. Is the client experiencing an overdose to a drug/alcohol that warrants immediate medical attention? For example, opioids or depressants can cause respiratory depression,

coma, and death. Refer to Table 10-2 for symptoms of drug overdose and treatments.

3. Does client have any physical complications related to drug abuse (e.g., AIDS, abscess, tachycardia, hepatitis)?
4. Does client have suicidal thoughts or indicate, through verbal or nonverbal cues, a potential for self-destructive behaviors?
5. Does the client seem interested in doing something about his or her drug/alcohol problem?
6. Do the client and family have information about community resources for alcohol/drug withdrawal (detoxify safely) and treatment; for example:
   • Support groups
   • Treatment for psychiatric comorbidities
   • Family treatment to address enabling behaviors, support adaptive behaviors, and provide support for families and friends

# NURSING DIAGNOSES WITH INTERVENTIONS

Nurses care for chemically impaired clients in a variety of settings and situations. Some interventions call for medical interventions and skilled nursing care, whereas others call for effective use of communication and counseling skills. The following sections offer the nurse guidelines for treatment.

## Discussion of Potential Nursing Diagnoses

### Overdose

**Drug overdoses** can be medical emergencies needing timely medical interventions. Drug overdoses most often seen in hospital emergency rooms are CNS depressants (e.g., barbiturates, benzodiazepines, alcohol), stimulants (e.g., crack/cocaine), opiates (e.g., heroin), and, to a lesser extent, hallucinogens (e.g., PCP). Table 10-2 lists the signs and symptoms of overdose for these drugs and identifies possible treatments.

### Withdrawal

**Withdrawal from alcohol and other CNS-depressant drugs** is associated with severe morbidity and mortality, unlike withdrawal from other drugs. For example, a person experiencing severe alcohol withdrawal might have delirium tremens (DTs). Death from DTs can be caused by volume depletion, electrolyte imbalance, cardiac arrhythmias, or suicide. Mortality rates range between 5% and 10%, even with treatment (Dunner, 1997).

Therefore, individuals with severe alcohol withdrawal syndrome or withdrawal from a CNS depressant might need hospitalization and close medical attention. Other drug withdrawals might not hold the same dangers; however, the client might benefit from titrating the dose under medical supervision. The major nursing diagnosis that applies for an individual going through withdrawal of a substance of abuse is **Risk for Injury.**

## Initial Drug Treatment and Active Treatment

People who are addicted to alcohol or drugs come from various environments, cultures, and sociologic backgrounds. Therefore, people seeking treatment for drug addictions and related problems present with a variety of personal strengths and social backgrounds and have different economic supports. Many clients have legal problems, and certainly possible medical complications from the drug, as well as coexisting psychiatric problems. Therefore, one form of treatment for a specific substance will not be effective for everyone addicted to that specific substance. It is probably best to take a long-term view of addictions and remember that lapses or relapses are often part of the long-term course of recovering (Vaillant, 1988).

However, many nursing diagnoses apply to the majority of clients with substance abuse problems. For example, individuals who have been abusing drugs for a long period of time most likely have poor general health. These clients might have nutritional deficits, be susceptible to infections, or be at risk for AIDS and hepatitis. **Ineffective Health Maintenance** is often a nursing focus, and an initial priority for clients when they present with life-threatening situations.

A common phenomenon shared among many addicted individuals is that people minimize their drug problems and have a tendency to deny having a "problem" (denial) or minimize the problem by blaming others (projection), rationalizing why they need the drug, or using other methods to deny responsibility for their drug-related behavior. Therefore, **Ineffective Denial** is present. Denial should be broken down so that the client can begin to perceive how his or her life has changed in a negative way because of his or her drug use, and find motivation for change. Until individuals can admit that they have a problem, and are ready to start to take responsibility for their drug use, there is little incentive for change as long as they blame others for their problems and think their behavior is justified.

## Relapse Prevention

Relapse prevention is part of most treatment planning for medical as well as psychiatric mental health disorders. For people with addictions, the main thrust of relapse prevention is recognizing triggers for abuse and learning different ways to respond to these cues. Because new coping skills are needed, the nursing diagnosis **Ineffective Coping** is used for relapse prevention.

There are many nursing diagnoses that can be a priority for your clients. One important area for assessment is **Risk for Other-Directed or Self-Directed Violence.** Assessment and intervention for **suicide** is addressed in **Chapter 16.** Suggestions for working with clients who are **angry and violent** are found in **Chapter 17.**

Addicted clients often have a lack of concern for the feelings of others and often act entitled or have a sense of grandiosity about them. Many clients who abuse substances learn to manipulate others (family, friends, and institutions) to get their needs met (e.g., money for drugs, shift blame to others, make false promises). Setting limits is key to working with an addicted client or clients with dual diagnoses. Interventions for **manipulative behaviors** are addressed in **Chapter 19.**

People with a history of long-term substance abuse often have many other needs as well (e.g., medical, social, legal, job-related, personal), warranting a variety of nursing diagnoses. See Table 10-3 for potential nursing diagnoses.

Table 10-3 **Potential Nursing Diagnoses for Substance Abuse**

| Signs and Symptoms | Nursing Diagnoses |
| --- | --- |
| Vomiting, diarrhea, poor nutritional and fluid intake | **Imbalanced Nutrition** <br> **Risk for Deficient Fluid Volume** |
| Audiovisual hallucinations, impaired judgment, memory deficits, cognitive impairments related to substance intoxication/withdrawal (problem-solving, ability to attend to tasks, grasp ideas) | **Disturbed Thought Processes** <br> **Disturbed Sensory Perception: Auditory/Visual** |
| Changes in sleep-wake cycle, interference with stage IV sleep, not sleeping or long periods of sleeping related to effects or withdrawal from substance | **Disturbed Sleep Pattern** |
| Lack of self-care (hygiene, grooming), not caring for basic health needs | **Ineffective Health Maintenance** <br> **Self-Care Deficit** <br> **Noncompliance (nonadherence to health care regimen)** |
| Feelings of hopelessness, inability to change, feelings of worthlessness, life has no meaning or future | **Hopelessness** <br> **Impaired Religiosity** <br> **Spiritual Distress** <br> **Chronic Low Self-Esteem** <br> **Risk for Self-Directed Violence** |
| Family crises and family pain, ineffective parenting, emotional neglect of others, increased incidence of physical and sexual abuse toward others, increased self-hate projected to others | **Interrupted Family Processes** <br> **Impaired Parenting** <br> **Risk for Other-Directed Violence** |
| Excessive substance abuse affects all areas of person's life: loses friends, has poor job performance, illness rates increase, prone to accidents and overdoses | **Ineffective Coping** <br> **Impaired Verbal Communication** <br> **Social Isolation** <br> **Risk for Loneliness** <br> **Anxiety** <br> **Risk for Suicide** |

*Continued*

Table 10-3 **Potential Nursing Diagnoses for Substance Abuse—cont'd**

| Signs and Symptoms | Nursing Diagnoses |
|---|---|
| Increased health problems related to substance used and route of use, as well as overdose | **Activity Intolerance** **Ineffective Airway Clearance** **Ineffective Breathing Pattern** **Impaired Oral Mucous Membranes** **Risk for Infection** **Decreased Cardiac Output** **Sexual Dysfunction** |
| Total preoccupation and time consumed with taking and withdrawing from drug | **Delayed Growth and Development** **Ineffective Coping** **Impaired Social Interaction** **Disabled Family Coping** |

## Overall Guidelines for Nursing Interventions

*Substance Abuse*

1. Detoxify the client.
2. Assess for feelings of hopelessness, helplessness, and suicidal thinking.
3. Ascertain that the client is getting interventions for any comorbid medical and/or psychologic condition (e.g., liver toxicity, infections, depression, anxiety attacks).
4. Intervene with the client's use of denial as well as rationalization, projection, and other defenses that stall motivation for change.
5. Enlist support of family members; confront any tendency on their part to minimize the problem or enable the client in maintaining his or her addiction.
6. Insist on abstinence.
7. Refer the client to self-help groups (e.g., AA, NA, CA) early on in treatment.
8. Teach client to avoid medications that promote dependence.
9. Encourage participation in psychotherapy (e.g., cognitive-behavioral strategies, motivational interviewing, solution-focused therapy).
10. Emphasize personal responsibility—placing control within the client's grasp removes the nurse from the all-knowing rescuer (Finfgeld, 1999).

11. Support residential treatment when appropriate, particularly for clients with multiple relapses.
12. Expect relapses.
13. Educate the client and the family on the medical and psychologic consequences of drug abuse.
14. Educate the client and family regarding pharmacotherapy for certain addictions (e.g., naltrexone or methadone to help prevent relapse in alcoholism and narcotic addiction).
15. Educate the client about the physical and developmental effects that taking the drug can have on future children (e.g., fetal alcohol syndrome, problems with school, social role performance) (Zerbe, 1999).

## Selected Nursing Diagnoses and Nursing Care Plans

### WITHDRAWAL

Abrupt withdrawal from some drugs can elicit a medical emergency. Overdose of some drugs is also a medical emergency. See Table 10-2 for common drugs of abuse in which withdrawal or overdose might require immediate nursing and medical attention. **NOTE: Refer to the nursing care plan for violence in Chapter 17, or suicide from Chapter 16 if these apply. If interventions for manipulation are needed, see Chapter 19.**

### RISK FOR INJURY

At risk of injury as a result of environmental conditions interacting with the individual's adaptive and defensive resources

## Related To (Etiology)

▲ Psychologic (affective orientation)
▲ Sensory dysfunction
▲ Developmental age (psychologic)
● Excess alcohol ingestion pattern

---

▲ NANDA International accepted; ● In addition to NANDA International

- Impaired judgment (disease, drugs, reality testing, risk-taking behaviors)
- Sensory-perceptual loss or disorientation
- Substance withdrawal
- Panic levels of anxiety and agitation
- Potential for electrolyte imbalance or seizures
- Unstable vital signs and temperature

## As Evidenced By
## (Assessment Findings/Diagnostic Cues)

- Signs and symptoms of specific drug withdrawal
- Evidence of hallucinations (bugs, animals, snakes)
- Poor skin turgor
- Elevated temperature, pulse, respirations
- Agitation, trying to "get away" or climb out of bed
- Combative behaviors
- Misrepresentation of reality (illusions)

## Outcome Criteria

- Safe withdrawal
- Free of physical injuries secondary to withdrawal

## Long-Term Goals

Client will:
- Remain free from injury while withdrawing from substance
- Be free of withdrawal symptoms within given time period for particular drug

## Short-Term Goals

- Client's condition will stabilize within 72 hours
- Client will be oriented during times of lucidity
- Client will demonstrate decreased aggressive and threatening behavior within 24 hours (using a scale of 1 to 5)

---

▲ NANDA International accepted; ● In addition to NANDA International

## Interventions and Rationales

| Intervention | Rationale |
|---|---|
| 1. Vital signs should be taken frequently, at least every 15 minutes until stable, then every hour for 4 to 8 hours according to hospital protocol or physician's order. | 1. Pulse is the best indicator of impending DTs, signaling the need for more rigorous sedation. |
| 2. Provide client with a quiet room free of environmental stimulation, a single room near the nurse's station if possible. | 2. Lowers irritability and confusion. |
| 3. Approach the client with a calm and reassuring manner. | 3. Clients need to feel that others are in control and that they are safe. |
| 4. Use simple, concrete language and directions. | 4. Client is able to follow simple commands, and unable to process complex or abstract ideas. |
| 5. Orient client to time/ place and person during periods of confusion; inform client of his or her progress during periods of lucidity. | 5. Fluctuating level of consciousness is the hallmark of delirium. Orientation can help reduce anxiety. |
| 6. Institute seizure precautions according to hospital protocol. | 6. Seizures might occur, and precautions for client safety are a priority. |
| 7. Carefully monitor intake and output. Check for dehydration or overhydration. | 7. Dehydration can aggravate electrolyte imbalance. Overhydration can lead to congestive heart failure. |

**Intervention**

8. If the client is having **hallucinations**, reassure client that you do not see them, that you are there and you will see that he remains safe (e.g., "I don't see rats on the wall jumping on your bed. You sound frightened right now. I will stay with you for a few minutes.").

9. If client is experiencing illusions, correct the client's misrepresentation in a calm and matter-of-fact manner (e.g., "This is not a snake around my neck ready to strike you, it is my stethoscope . . . let me show you.").

10. Maintain safety precautions at all times; for example:
    a. Provide electric shaver.
    b. Take away all matches and cigarettes.
    c. Keep side-rails up at all times.
    d. Have client in private room where possible, near nurse's station.

11. Administer medications ordered for safe withdrawal.

**Rationale**

8. Do not argue with the client, but share your experience that you do not see anything frightening. Address the fear and let the client know that you and the staff are here to help him or her remain safe.

9. Illusions can be explained to a client who is misinterpreting environmental cues. When client recognizes normal objects for what they are, anxiety is lessened.

10. During withdrawal, physical safety is the main priority.

11. Abrupt withdrawal from a CNS depressant can be fatal.

| Intervention | Rationale |
|---|---|
| 12. Use restraints with caution if client is combative and dangerous to others. Try to avoid mechanical restraints whenever possible. Always follow unit protocols. | 12. Myocardial infarctions, cardiac collapse, and death have occurred when clients have fought against the restraints during experiences of terror. |
| 13. Keep frequent, accurate records of client's vital signs, behaviors, medication, interventions, and effects of interventions. | 13. Monitor progress; identify what works best; identify potential complications. |

## *Initial and Active Drug Treatment*

### INEFFECTIVE HEALTH MAINTENANCE

Inability to identify, manage, and/or seek out help to maintain health

## *Related To (Etiology)*

- ▲ Lack of ability to make deliberate and thoughtful judgments
- ▲ Ineffective coping
- ▲ Perceptual/cognitive impairment
- All activities of life focused on obtaining and taking drug
- Money spent on substance of abuse and none left for health care, nourishing food, or safe shelter
- Poor nutrition related to prolonged drug binges, taking drug instead of eating nourishing food, or diminished appetite related to choice of drug (e.g., cocaine)
- Inability to make or keep health care appointments (e.g., mammograms, dentist, yearly physicals) because of either being intoxicated, being hung over, or withdrawing from an illicit substance
- Sleep deprivation related to decreased rapid eye movement (REM) sleep as a result of long-term stimulant, alcohol, or CNS depressant abuse

---

▲ NANDA International accepted; ● In addition to NANDA International

● Malabsorption of nutrients related to chronic alcohol abuse

*As Evidenced By*
*(Assessment Finding/Diagnostic Cues)*

▲ History of lack of health-seeking behaviors
▲ Reported or observed inability to take responsibility for meeting basic health practices in any or all functional pattern areas
● Physical exhaustion
● Sleep disturbances
● Unattended physical symptoms, for example:
  • Gastrointestinal problems
  • Extreme weight loss
  • Edema of extremities
  • Muscle weakness
  • Ascites
  • Abscesses on extremities
  • Bronchitis

*Outcome Criteria*

• Obtain stable health status meeting minimal requirements for:
  ○ Sleep
  ○ Nutrition
  ○ Weight
• Adheres to medication and treatment regimen

*Long-Term Goals*

• Client will demonstrate responsibility in taking care of health care needs as evidenced by keeping appointments by (date)
• Client's medical tests will demonstrate a reduced incidence of medical complications related to substance abuse after 6 months
• Client's weight is within normal range by (date)

---

▲ NANDA International accepted; ● In addition to NANDA International

- Client's daily nutritional intake will include 5 servings from fruit and vegetables, 2 to 3 from dairy, 2 to 3 from meat/poultry/fish, and 6 from grains (pasta, bread, rice) with help of nurse/nutritionist/family/support group
- Client will sleep at least 6 hours a night by (date)
- Client keeps appointments for medical treatment and follow-up within 2 months of treatment

*Short-Term Goals*

Client will:
- Go for medical checkup and treatment of any medical problems within 2 to 3 weeks of starting treatment
- Agree to go for nutritional counseling
- Identify three bodily effects of his or her substance abuse, and how these effects can affect self, loved ones, and unborn children within 1 to 2 weeks

*Interventions and Rationales (if Hospitalized)*

| Intervention | Rationale |
|---|---|
| 1. Encourage small feedings if appropriate. Check nutritional status (e.g., conjunctiva, body weight, eating history). | 1. If client is anorexic, small feedings will be better tolerated. Bland foods are often more appealing. Pale conjunctiva can signal an anemia. |
| 2. Monitor fluid intake and output. Check skin turgor. Check for ankle edema. Do urine specific gravity if skin turgor is poor. | 2. Clients can have potentially serious electrolyte imbalances. Too few fluids can cause or signal renal problems. If client is retaining too much fluid, there can be a danger of congestive heart failure. |
| 3. When skin turgor is poor, offer fluids frequently, containing protein and vitamins (e.g., milk, malts, juices). | 3. Proteins and vitamins help build nutritional status. |

| Intervention | Rationale |
|---|---|
| 4. Promote rest and sleep by placing client in a quiet environment. | 4. Provide the client with long rest periods between medical interventions. |
| 5. Identify client's understanding of how the alcohol/drugs they are taking can cause possible future problems (e.g., fetal alcohol syndrome, hepatitis/AIDS, fertility issues). | 5. Before teaching, nurse needs to identify what the client knows about the drugs, and evaluate his or her readiness to learn. |
| 6. With physician's approval, review client's blood work and physical examination with him or her. | 6. Lab results help the nurse identify possible causes of symptoms (e.g., infection) and initiate early counseling. |
| 7. Set up an appointment for medical follow-up in the clinic or community. | 7. Follow-up calls are important reminders. |

## INEFFECTIVE DENIAL

Conscious or unconscious attempt to disavow the knowledge or meaning of an event to reduce anxiety/fear, but leading to the detriment of health

### *Related To (Etiology)*

- Physical and/or emotional dependence on substance of abuse and a need to maintain the status quo
- Fear of having to change and give up substance of dependence and take responsibility for maladaptive past behaviors and chaotic life situations (legal, family, job problems)

---

▲ NANDA International accepted; ● In addition to NANDA International

- Underlying feelings of hopelessness and helplessness at having to cope with life without substance
- Long-term self-destructive patterns of behavior and lifestyle

## As Evidenced By
### (Assessment Findings/Diagnostic Cues)

▲ Displays inappropriate affect
▲ Minimizes symptoms and substance use
▲ Does not perceive personal relevance of symptoms or danger
  - Continues to use substance/drug, knowing it contributes to impaired functioning and exacerbation of physical symptoms
  - Uses substance/drug in potentially dangerous situations (e.g., driving while intoxicated)
- Uses rationalization and projection to explain irresponsible, aggressive, manipulative, and other maladaptive behaviors
- Fails to accept responsibility for behaviors that result in disrupted family life, legal problems, serious problems at work/lack of work, disrupted relationships with others
- Reluctant to discuss self or problems

## Outcome Criteria

- Maintains abstinence from chemical substances
- Continues attendance for treatment and maintenance of sobriety (e.g., AA, CA, NA, or group therapy, cognitive-behavioral psychotherapy, or other)

## Long-Term Goals

Client will:
- Demonstrate acceptance or responsibility for own behavior at the end of 3 months
- Demonstrate three alternative adaptive responses to stress in family, job, legal, and social situations within 1 month
- Demonstrate three strategies to use in vulnerable situations by (date)

---

▲ NANDA International accepted; ● In addition to NANDA International

- Identify maladaptive behaviors used in the past and demonstrate three new adaptive behaviors used in the present by (date)
- Attend a relapse program during active course of treatment

*Short-Term Goals*

Client will:
- Acknowledge that addiction does not cure itself, and it will worsen until it is treated, by third/fourth week of treatment
- Make a written contract to stay drug-free 1 day at a time within the first week of treatment
- Participate in a support group at least three times a week by second week of treatment
- Agree to contact a support person when he or she feels the need to use substance by the end of the first session
- Recognize and state when using denial, rationalization, and projection when speaking of drug use within the first month of treatment
- Identify at least three areas of his or her life that drugs have negatively affected within the first week
- Work with nurse, sponsor, chemical dependency counselor, therapist, or support group members on ways to change negative situations in his or her life
- Identify at least three positive role models, especially those that have overcome the same addiction themselves, within the first week
- Identify three vulnerable situations, and give three strategies to employ
- Take advantage of cognitive-behavioral therapy to increase coping skills during active phase of treatment
- Work with nurse, therapist, chemical dependency counselor, sponsor (in support group) to develop a relapse program
- Become a member of a relapse-prevention group

*Interventions and Rationales*

| Intervention | Rationale |
|---|---|
| **Initial Interventions** | |
| 1. Initially, work with client on crisis situations and establishing a rapport with client. | 1. People cannot work on issues when in crisis situations (e.g., practical living problems, family crisis). |

| Intervention | Rationale |
|---|---|
| 2. Refer the client to appropriate social services, occupational rehabilitation, or other resources as indicated. | 2. Client might need help that the nurse cannot provide, but assistance that is needed if client is to focus on and make changes in drug-related problems and behaviors. |
| 3. Maintain an interested, nonjudgmental, supportive approach. | 3. A nonjudgmental, supportive approach based on medical concern is most effective. |
| 4. Refrain from being pulled into power struggles, defending your position, preaching, or criticizing client's behaviors. | 4. Will only make the client more defensive. |
| 5. Continue to empathetically confront denial. | 5. Denial is the primary obstacle to receiving treatment. |
| 6. Forge an alliance with the client on some initial goals and what client wants to change in his or her life. | 6. Initially, the client's goal might not be total abstinence. Identifying areas that the client wants to change gives both client and nurse a basis for working together. |
| 7. Use of *miracle questions* can help identify what clients want to change (e.g., "What if your worst problem were miraculously solved overnight. What would be different about your life the next day?"). | 7. Helps clients perceive their future without some of their problems. Gives direction to moving forward and identifying long- and short-term goals. |

| **Intervention** | **Rationale** |
|---|---|
| 8. Help clients analyze specific pro's and con's of substance use/abuse. | 8. Helps clients look at what substances do and do not do for them in a clear light. Can help strengthen motives for change. |
| 9. Discourage the client's attempts to focus on only external problems (relationships, job related, legal) without relating them to substance use/abuse. | 9. Helps clients see the relationship between their problems and their drug use. Helps break down denial. |
| 10. Work with client to identify behaviors that have contributed to life problems (e.g., family problems, social difficulties, job-related problems, legal difficulties). | 10. When clients take responsibility for maladaptive behaviors, they are more prepared to take responsibility for learning effective and satisfying behaviors. |
| 11. Encourage client to stay in the "here and now" (e.g., "You can't change the fact that your mother put you down all your life." "Let's focus on how you want to respond when you perceive that your boss puts you down."). | 11. Dwelling on past disappointments and hurt is not useful to working on new and more adaptive coping behaviors. |
| 12. Refer and encourage client to attend a 12-step support group. | 12. Research shows that such involvement is the most effective tool in countering addiction (Zerbe, 1999). |
| 13. Encourage client to find a sponsor within the 12-step program, or other therapeutic mode. | 13. Having a sponsor and being a sponsor, according to some research, is important for success (Harvard Mental Health Letter, 1996). |

| Intervention | Rationale |
|---|---|
| 14. Work with clients to identify times they might be vulnerable to drinking/drugs and strategies to use at those times. | 14. Having thought out alternative strategies to drinking/drugs in vulnerable situations gives client ready choice. |
| 15. Encourage family and friends to seek support, education, and ways to recognize and refrain from enabling client. | 15. Enabling behavior supports the client's use of drugs by taking away incentive for change. |
| 16. Educate family and client regarding the physical and psychologic effects of the drug, the process of treatment, and aftercare. | 16. An addicted family member greatly changes the dynamics and roles within families. Family and client need to make decisions based on facts. |
| 17. Attend several open meetings in your local community. | 17. Helps nurse understand how 12-step fellowship process works. |
| 18. Realize that several sessions over weeks or months might pass before client accepts there is a problem and need for treatment. | 18. When helpers push too hard and become impatient, the client might leave treatment before making a commitment. |

**Active Treatment**

| | |
|---|---|
| 1. Expect sobriety. Work with clients to view their commitment to *one day at a time*. Thinking that he or she can never take the drug again might seem like an overwhelming responsibility. | 1. Client is not able to think rationally, make informed decisions, or learn while drug/alcohol impaired. |

| Intervention | Rationale |
|---|---|
| 2. Give feedback constantly when client tries to rationalize, blame, or minimize effects of drug use. | 2. As long as client believes that others are responsible or that his or her behavior is normal, or that there is really nothing wrong with his or her drug use, there will be no motivation for change. |
| 3. Teach client alternative ways to deal with stress:<br>  a. Relaxation techniques<br>  b. Exercise<br>  c. Taking "time out"<br>  d. Getting proper rest and nutrition<br>  e. Strategies for vulnerable situations | 3. Helps both client and nurse articulate what alternative skills can be identified, rehearsed, and practiced in social situations. |
| 4. Have clients identify their stress level on a scale of 1 to 10. Then have them reevaluate stress after using stress reduction techniques, and discuss next session. | 4. Helps client identify what works and what does not work. Nurse then works with client to learn and try alternative techniques. |
| 5. Assess other coping skills that will help client maintain sobriety/abstinence: for example:<br>  a. Anger management<br>  b. Impulse control<br>  c. Maintaining relationships<br>  d. Problem-solving skills | 5. Addicted client's usual method of getting all emotional needs met was through drugs. Problems with impulse control, anger and problem-solving are usually present. Relating to people in a drug-free environment can be very frightening. |

| Intervention | Rationale |
|---|---|
| 6. Refer the client to social services, vocational rehabilitation, workshops, skills groups, or other resources, when appropriate. | 6. Client recovering from addictions might have a myriad of needs that must be addressed, which can be key for maintaining sobriety. |
| 7. Continue to encourage group participation. | 7. Group participation provides people with: <br> a. Sense of belonging <br> b. Source of friendships <br> c. Reduction in feelings of isolation <br> d. Reduction in feelings of despair and shame <br> e. Alternatives to dealing with common situations and problems <br> f. Increased motivation toward sobriety |
| 8. Problem-solve with client realistic future goals, and identify life changes needed to meet these goals. | 8. Drug-free activities and companions need to be established to take the place of usual drug-related activities and drug-abusing companions. |
| 9. Discuss with client potential difficulty client might have relating to family and friends who continue to use substances of abuse. | 9. Client needs to be prepared to communicate with impaired friends and family differently. Client also needs to identify ways to meet new friends to continue a drug-free lifestyle. |

*RELAPSE PREVENTION*

## INEFFECTIVE COPING

Inability to form a valid appraisal of the stressors, inadequate choices of practiced response, and/or inability to use available resources

### Related To (Etiology)

- ▲ Inadequate opportunity to prepare for stressor
- ▲ Disturbance in pattern of appraisal of threat
- ▲ Disturbance in pattern of tension release
- ▲ Inadequate level of or perception of control
- ● Knowledge deficit
- ● Old coping styles no longer adaptive in present situations

### As Evidenced By
### (Assessment Findings/Diagnostic Cues)

- ▲ Abuse of chemical agents
- ▲ Inadequate problem-solving
- ▲ Destructive behavior toward self or others
- ▲ Inability to meet role expectations
- ▲ Risk taking
- ▲ Use of forms of coping that impede adaptive behavior
- ▲ Poor concentration

### Outcome Criteria

- • Continues counseling, cognitive-behavioral, interpersonal, or other therapy to deal with arising issues faced in sobriety
- • Continues to learn and practice effective coping skills
- • Continues to modify lifestyle as needed to maintain sobriety
- • Maintains total abstinence from all substances of abuse

### Long-Term Goals

Client will:
- • Participate at least weekly in a relapse prevention program and/or 12-step program

---

▲ NANDA International accepted; ● In addition to NANDA International

- Continue to verbalize cues or situations that pose increased risk of drug use
- Demonstrate strategies for avoiding and managing these cues
- State that he or she has a stable group of drug-free friends and socialize with them at least three times a week by (date)
- Participate routinely in at least four drug-free activities that give satisfaction and pleasure by (date)
- State that relationships with family members are more enjoyable and stable; family members will agree

### Short-Term Goals

- Client will identify at least three situations or events that serve as a source of vulnerability to relapse by (date)
- Client will demonstrate at least three cognitive-behavioral strategies to deal with sources of vulnerability to relapse by (date)
- Client will form relationships with at least four drug-free individuals that he or she enjoys spending time with in social activities by (date)
- Client will increase his or her drug-free social circle by two new people by the end of each month within the first month of treatment
- Client will identify at least two drug-free activities that he or she enjoys that do not trigger drug cravings
- Client will remain drug-free one day at a time
- Family members will state they feel supported in family counseling

### Interventions and Rationales

| Intervention | Rationale |
|---|---|
| 1. Work with client to keep treatment plan simple in the beginning. | 1. Approximately 40% to 50% of clients with substance abuse problems have mild to moderate cognitive problems while using substances. |
| 2. Have clients write notes and self-memos in order to keep appointments and follow treatment plan. | 2. Cognition usually gets better with long-term abstinence, but initially memory aids prove helpful. |

| Intervention | Rationale |
|---|---|
| 3. Encourage client to join relapse prevention groups (Box 10-3). | 3. Helps client anticipate and rehearse healthy responses to stressful situations. |
| 4. Encourage client to find role models (counselors or other recovering people). | 4. Role models serve as examples of how client can learn effective ways to make necessary life changes. |
| 5. Work with client on identifying triggers (people, feelings, situations) that help drive the client's addiction. | 5. Mastering the issues that perpetuate substance use allows for effective change and targets areas for acquiring new skills. |
| 6. Practice and role play with client alternative responses to triggers. | 6. Increases client confidence of handling drug triggers effectively. |
| 7. Give positive feedback when client applies new and effective responses to difficult "trigger" situations. | 7. Validates client's positive steps toward growth and change. |
| 8. Continue to empathetically confront denial throughout recovery. | 8. Denial can surface throughout recovery, and can interfere with sobriety during all stages of recovery. |
| 9. Continue to work with client on the following three areas: <br> a. **Personal issues** (relationship issue) <br> b. **Social issues** (issues of family abuse) <br> c. **Feelings of self-worth** | 9. These areas of human life need to find healing so that growth and change can take place. |
| 10. Recommend family therapy. | 10. Enhanced strategies for dealing with conflict in client's family are essential to recovery. |

| Intervention | Rationale |
|---|---|
| 11. Stress the fact that substance abuse is a disease the entire family must conquer. | 11. Family members also need encouragement to face their own struggles (Zerbe, 1999). |
| 12. Expect slips to occur. Reaffirm that sobriety can be achieved as emotional pain becomes endurable. | 12. Helps minimize shame and guilt, and rebuild self-esteem. |

# MEDICAL TREATMENTS

## Psychopharmacology

In the formulation of a treatment plan for individual drug-dependent clients, treatment for comorbid psychiatric or medical disorders must be included. Some clients, for example, might benefit from an antidepressant for secondary depressive disorder. The effectiveness of some pharmacologic treatments of drug dependencies is not necessarily well established. However, some drugs can be useful in clients with the following dependencies (APA, 2000b). Please keep in mind, *these agents* should be part of a comprehensive treatment program that includes psychosocial support such as counseling and support groups.

**Alcohol:**
A. **Disulfiram** (Antabuse) is an effective adjunct to a comprehensive treatment program for reliable, motivated clients whose drinking is triggered by events that can suddenly increase alcohol cravings.

B. **Naltrexone** (Revia), an opiate antagonist, can attenuate some of the reinforcing affects of alcohol and decrease cravings. Alcohol sensitivity drug.

C. **Nalmefine** (Revex) is an opiate antagonist similar to naltrexone. Effective in heavy drinkers with fewer side effects than naltrexone.

D. **Acamprosate** (Campral) is an amino acid derivative that has a benign side effect profile and shows value in alcohol dependence. Acamprosate affects both gamma-aminobutyric acid (GABA) and excitatory amino acid (e. g., glucamate) neurotransmission.

---

### Box 10-3 Relapse Prevention Strategies

**Basics**
1. Keep the program simple at first; 40% to 50% of clients who abuse substances have mild to moderate cognitive problems while actively using.
2. Review instructions with health-team members.
3. Use a notebook and write down important information and telephone numbers.

**Skills**
Take advantage of cognitive-behavioral therapy to increase your coping skills. Identify which important life skills are needed:
1. What situations do you have difficulty handling?
2. What situations are you managing more effectively?
3. For which situations would you like to develop more effective coping skills?

**Relapse Prevention Groups**
Become a member of a relapse prevention group. These groups work on:
1. Rehearsing stressful situations using a variety of techniques
2. Finding ways to deal with current problems or ones that are likely to arise as you become drug free
3. Providing role models to help you make necessary life changes

**Increase Personal Insight**
Therapy—group therapy, individual therapy, family therapy—can help you gain insight and control over many psychologic concerns—for example:
1. What drives your addictions?
2. What constitutes a healthy supportive relationship?
3. Increasing your sense of self and self-worth.
4. What does your addictive substance give you that you think you need and cannot find otherwise?

---

Adapted from Zerbe, K.J. (1999). *Women's mental health in primary care.* Philadelphia: WB Saunders, pp. 94–95; reprinted with permission.

**Cocaine:** A. Pharmacologic treatment is not usually indicated as an initial treatment, although clients with more severe dependence might be considered for treatment with dopaminergic medications.

**Opioids:** A. Detoxification may include use of opioid agonists (e.g., methadone), partial agonists (e.g., buprenorphine), antagonists (e.g., naloxone, naltrexone), or nonopoid alternative such as clonidine or a benzodiazepine.

B. Maintenance on methadone (suppresses withdrawal for 24 to 36 hours) or Levo-alpha-acetyl-methadol (LAAM) (suppresses withdrawal for 48 to 72 hours) can reduce the morbidity in clients with prolonged opioid dependence.

C. **Buprenorphine** is an opiate approved for the treatment of opioid addiction. Buprenorphine monotherapy **(Subutex)** and a buprenorphine combination product, **Suboxone,** a buprenorphine/naloxone derivative, are the two FDA-approved forms at this writing. Buprenorphine's potential for abuse is lessened when combined with naloxone. Advantages include less risk of respiratory arrest in overdose, less severe withdrawal symptoms, and the use of a buprenorphine/naloxone combination can be administered in an office-based setting.

D. Maintenance on naltrexone used in abstinence therapy is beneficial except for lack of client compliance and low treatment retention.

### *Management of Drug Intoxication and Withdrawal*

The medical treatment for intoxication and overdose for common drugs of abuse are outlined in Table 10-2.

### *Psychosocial*

Psychosocial therapies are helpful to many motivated clients with substance-use dependencies. Therapies that can be effective in some clients include cognitive behavioral therapies, interpersonal therapy, brief interventions, marital and family therapy, and group therapy, and extremely useful for many are self-help groups such as AA, NA, and PA.

## CLIENT AND FAMILY TEACHING

Clients, families, and significant others all need support and information to guide them during early and middle phases of treatment. Box 10-4 offers the nurse some guidelines.

---

**Box 10-4** Client and Family Teaching: Chemical Dependence

- Teach clients and families that alcoholism and substance abuse are diseases, not moral weaknesses.
- Like diseases, addictions can be treated through a variety of therapeutic and pharmacologic approaches.
- Recognize that substance-related disorders affect all family members.
- Identify "enabling" behaviors, and teach families how to substitute healthier patterns.
- Tell families that they are not responsible for their member's substance abuse.
- Tell the client and family to report any worsening signs of depression or suicidal thoughts.
- Educate about the detrimental effects of alcohol and substance abuse, including depression and sleep disruption.
- Help the client and family identify community resources such as Adult Children of Alcoholics (ACOA), Al-Anon, and other self-help groups.
- Encourage clients to reveal their urges to use substances before they can act on them.
- Educate clients about the risk of HIV, hepatitis, and other diseases associated with substance abuse.

---

Adapted from Gorman, L.M., Sultan, D.F., & Raines, M.L. (1996). *Davis's manual of psychosocial nursing for general patient care.* Philadelphia: FA Davis, pp. 283–289; reprinted with permission.

# NURSE, CLIENT, AND FAMILY RESOURCES

## ASSOCIATIONS

**Alcoholics Anonymous World Services**
475 Riverside
New York, NY 10115
(212) 870-3400

**Narcotics Anonymous World Services Office**
PO Box 9999
Van Nuys, CA 91409
(818) 773-9999

**Al-Anon Family Group Headquarters, Inc. (for Al-Anon, Alateen, Alatots, ACOA)**
1600 Corporate Landing Parkway
Virginia Beach, VA 23454-5617
(757) 563-1600; (800) 4AL-ANON

**National Clearinghouse for Alcohol and Drug Information**
PO Box 2345
Rockville, MD 20856
http://www.health.org

**Center for Substance Abuse Treatment (CSAT)**
National Drug Hotline (bilingual)
(800) 662-4357
http://samsha.gov/

**National Institute on Drug Abuse (NIDA)**
American Self-Help Clearinghouse
(201) 625-7101
http://mentalhelp.net/selfhelp

## INTERNET SITES

**Addiction Technology Transfer Center**
http://www.nattc.org

**Centre for Addiction and Mental Health**
http://www.camh.net

# CHAPTER 11

# Eating Disorders

## OVERVIEW

**Anorexia nervosa** and **bulimia nervosa** are both potentially fatal eating disorders. These disorders are severe and disabling, and successful treatment entails long-term care and follow-up. Unlike most psychiatric conditions, these disorders can cause severe physiologic damage. (Refer to Table 11-1 for some medical complications of eating disorders.) Because anorexia nervosa and bulimia nervosa are chronic, complex disorders, nursing interventions need to include actions to help minimize harm during the acute phase and help prevent relapse. Predominantly, these disorders affect adolescents, and cause great suffering and frustration to the families, friends, and loved ones. Treating these disorders can pose a formidable challenge to the health care system. The two primary categories of eating disorders discussed in this section are anorexia nervosa and bulimia nervosa. When there is evidence that psychologic factors are important to the etiology or cause of a particular case of obesity, it is noted as **psychological factors affecting medical condition** (American Psychiatric Association [APA], 2000b). Comorbid personality disorders are frequent among clients with eating disorders (42% to 75%), along with comorbid major depression or dysthymia (50% to 75%) (APA, 2000b). Therefore, an understanding of cognitive development, psychologic defenses, and complexity of family relationships, as well as the presence of other psychiatric disorders should be incorporated into the treatment plan (APA, 2000b). **Eating disorders not otherwise specified (NOS)** is the diagnosis often given when clients have signs and symptoms of both categories.

# Anorexia Nervosa

The diagnosis of anorexia nervosa is based on psychologic and physical criteria. Psychologic criteria include an intense fear of gaining weight or becoming fat and a gross disturbance in body image. Physiologic requisites for the diagnosis of anorexia nervosa are maintenance of body weight less than 85% of that expected. Box 11-1 presents the *Diagnostic and Statistical Manual of Mental Disorders* (4th edition, text revision) (DSM-IV-TR) diagnostic criteria for anorexia nervosa.

Most cases of anorexia nervosa are seen in adolescent women, with approximately 85% of cases developing between the ages of 13 and 20. Although most individuals with anorexia nervosa are adolescents, anorexia is being diagnosed in preadolescents, in adults, and even in the elderly. Males account for approximately 19% to 30% of the younger patients diagnosed with anorexia nervosa (APA, 2000b). The issues and the treatment modalities remain the same for both men and women.

Characteristically, anorectics are emaciated, but they still feel "fat" and want to hide their "ugly, fat body." Anorectics might have ritualistic eating patterns and compulsive behaviors; often feel hopeless, helpless, and depressed; and might feel the only control they can exert in their life is through what food they will eat. Suicide is a real concern.

People with this disorder use two methods to control weight:

1. **Bulimic** approach alternates bingeing and starvation (including purging and laxative and/or diuretic abuse). Purging might occur in up to 70% of young clients (binge eating/purging type).
2. **Restrictive** approach uses low calorie intake and exercise (restricting type).

The course of anorexia varies from (Hoffman & Halmi, 1997):

- A single episode with weight and psychologic recovery, to
- Nutritional rehabilitation with relapses, to
- An unremitting course resulting in death.

The disease has a mortality rate of 5% (most studies) to 20% (long-term studies looking at ultimate mortality rate over

| Box | DSM-IV-TR |
| 11-1 | Criteria for Anorexia Nervosa |

1. Refusal to maintain body weight over a minimum normal weight for age and height (e.g., weight loss leading to maintenance of body weight less than 85% of that expected, or failure to make expected weight gain during period of growth, leading to body weight less than 85% of that expected).
2. Intense fear of gaining weight or becoming fat, although underweight.
3. Disturbance in the way in which one's body weight or shape is experienced, undue influence of body weight or shape on self-evaluation, or denial of the seriousness of the current low body weight.
4. In females, postmenarchal amenorrhea (i.e., the absence of at least three consecutive menstrual cycles). (A woman is considered to have amenorrhea if her periods occur only following hormone [e.g., estrogen] administration.)

*Specify type:*

**Binge eating/purging type:** During the episode of anorexia nervosa, the person engages in recurrent episodes of binge eating or purging behaviors.

**Restricting type:** During the episode of anorexia nervosa, the person does not engage in recurrent episodes of binge eating or purging behaviors.

Adapted from American Psychiatric Association. (2000). *Diagnostic and statistical manual of mental disorders* (4th ed., text revision). Washington, DC: American Psychiatric Association, p. 589; reprinted with permission.

20 years or longer). Death occurs from starvation, fluid and electrolyte imbalance, or suicide in chronically ill clients. Goldberg (1998) has identified favorable and negative prognostic indicators for anorexia nervosa:

1. **Favorable prognostic indicators:**
   a. Earlier age at onset
   b. Return of menses
   c. Good premorbid school/work history
2. **Negative prognostic indicators:**
   a. Recurrent illness
   b. Multiple hospitalizations
   c. Male

d. Family pathology
e. Premorbid personality difficulties and poor social adjustment in childhood

## ASSESSMENT

### Presenting Signs and Symptoms

*Psychosocial*

- Extreme fear of gaining weight
- Poor social adjustment with some areas of high functioning (e.g., intellectual)
- Odd food habits (hoarding, hiding food [e.g., in pockets, under plate])
- Hyperactivity (compulsive and obsessive exercise and/or secretive physical activity in an attempt to burn calories)
- Mood and/or sleep disturbances
- Obsessive-compulsive behaviors (e.g., eating only one pea at a time, arranging and rearranging food on plate before each bite, cutting food into tiny pieces and chewing each piece excessively)
- Perfectionist
- Introverted; avoids intimacy and sexual activity
- Denies feelings of sadness or anger and will often appear pleasant and compliant
- Although cachectic, clients see themselves as fat, underlying an unrealistic body image
- Families often have rigid rules and have high expectations for their members

*Physiologic and Endocrine Symptoms*

- Emaciated physical appearance
- Changes in cardiac status (e.g., bradycardia, hypotension, dysrhythmia)
- Dry, yellowish skin
- Amenorrhea, infertility
- Hair loss, possible presence of lanugo (fine body hair covering)
- Decreased metabolic rate
- Chronic constipation
- Fatigue and lack of energy

- Insomnia
- Loss of bone mass, osteoporosis
- In clients who vomit or use laxatives to purge, loss of tooth enamel and scarring of the back of the hand from inducing vomiting, and enlarged salivary glands might be seen. Serum amylase level is often elevated.
- Dehydration, edema
- Laboratory abnormalities and medical complications (Table 11-1)

## Assessment Tools

The nurse must be able to make a comprehensive nursing assessment as well as be able to assess when a medical or psychologic emergency warrants hospitalization and alert the medical staff. Refer to Appendix D-8 for a guide that will help the nurse assess if the client with an eating disorder warrants hospitalization.

## Assessment Guidelines
### Anorexia Nervosa

Determine if:
1. The client has a medical or psychiatric situation that warrants hospitalization (see Appendix D-8).
2. The family has information about the disease and knows where to get support.
3. The client is amenable to attending, or compliant with appropriate therapeutic modalities.
4. Family counseling has been offered to the family or individual family members for support, or to target a family or individual family member's problem.
5. A thorough physical examination with appropriate blood work has been done.
6. Other medical conditions have been ruled out.
7. The family and client need further teaching or information regarding client's treatment plan (e.g., psychopharmacologic interventions, behavioral therapy, cognitive therapy, family therapy, individual psychotherapy). If the client is a candidate for partial hospitalization, can the family/client discuss their function?
8. The client and family desire a support group; if yes, provide referrals.

Table 11-1 **Some Medical Complications of Eating Disorders**

| Complication | Laboratory Findings |
|---|---|
| Cardiovascular | Electrocardiographic abnormalities |
|   Bradycardia | |
|   Postural hypotension | |
|   Dysrhythmias | |
| Metabolic | |
|   Acidosis (laxatives) | $\downarrow K^+$ |
|   Alkalosis (vomiting) | $\uparrow$ Cholesterol |
|   Hypokalemia | $\uparrow$ Liver function tests |
|   Hypocalcemia | $\downarrow Mg^{2+}$ |
|   Hypomagnesemia | $\downarrow Na^+$ |
|   Osteoporosis | $\downarrow Ca^{2+}$ |
|   Dehydration | $\downarrow$ Bone density |
| Renal | |
|   Hematuria | $\uparrow$ Blood urea nitrogen |
|   Proteinuria | |
| Gastrointestinal | |
|   Hyperamylasemia | $\uparrow$ Serum amylase |
|   Parotid swelling—hypertrophy | |
|   Dental erosion (vomiting HCL) | |
|   Esophagitis, esophageal tears (vomiting) | |
|   Pancreatitis | |
|   Diarrhea (laxative abuse) | |
|   Gastric dilation—bingeing | |
| Hematologic | |
|   Leukopenia | $\downarrow$ Erythrocyte sedimentation rate |
|   Lymphocytosis | Abnormal complete blood count |
|   Anemias (iron and vitamin $B_{12}$ deficiency) | |
| Endocrine | |
|   Amenorrhea | $\downarrow$ Follicle-stimulating hormone, luteinizing hormone, estradiol levels |
|   Urinary and plasma gonadotropins | |
|   Hypercortisolism | $\uparrow$ Corticotropin-releasing hormone |
|   Abnormal thyroid function test | $\downarrow$ Triiodothyronine |

# NURSING DIAGNOSES WITH INTERVENTIONS

## Discussion of Potential Nursing Diagnoses

Eating disorders have both physiologic and psychologic components. The aims of treatment are survival based (Hill, 1998):

- Regain a healthy weight.
- Restore healthy eating habits.
- Treat physical complications.
- Address dysfunctional beliefs.
- Intervene in those dysfunctional thoughts, feelings, and beliefs.
- Deal with affective and behavioral issues.
- Include family therapy when appropriate and possible.
- Teach relapse prevention.

The first steps in treating the anorexic client include nutritional rehabilitation and weight restoration. Psychotherapy is not appropriate at this phase because there are profound psychologic effects on mood and behavior from self-starvation. Hospitalization is warranted when emaciation is severe, vomiting is present, outpatient treatment has failed, or there is severe depression or suicidal feelings or physical complications (see Appendix D-8).

During hospitalization, treatment goals include the following:

- Weight restoration
- Normalization of eating behavior
- Change in the pursuit of thinness
- Prevention of relapse

Therefore, **Imbalanced Nutrition: Less Than Body Requirements** is a primary nursing diagnosis.

Because clients with anorexia have extreme distortions of their body (seeing themselves as fat when emaciated) and an intense fear of being fat, **Disturbed Body Image** is an important nursing diagnosis; a realistic perception of body size is important to help the client refrain from the compulsive need to lose weight. There is real threat for self-harm; therefore, **Risk for Self-Mutilation** or **Risk for Self-Directed Violence** might be appropriate diagnoses for some young clients. **Refer to Chapter 16 for guidelines to assessment and care.** Clients with anorexia are terrified about gaining weight and will do anything to prevent gaining weight.

Therefore, they frequently try to manipulate staff. Although briefly addressed here, **refer to Chapter 19 for dealing with manipulative behaviors**, because anorectic clients are desperate in their quest to avoid gaining weight.

**Understand that anorectics are notoriously disinterested in treatment. Gaining trust and cooperation can be difficult.** Table 11-2 offers potential nursing diagnoses for people with eating disorders.

Table 11-2 **Potential Nursing Diagnoses for Eating Disorders**

| Symptoms | Nursing Diagnoses |
|---|---|
| Emaciated, dehydrated, fatigued and lacking energy, edema | **Imbalanced Nutrition: Less Than Body Requirements**<br>**Deficient Fluid Volume**<br>**Impaired Skin Integrity**<br>**Risk for Imbalanced Body Temperature**<br>**Activity Intolerance**<br>**Fatigue**<br>**Risk for Infection**<br>**Decreased Cardiac Output** |
| Chronic constipation or diarrhea, abuse of laxatives | **Constipation**<br>**Diarrhea** |
| Sees self as fat (even when emaciated), has extreme fear of gaining weight, denies feelings of sadness or anger, has obsessive thoughts around food | **Disturbed Thought Processes**<br>**Ineffective Denial**<br>**Disturbed Body Image** |
| Poor social adjustment, introverted, compulsive behaviors (sexual acting out, shoplifting, bingeing, substance use), perfectionistic, manipulates to avoid calorie intake | **Ineffective Coping**<br>**Social Isolation**<br>**Impaired Social Interaction** |
| Feelings of helplessness, worthlessness, being out of control; mood and sleep disturbances | **Hopelessness**<br>**Powerlessness**<br>**Chronic Low Self-Esteem**<br>**Risk for Self-Directed Violence**<br>**Risk for Self-Mutilation**<br>**Spiritual Distress**<br>**Risk for Loneliness**<br>**Anxiety** |

*Continued*

Table 11-2 **Potential Nursing Diagnoses for Eating Disorders—cont'd**

| Symptoms | Nursing Diagnoses |
|---|---|
| Disrupted family, family in crisis, family confusion | **Interrupted Family Processes** **Compromised Family Coping** **Disabled Family Coping** |
| Resistance to treatment, denial of problems, shame over bingeing, extreme fear of gaining weight, non-adherence to medications or treatment | **Deficient Knowledge** **Noncompliance** **Anxiety** |

## Overall Guidelines for Nursing Intervention

### *Anorexic Individual*

1. Gaining an anorexic individual's cooperation is best accomplished by acknowledging his or her desire for thinness and control and stimulating motivation for change.
2. Do a self-assessment and be aware of your own reactions that might hinder your ability to help the client. Some nurses might (Gorman et al., 1996):
   - Feel shocked or disgusted by the client's behavior or appearance.
   - Resent the client, believing that the disorder is self-inflicted.
   - Feel helpless to change the client's behavior, leading to anger, frustration, and criticism.
   - Become overwhelmed by the client's problems, leading to feelings of hopelessness or setting rigid limits to feel more in control of the client's behavior.
   - Be swept up into power struggles with the client, resulting in angry feelings in the nurse toward the client.
   When any of these or other negative feelings toward the client arise, supervision and/or peer review is needed to help shape the nurse's perspective, and lessen feelings of helplessness, guilt, need for control, frustration, or hopelessness.
3. When problems in the family contribute to the feeling of loss of control, family therapy has provided a significant improvement rate.

4. Individual therapy and group therapy are essential in treating clients with eating disorders. Treatment for anorectic clients often includes a behavior modification program, especially initially. Family therapy and family education are often key to a client's success.

5. Behavior therapy is often used to change the eating patterns of an anorexic who is seriously close to death. This is usually implemented after the anorexic has been tube-fed to prevent death.

6. Refrain from focusing on the person's need to eat; recognize that other, nonfood factors are the heart of the problem.

7. Monitor lab values, and report abnormal values to primary clinician.

## Selected Nursing Diagnoses and Nursing Care Plans

### IMBALANCED NUTRITION: LESS THAN BODY REQUIREMENTS

Intake of nutrients insufficient to meet metabolic needs

### Related To (Etiology)

▲ Inability to ingest or digest food or to absorb nutrients because of biologic, psychologic, or economic factors
● Excessive fear of weight gain
● Restricting caloric intake or refusing to eat
● Excessive physical exertion resulting in caloric loss in excess of caloric intake
● Self-induced vomiting related to self-starvation

### As Evidenced By (Assessment Findings/Diagnostic Cues)

▲ Weight loss (with or without adequate intake): 15% or more under ideal body weight
▲ Reported or observed food intake less than recommended minimum daily requirements

---

▲ NANDA International accepted; ● In addition to NANDA International

▲ Excessive hair loss or increased growth of hair on body (lanugo)
▲ Poor muscle tone
▲ Fatigue
▲ Diarrhea and/or steatorrhea, abdominal cramping, pain
● Emaciated appearance
● Serious medical complications resulting from starvation (e.g., electrolyte imbalances, hypothermia, bradycardia, hypotension, cardiac arrhythmias, edema)

## Outcome Criteria

- Food and fluid intake is within normal limits
- Weight is maintained within a medically safe range

## Long-Term Goals

- Client's electrolytes will be within normal limits by (date)
- Client's cardiac status will be within normal limits by (date)
- Client will achieve 85% to 90% of ideal body weight
- Client will commit to long-term treatment to prevent relapse by (date)
- Client will demonstrate regular, independent, nutritional eating habits by (date)

## Short-Term Goals

Client will:
- Increase caloric and nutritional intake, showing gradual increases on a weekly basis
- Gain no more than____in the first week of refeeding as decided by client and health team
- Exercise in limited amounts only when assessed to be both nutritionally and medically stable
- Formulate with the nurse a *nurse-client contract* facilitating a therapeutic alliance and a commitment on the part of the client to treatment

---

▲ NANDA International accepted; ● In addition to NANDA International

*Interventions and Rationales*

| Intervention | Rationale |
|---|---|

**The Severely Malnourished Client—Nutritional Rehabilitation**

| Intervention | Rationale |
|---|---|
| 1. When severely malnourished and refusing nourishment, client might require tube feedings, either alone or in conjunction with oral or parenteral nutrition. | 1. Tube feedings might be the only means available to maintain client's life. Client might not be able to tolerate solid foods at first. The use of nasogastric tube feedings decreases the chance of vomiting. |
| 2. Tube feedings or parenteral nutrition is often given at night. | 2. Using nighttime administration can diminish drawing attention or sympathy from other clients, and allows the client to participate more fully in daytime activities. |
| 3. After completion of tube feeding, it is best to supervise client for 90 minutes initially, then gradually reduce to 30 minutes, after administration of nasogastric tube feeding. | 3. Helps to minimize the client's chance of vomiting or siphoning off feedings. |
| 4. Vital signs at least tid until stable, then daily. Repeat electrocardiogram (ECG) and laboratory tests (electrolytes, acid-base balance, liver enzymes, albumin, and others) until stable. | 4. As client begins to increase in weight, cardiovascular status improves to within normal range, and monitoring is needed less frequently. |

| Intervention | Rationale |
|---|---|
| 5. Administer tube feedings in a matter-of-fact, nonpunitive manner. Tube feedings are not to be used as threats, nor are they to be bargained about. | 5. Tube feedings are medical treatments, not a punishment or a bargaining chip. Being consistent and enforcing limits lowers the chance of manipulation and the use of power struggles. |
| 6. Give the client the chance to take foods or liquid supplements orally, and supplement insufficient intake through tube feedings. | 6. Allows the client some control over whether he or she needs tube feedings or not. The client's life is the priority, however. |
| 7. Weigh the client weekly or biweekly at the same time of day each week. Use the following guidelines: <br> • Before the morning meal <br> • After the client has voided <br> • In hospital gown or bra and pants only | 7. Clients are terrified about gaining weight. Staff members should guard against clients trying to manipulate their weight by drinking excess water before being weighed, having a full bladder, and putting heavy objects in their pockets or on their person. |
| 8. Remain neutral, neither approving nor disapproving. | 8. Keep issues of approval and disapproval separate from issues of health. Weight gain/loss is a health matter, not an area that has to do with the staff's pleasure or disapproval. |

| Intervention | Rationale |
|---|---|

**The Less Severely Malnourished Client—Nutritional Maintenance**

| Intervention | Rationale |
|---|---|
| 1. When possible, set up a contract with the client regarding treatment goals and outcome criteria. | 1. When clients agree to take part in establishing goals, they are in a position to have some control over their care. |
| 2. Provide a pleasant, calm atmosphere at mealtime. Mealtime should be structured. Clients should be told the specific time and duration of a meal (e.g., 30 minutes). | 2. Mealtimes become episodes of high anxiety, and knowledge of regulations decreases tension in the milieu, particularly when the client has given up so much control by entering treatment. |
| 3. Observe client *during* meals to prevent hiding or throwing away food. Accompany to the bathroom if purging is suspected. Observe client for at least 1 hour *after* meals/snacks to prevent purging. | 3. These behaviors are difficult for the client to stop. A power struggle might emerge around issues of control. |
| 4. Observe client closely for using physical activity to control weight. | 4. Clients are often discouraged from engaging in planned exercise programs until their weight reaches 85% of ideal body weight. |
| 5. Closely monitor and record:<br>• Fluid and food intake<br>• Vital signs<br>• Elimination pattern: discourage the use of laxatives, enemas, or suppositories. | 5. Fluid and electrolyte balance is crucial to client's well-being and safety. Abnormal data should alert staff to potential physical crises. |

| Intervention | Rationale |
|---|---|
| 6. Continue to weigh client as described earlier. | 6. Monitor progress. |
| 7. As client approaches target weight, gradually encourage client to make own choices for menu selection. | 7. Fosters a sense of control and independence. |
| 8. Privileges are based on weight gain (or loss) when setting limits. When weight *loss* occurs, decrease privileges. Use this time to focus on circumstances sur-rounding the weight loss and feelings of the client. | 8. By not focusing on eating, physical activity, calorie counts, and the like, there is more emphasis on the client's feelings and perceptions. |
| 9. When weight gain occurs, increase privileges. | 9. Client receives positive reinforcements for healthy outcomes and behaviors. |

**Maintenance**

| | |
|---|---|
| 1. Continue to provide a supportive and empathetic approach as client continues to meet target weight. | 1. Eating regularly for the anorectic client, even within the framework of restoring health, is extremely difficult. |
| 2. The weight mainte-nance phase of treatment challenges the client. This is the ideal time to address more of the issues underlying the client's attitude toward weight and shape. | 2. At a healthier weight, client is cognitively better prepared to examine emotional conflicts and themes. |

| Intervention | Rationale |
|---|---|
| 3. Use a cognitive-behavioral approach to client's expressed fears regarding weight gain. Identify dysfunctional thoughts. | 3. Confronting dysfunctional thoughts and beliefs is crucial to changing eating behaviors. |
| 4. Emphasize social nature of eating. Encourage conversation that does not have the theme of food during mealtimes. | 4. Eating is a social activity, shared with others, and participating in conversation serves both as a distraction from obsessional preoccupation and as a pleasurable event. |
| 5. Focus on the client's strengths, including his or her good work in normalizing weight and eating habits. | 5. The client has achieved a major accomplishment and should be proud. Explore noneating activities as a source of gratification. |
| 6. Encourage client to apply all the knowledge, skills, and gains made from the various individual, family, and group therapy sessions. | 6. The client should have been receiving intensive therapy (cognitive-behavioral) and education, which have provided tools and techniques useful in maintaining healthy eating and living behaviors. |
| 7. Teach and role model assertiveness. | 7. Client learns to get his or her needs met appropriately. Helps lower anxiety and acting-out behaviors. |

| Intervention | Rationale |
|---|---|
| **Follow-Up Care** | |
| 1. Involve the client's family and significant others with teaching, treatment, and discharge and follow-up plans. Teaching includes nutrition, medication, if any, and the dynamics of the illness (Schultz & Videbeck, 2005). | 1. Family involvement is a key factor to client success. Family dynamics are usually a significant factor in the client's illness and distress. |
| 2. Make arrangements for follow-up therapy for both the client and the family. | 2. Follow-up therapy for both family and client is key to prevention of relapse. |
| 3. Offer referrals to the client and family to local support groups or national groups. (See list at end of chapter for suggestions.) | 3. Support groups offer emotional guidance and support, resources, and important information, and help minimize feelings of isolation, and encourage healthier coping strategies. |

## DISTURBED BODY IMAGE

Confusion in mental picture of one's physical self

*Related To (Etiology)*

▲ Cognitive/perceptual factors
▲ Psychosocial factors
● Morbid fear of obesity
● Low self-esteem
● Feelings of helplessness
● Chemical/biologic imbalances

---

▲ NANDA International accepted; ● In addition to NANDA International

## As Evidenced By
### (Assessment Findings/Diagnostic Cues)

- ▲ Verbalized negative feelings about body (e.g., dirty, big, unsightly)
- ▲ Verbalized feelings of helplessness, hopelessness, and/or powerlessness in relation to body and fear of rejection/reaction of others
- ▲ Self-destructive behavior (purging, refusal to eat, abuse of laxatives)
- ● Sees self as fat, although body weight is normal, or client is severely emaciated
- ● High to panic levels of anxiety over potential for slight weight gain, although grossly underweight to the point of starvation

## Outcome Criteria

- Comfortable with a weight that meets medically safe limits
- Demonstrates pride in self through dress and grooming

## Long-Term Goals

Client will:
- Describe a more realistic perception of body size and shape in line with height and body type by (date)
- Refer to body in a more positive way by (date)
- Improve grooming, dress, and posture and present self in more socially acceptable and appropriate manner by (date)

## Short-Term Goals

Client will:
- Challenge dysfunctional thoughts and beliefs about weight with help of nurse after acute phase of treatment has passed
- State three positive aspects about self

---

▲ NANDA International accepted; ● In addition to NANDA International

*Interventions and Rationales*

| Intervention | Rationale |
|---|---|
| 1. Establish a therapeutic alliance with client. | 1. Anorexic clients are highly resistant to giving up their distorted eating behaviors. |
| 2. Give the client factual feedback about the client's low weight and resultant impaired health. However, do not argue or challenge the client's distorted perceptions (Ibrahim, 2005). | 2. Focuses on health and benefits of increased energy. Arguments or power struggles will only increase the client's need to control. |
| 3. Recognize that the client's distorted image is real to him/her. Avoid minimizing client's perceptions (e.g., "I understand you see yourself as fat. I do not see you that way.") | 3. Acknowledges client's perceptions, and the client feels understood, although your perception is different. This kind of feedback is easier to hear than a negation of client's beliefs. |
| 4. Encourage expression of feelings regarding how the client thinks and feels about self and body. | 4. Promotes a clear under-standing of client's perceptions and lays the groundwork for working with client. |
| 5. Assist the client to distinguish between thoughts and feelings. Statements such as "I feel fat" should be challenged and reframed. | 5. It is important for the client to distinguish between feelings and facts. The client often speaks of feelings as though they are reality. |

| Intervention | Rationale |
|---|---|
| 6. Nurses who have training in cognitive-behavioral therapeutic interventions can encourage client to keep a journal of thoughts and feelings and teach client how to identify and challenge irrational beliefs. | 6. Cognitive and behavioral approaches can be very effective in helping client challenge irrational beliefs about self and body image. |
| 7. Encourage client to identify positive personal traits. Have client identify positive aspects of personal appearance. | 7. Helps client refocus on strengths and actual physical and other attributes. Encourages breaking negative rumination. |
| 8. Educate family regarding the client's illness and encourage attendance at family and group therapy sessions. | 8. Reactions of others often become triggers for dysphoric reactions and distorted perceptions. Relationships with others, although not causal, are the context in which the eating disorder exists and thrives. |
| 9. Encourage family therapy for family members and significant others. | 9. Families and significant others need assistance in how to communicate and share a relationship with the anorexic client (Ibrahim, 2005). |

## MEDICAL TREATMENTS

### Psychopharmacology

Although there have been many drugs used to treat anorexia nervosa, no medication has been shown to be effective in maintaining weight gain, in changing anorectic attitudes, or in preventing relapse either by itself or as an adjunct for treating anorexia nervosa (APA, 2000b).

SSRI *antidepressants* have provided some success with anorectic clients. Neuroleptics (olazapine/haloperidol) at very low doses look promising in open trials (Stern et al, 2004).

Cyproheptadine hydrochloride (Periactin), an *antihistamine*, has also been found to be effective in emaciated anorectic clients in decreasing depression and in inducing weight gain among the anorexic restrictors (but not the bulimic subgroups).

One challenge is that often teenagers are nonadherent to medication regimens and treatment. This knowledge is best factored into the nurse's approach to the anorectic.

### Psychosocial

As mentioned in the opening paragraph, a number of factors should be known when formulating the treatment plan. Box 11-2 summarizes some of the more successful psychosocial approaches with anorexia nervosa.

# Bulimia Nervosa

People with bulimia might be slightly overweight, normal weight, or slightly below. The hallmark feature of bulimia nervosa is an excessive intake of food (binge eating) with purging behaviors to maintain body weight. Purging behaviors can include self-induced vomiting or the excessive use of laxatives, diuretics, or enemas. Other behaviors directed at maintaining body weight might include prolonged fasting, excessive exercise, or misuse of diet pills. Purging is used by 80% to 90% of individuals who present for treatment at eating disorder clinics (APA, 2000b).

People with bulimia who use purging behaviors are referred to as having **bulimia nervosa—purging type**. Similarly, **bulimia nervosa—nonpurging type** represents people who use inappropriate compensatory behaviors (fasting, excessive exercise, misuse of diet pills), but do not engage in the previously mentioned purging behaviors. (See the DSM-IV-TR diagnostic criteria in Box 11-3.)

## Box 11–2 Effective Therapeutic Modalities for People Suffering From Anorexia Nervosa

### Behavioral Therapy

Behavioral therapy is effective in inducing short-term weight gain in anorectic clients; this approach is incorporated into most structured treatment programs for anorexia using an operant conditioning paradigm.

### Cognitive Therapy

Cognitive therapy helps clients challenge the validity of distorted beliefs and perceptions that are perpetuating their illness. The modification of cognitive techniques for the treatment of anorexia nervosa includes examining underlying assumptions, modifying basic assumptions, reinterpreting body image misperceptions, and using the "what if" technique (Dunner, 1997).

### Family Therapy

Family therapy is advocated not as a single mode of treatment, but as an adjunct therapy, especially for anorectic clients with an early age of onset (younger than 18 years). The most commonly found dysfunctional difficulties are enmeshment, rigidity, and failure to resolve conflict. These issues are usually compounded by the pathologic family dynamics that usually develop around the eating problems.

### Individual Psychotherapy

Although most therapists who work with anorectic clients advocate some form of individual psychotherapy, the traditional psychoanalytic approach is thought to be *ineffective* with these clients. Successful psychotherapy needs to be highly interactive, explore relevant issues, educate, negotiate, challenge assumptions underlying anorectic behavior, and encourage the client directly and openly (Dunner, 1997). Themes that are common when treating anorectic clients are:

- Low self-esteem
- Self-hatred
- Perfectionist strivings
- Inner emptiness
- Profound sense of ineffectiveness

| Box 11-3 | DSM-IV-TR Criteria for Bulimia Nervosa |
|---|---|

1. Recurrent episodes of binge eating. An episode of binge eating is characterized by both of the following:
   - Eating in a discrete period of time (e.g., within any 2-hour period) an amount of food that is definitely larger than most people would eat during a similar period of time and under similar circumstances.
   - A sense of lack of control over eating during the episode (e.g., a feeling that one cannot stop eating or control what or how much one is eating).
2. Recurrent inappropriate compensatory behavior in order to prevent weight gain, such as self-induced vomiting; misuse of laxatives, diuretics, enemas, or other medications; fasting; or excessive exercise.
3. The binge-eating and inappropriate compensatory behaviors both occur, on average, at least twice a week for 3 months.
4. Self-evaluation is unduly influenced by body shape and weight.
5. The disturbance does not occur exclusively during episodes of anorexia nervosa.

*Specify Type:*

**Purging type:** During the current episode of bulimia nervosa, the person has regularly engaged in self-induced vomiting or the misuse of laxatives, diuretics, or enemas.

**Nonpurging type:** During the current episode of bulimia nervosa, the person has used other inappropriate compensatory behaviors, such as fasting or excessive exercise, but has not regularly engaged in self-induced vomiting or the misuse of laxatives, diuretics, or enemas.

---

Adapted from American Psychiatric Association. (2000). *Diagnostic and statistical manual of mental disorders* (4th ed., text revision). Washington, DC: American Psychiatric Association, p. 594; reprinted with permission.

Women considered most at risk for bulimia in the United States are Caucasian females between the ages of 14 and 40 years old, although most are in late adolescence or their early 20s. Only 5%–10% of the eating disorder population are males (Stern et al., 2004).

Depressive symptoms often complicate the picture. Suicidal behaviors or self-mutilation behaviors can be associated with depression. Depression usually follows the development of bulimia nervosa (up to 70% of the time). However, in some cases, depression precedes bulimia. Substance abuse (particularly alcohol and stimulants such as cocaine) are often present. A substantial number of bulimic clients have personality features of one or more personality disorders, frequently borderline personality disorder (APA, 2000a). This might account for the prevalence of bulimic individuals who present with dysfunctional personal relationships.

Individuals with bulimia are often more socially skilled and sexually active than clients with anorexia nervosa. The bulimic's bingeing is usually done alone and in secret. In one episode of bingeing, a bulimic can consume more than 5000 calories. Excessive vomiting can lead to severe dehydration and electrolyte imbalance, particularly hypokalemia. Teeth might be discolored or rotten as a result of erosion by gastric acid related to excessive vomiting. Calluses on fingers result from inducing vomiting.

A sense of being out of control accompanies the excessive and/or compulsive consumption of large amounts of food. Binges are usually recurrent and are only interrupted when there is a social interruption, physical pain, or nausea. Poor impulse control can manifest itself in other impulsive behaviors as well (e.g., shoplifting and promiscuity). Following a binge, individuals often experience tremendous guilt, depression, or disgust with themselves. Young women with bulimia nervosa have an obsessive and persistent overconcern with body shape and weight and experience a distortion of body image. That is, they see themselves as too fat or large even when they are near or below normal body weight.

Treatment is provided in an outpatient setting unless there is a physical or psychologic emergency. (Refer to Appendix D-18 for criteria for hospital admittance.)

The clinical course of bulimia nervosa can be either chronic or intermittent, with waxing and waning of symptoms. Many individuals experience the development of other psychiatric or medical problems. Up to 50% of bulimics recover; approximately 25% remain unimproved in follow-up. In addition to suicide, death can occur after severe binging.

# ASSESSMENT

## Presenting Signs and Symptoms

- Enlarged parotid glands
- Dental erosion, caries
- Calluses on dorsum of hands (from manually stimulating vomiting) and/or finger calluses
- Electrolyte imbalance, especially hypokalemia
- Irregular menses
- Fluid retention and/or dehydration
- Hypotension
- Ulcerations around mouth and cheeks (from emesis splashback)
- Chronic hoarseness, chronic sore throat
- Possible cardiac arrhythmias secondary to electrolyte imbalance
- Fatigue and lack of energy
- Gastrointestinal problems (e.g., constipation, diarrhea, reflux, and esophagitis)
- Alkalosis

## Assessment Tools

Refer to Table 11-3 for a comparison of assessment features between anorexia and bulimia.

## Assessment Guidelines

### Bulimia Nervosa

1. Medical stabilization is the first priority. Problems resulting from purging are disruptions in electrolyte and fluid balance and cardiac function. Therefore, a thorough medical examination is vital.
2. Medical evaluation usually includes a thorough physical, as well as interpretation of pertinent laboratory values:
   - Electrolytes
   - Glucose
   - Thyroid function tests
   - Neuroimaging of pituitary gland
   - Complete blood count
   - Electrocardiogram
3. Psychiatric evaluation is advised because treatment of psychiatric comorbidity is important to outcome.

Table 11-3 **Comparison of Characteristics of Anorexia and Bulimia**

| Characteristic | Anorexia— Restricting Type | Bulimia |
|---|---|---|
| Prevalence | Approximately 0.5%-1% for presentations that meet full criteria. Those who are subthreshold for the disorder (eating disorder NOS) are more common. | Approximately 1%-3% among adolescent and young adult females. The disorder in males is about 10% that in females. |
| Appearance | Below 85% of ideal body weight | Normal weight range; might be slightly above or below |
| Onset of illness | Early adolescence with peaks at 14 and 17 years of age | Late adolescence, early adult |
| Physical signs | Thin, emaciated Amenorrhea Slight yellowing of skin Bradycardia Hypotension, hypothermia Peripheral edema Bradycardia, electrocardiogram (ECG) abnormalities | Altered thyroid and cortisol function Enlarged parotid glands Dental erosion, caries Calluses on dorsum of hands from inducing vomiting Electrolyte imbalance, especially hypokalemia Fluid retention Cardiac problems (heart failure, ECG change, cardiomyopathy) Increased blood urea nitrogen |
| Familial patterns | Increased incidence of mood disorders in first-degree relatives | Increased incidence of mood disorders, substance abuse, dependence in first-degree relatives |

Data from American Psychiatric Association. (2000). *Practice guidelines for the treatment of psychiatric disorders: Compendium* 2000. Washington, DC: American Psychiatric Association.

*Continued*

Table 11-3 **Comparison of Characteristics of Anorexia and Bulimia—cont'd**

| Characteristic | Anorexia— Restricting Type | Bulimia |
|---|---|---|
| **Personality traits** | Perfectionism Social isolation | Poor impulse control Low self-esteem |
| **Insight into illness** | Denies seriousness of illness; eating disordered behaviors are egosyntonic | Aware of illness; disturbed behaviors are egodystonic |

# NURSING DIAGNOSES WITH INTERVENTIONS

Individuals with uncomplicated bulimia nervosa are usually treated as outpatients in a clinic setting, a partial hospitalization program, or in private practice. However, hospitalization might be necessary when purging is so severe that it is out of the client's control, or it is causing severe electrolyte and metabolic disturbances. Psychiatric emergencies such as suicidal ideation or uncontrolled substance abuse might also indicate a need for hospitalization.

## Discussion of Potential Nursing Diagnoses

Because electrolyte and fluid balance and cardiac function can be affected, there is a serious potential for **Risk for Injury.** Because bingeing and purging are often felt to be out of the individual's ability to control, **Powerlessness** is an area that needs to be targeted. **Comorbidity with personality disorders** might play a part in treatment, and the reader is encouraged to refer to Chapter 9. If there are issues of **substance abuse,** Chapter 10 might offer some guidelines for care. Because depression is usually present, there is always the concern with the **potential for suicide.** Refer to Chapter 16 for intervention strategies. Refer to Table 11-2 for potential nursing diagnoses for people with eating disorders.

## Overall Guidelines for Nursing Interventions
### Bulimic Individual

1. Often coexisting disorders complicate the clinical picture (depression, substance use, personality disorders), and these might warrant additional psychotherapy (psychodynamic, interpersonal, family therapy).
2. Cognitive-behavioral psychotherapy has been shown to be useful.
3. Group therapy with other individuals suffering from bulimia is often part of successful therapy.
4. Because anxiety and feelings of stress often precede bingeing, alternative ways of dealing with anxiety and alternative coping strategies to lessen anxiety are useful tools.
5. Family therapy is helpful and encouraged.

## Selected Nursing Diagnoses and Nursing Care Plans

### RISK FOR INJURY

At risk of injury as a result of environmental conditions interacting with the individual's adaptive and defensive resources

### Related To (Etiology)

- Uncontrollable binge-purge cycles
- Inadequate coping mechanisms to deal with anxiety and stress
- Coexisting conditions, when not addressed, could cause injury or self-injury (suicidal thoughts, self-multilation, substance abuse)
- Poor impulse control

---

●In addition to NANDA International

## As Evidenced By
## (Assessment Findings/Diagnostic Cues)

- Medical complications
  - ○ Electrolyte imbalances (hypokalemia, hypomagnesemia, hyponatremia, hypocalcemia)
  - ○ Esophageal tears
  - ○ Cardiac problems
  - ○ Altered thyroid and cortisol function
- Overuse of laxatives, diet pills, or diuretics
- Self-destructive behaviors
- Denial of feelings, illness, or problems

## Outcome Criteria

- Binge-purge cycle has ceased
- Normal electrolyte balance is maintained
- Uses supports (individual/group therapy, support groups, etc.) when stressed, to help prevent relapse

## Long-Term Goals

Client will:
- Demonstrate at least four newly learned skills for managing stress and anxiety, shame and guilt, and other triggers that induce compulsive eating
- Abstain from binge-purge behaviors
- Be free of self-directed harm
- Demonstrate ability to recognize and refute dysfunctional thoughts and record in journal
- Obtain and maintain normal electrocardiogram readings
- Verbalize a desire to participate in an ongoing treatment program (support groups or therapy as indicated)
- Express feelings in non–food-related ways

## Short-Term Goals

Client will:
- Remain free of self-directed harm
- Identify and role-play with nurse three alternative ways to deal with anxiety and stress by (date)

---

- In addition to NANDA International

- Identify dysfunctional thoughts that might precede a binge-purge episode, and learn to challenge and refute these thoughts with aid of nurse within 2 weeks
- Identify signs and symptoms of low potassium level and other medical complication that would warrant immediate medical attention within 2 days

## Interventions and Rationales

| Intervention | Rationale |
|---|---|
| 1. Assess for suicidal thoughts and other self-destructive behaviors. | 1. Always be on guard for psychiatric and medical thoughts and emergencies, which take precedence over other forms of treatment. |
| 2. Educate the client regarding the ill effects of self-induced vomiting (low potassium level, dental erosion, cardiac problems). | 2. Health teaching is crucial to treatment. The client needs to be reminded of the benefits of normal eating behavior. |
| 3. Educate the client about the binge-purge cycle and its self-perpetuating nature. | 3. The compulsive nature of the binge-purge cycle maintained by the cycle of restricting, hunger, bingeing, and then purging accompanied by feelings of guilt. Then the cycle begins again. |
| 4. Identify client triggers that induce compulsive eating and purging behaviors. | 4. Work with client to find alternative ways to think and behave when triggers are present. |

| Intervention | Rationale |
|---|---|
| 5. Explore with the client dysfunctional thoughts that precede the binge-purge cycle. Teach clients to refute these thoughts and to reframe them in healthier ways. | 5. Strong rebuttals and nonjudgmental reframing can balance and combat distorted thinking. More rational thinking can lead to healthier behaviors to combat issues of self-esteem, body image, self-worth, and feelings of alienation. |
| 6. Have client record thoughts and refutes in journal and share with nurse. | 6. Recognizing and reviewing with nurse helps reinforce learning. |
| 7. Work with the client to identify problems, and mutually establish short- and long-term goals. | 7. Clients need to develop tools for dealing with personal problems, rather than turning to automatic binge-purge behaviors. |
| 8. Assess and teach problem-solving skills when dealing with client's problem. | 8. Gives the client alternative means of dealing with problems other than binge-purge behaviors. |
| 9. Arrange for the client to learn ways to increase interpersonal communication, socialization, and assertiveness skills. | 9. Client is often isolated from close relationships, and lacks appropriate skills for getting needs met. |
| 10. Encourage attendance at support groups or therapy groups or therapy groups with other bulimic individuals. Provide information for family members as well. | 10. The eating disorders are chronic diseases, and long-term follow-up therapy is critical for success. |

## POWERLESSNESS

Perception that one's own actions will not significantly affect an outcome; a perceived lack of control over a current situation or immediate happening

### Related To (Etiology)

- ▲ Lifestyle of helplessness
- ▲ Interpersonal interaction
- ● Inability to control binge-eating and purging behavior
- ● Severe distortion of body image that perpetuates dysfunctional behavior
- ● Feelings of low self-worth
- ● Insufficient coping skills in dealing with stress and anxiety

### As Evidenced By
### (Assessment Findings/Diagnostic Cues)

- ▲ Verbal expressions of having no control or influence over situations
- ▲ Nonparticipation in care or decision making when opportunities are provided
- ▲ Expression of doubt regarding role performance
- ● Reluctance to express true feelings
- ● Guilt over uncontrollable behavior
- ● Distorted perceptions and beliefs regarding eating and self-image (e.g., "If I gain an ounce, I'll feel fat. Being thin is crucial to my success")

### Outcome Criteria

- • Has a sense of control over life
- • Has a sense of control over personal choices
- • Seeks solution to comorbid issues (e.g., depression, substance abuse) through therapeutic channels

---

▲ NANDA International accepted;  ● In addition to NANDA International

## Long-Term Goals

Client will:
- Verbalize increased feelings of security and autonomy over his/her life
- Identify people and resources in the community for support and follow-up
- State that he/she feels better able to cope with stress and anxiety
- Demonstrate ability to refrain from binge-purge behaviors

## Short-Term Goals

Client will:
- Keep a journal of thoughts and feelings and learn to identify automatic thoughts and beliefs that trigger binge-purge behaviors by (date)
- Review journal with nurse/counselor on a weekly basis (clinic)
- Demonstrate the ability to dispute dysfunctional negative thoughts about self and abilities by (date)
- Demonstrate ability to do a realistic self-appraisal of strengths by (date)

## Interventions and Rationales

| Intervention | Rationale |
|---|---|
| 1. Explore the client's experience of out-of-control eating behavior. | 1. Listening in an empathetic, nonjudgmental manner helps clients feel that someone understands their experience. |
| 2. Encourage the client to keep a journal of thoughts and feelings surrounding binge-purge behaviors. | 2. Automatic thoughts and beliefs maintain the binge-purge cycle. A journal is an excellent way to identify these dysfunctional thoughts and underlying assumptions. |

| Intervention | Rationale |
|---|---|
| 3. Teach or refer to a counselor who can teach client how to challenge dysfunctional thoughts and beliefs in a systematic manner. | 3. These automatic dysfunctional thoughts must be examined and challenged if change in client thinking and behavior is to occur. |
| 4. Review with the client the kinds of cognitive distortions that affect feelings, beliefs, and behavior. | 4. Cognitive distortions reinforce unrealistic views of self in terms of strengths and future potential. Realistic self-views are necessary for change to occur. |
| 5. Encourage client's participation in decisions and client's responsibility in his or her care and future. | 5. Helps clients gain a sense of control over their lives, and realize that they have options to make important changes in their lives. |
| 6. Teach client alternative stress-reduction techniques and visualization skills to improve self-confidence and feelings of self-worth. | 6. Visualizing a positive self-image and positive outcomes for life goals stimulates problem-solving toward desired goals. |
| 7. Role-play new skills. Encourage client to apply new skills in individual and group therapy in communications with others, particularly family. | 7. Role-play allows the opportunity for client to become comfortable with new and different ways of relating and responding to others in a safe environment. |
| 8. Teach the client that one lapse is not a relapse. One slip of control does not eliminate all positive accomplishments. | 8. At time of lapse, it is helpful to examine what led to the lapse, knowing that one lapse does not eliminate all positive accomplishments. |

# MEDICAL TREATMENTS

## Psychopharmacology

No drug has been proven effective by itself or as an adjunct for treating bulimia nervosa. *Antidepressants* have been used with bulimia nervosa. In particular, the selective serotonin reuptake inhibitors (SSRIs) have been well studied, and are currently considered the safest. They are particularly helpful for those clients who suffer with depression, anxiety, obsessions, or certain impulse disorder symptoms (APA, 2000b). Fluoxetine has been shown to positively affect the binge-purge cycle in some bulimic clients. In particular, the SSRIs can be effective with highly obsessional clients as well as clients who are depressed. The SSRIs can also help carbohydrate cravings and mood disturbances that are associated with bulimia nervosa and obesity (Schatzberg et al., 1997).

It is now believed that a combination of psychotherapeutic intervention and medication results in higher remission rates (APA, 2000b).

## Psychosocial

Currently, cognitive behavioral psychotherapy is the psychosocial treatment that is the most useful. Controlled trials have shown that interpersonal psychotherapy has also been effective. Also, an important intervention modality is family therapy, especially for adolescents who still live with parents (APA, 2000b).

---

Box 11-4 **Do's and Don'ts of Helping Someone Recover from an Eating Disorder**

*This information is provided by the National Association of Anorexia Nervosa and Associated Disorders (ANAD).*
Do:

- Gently encourage her to eat properly.
- Express your love and support.
- Try to understand, although this seems impossible.
- Take time to listen, although the talk might seem trivial or insignificant to you.
- Try to see how she (and each family member) perceives the situation.

## Box 11-4 Do's and Don'ts of Helping Someone Recover from an Eating Disorder—cont'd

- Realize that she is terrified of gaining weight and being fat, although she might actually be underweight. These irrational fears are real to her.
- Emphasize her positive, good characteristics, and compliment her on all the things she does right.
- Encourage her to accept support and honestly express her feelings.
- Talk honestly and sincerely, with love and understanding.
- Recognize that other, nonfood factors are at the heart of the problem.
- Help her find someone to support her, who knows what she is going through.
- Realize that, although she must have help from others, she must want to get better, and she needs to love herself.

Don't:

- Try to force her to eat or stop exercising.
- Get angry or punish her.
- Be impatient (this is really tough).
- Lecture.
- Be too busy, even if you have to give up "important" things.
- Jump to conclusions or see things only through your eyes and mind.
- Make her feel bad or guilty for having an eating disorder.
- Spy on her.
- Place the blame on anyone.
- Be afraid to talk about problems.
- Pretend it will all just go away.
- Expect an instant recovery.
- Let her feel she is the only one with this problem.

Do all that you can to help her realize what a beautiful person she really is.

## CLIENT AND FAMILY TEACHING

The National Association of Anorexia Nervosa and Associated Disorders (ANAD) has provided information that families and friends might find helpful in their dealings with a person with an eating disorder (Box 11-4).

### NURSE, CLIENT, AND FAMILY RESOURCES

## ASSOCIATIONS

**American Anorexia/Bulimia Association**
165 West 46th Street, Suite 1108
New York, NY 10036
(212) 575-6200
For people with eating disorders

**National Association of Anorexia Nervosa and Associated Disorders (ANAD)**
PO Box 7
Highland Park, IL 60035
(847) 831-3438
For people with eating disorders

**National Eating Disorders Association**
603 Stewart Street, Suite 803
Seattle, WA 98101
(206) 382-3438
http://www.nationaleatingdisorders.org
For people with eating disorders, their families, and their friends

## INTERNET SITES

**Mirror Mirror Eating Disorders Home Page**
http://www.mirror-mirror.org/eatdis.htm

**Anorexia Nervosa and Related Eating Disorders, Inc.**
http://www.anred.com

**Healthtouch Online**
http://www.healthtouch.com

# CHAPTER 12

# Cognitive Disorders: Delirium and Dementia

## OVERVIEW

**Delirium** is usually characterized by a sudden disturbance of consciousness and a change in cognition, such as impaired attention span and disturbances of consciousness (American Psychiatric Association [APA], 2000). Delirium is always secondary to another condition, such as a general medical condition (i.e., infections, diabetes), or is substance induced (drugs, medications, or toxins); delirium can also have multiple causes. Delirium is usually a transitory condition and reversed when interventions are timely. Prolonged delirium can lead to dementia.

**Dementia** develops more slowly and is characterized by multiple cognitive deficits that include impairment in short-term and long-term memory. Dementia is usually irreversible. Dementia can be primary, or secondary to another condition. Refer to Table 12-3 for a side-by-side comparison of the characteristics of delirium and dementia.

## Delirium

Box 12-1 presents the *Diagnostic and Statistical Manual of Mental Disorders* (4th edition, text revision) (DSM-IV-TR) diagnostic criteria for delirium.

| Box 12-1 | DSM-IV-TR Criteria for Delirium |
|---|---|

1. Disturbance of consciousness (i.e., reduced clarity of awareness of the environment with reduced ability to focus, sustain, or shift attention).
2. A change in cognition (memory deficit, disorientation, language disturbance) or the development of a perceptual disturbance that is not better accounted for by a preexisting, established, or evolving dementia.
3. The disturbance develops over a short period of time (usually hours to days) and tends to fluctuate during the course of the day.
4. The disturbance is due to:
   • A general medical condition, *or*
   • Substance-induced (intoxication or withdrawal), *or*
   • Multiple etiologies (both of the above causes), *or*
   • Not known (not otherwise specified).

Adapted from American Psychiatric Association. (2000). *Diagnostic and statistical manual of mental disorders* (4th ed., text revision). Washington, DC: American Psychiatric Association, pp. 143-147; reprinted with permission.

Because delirium is always secondary to medical disorder or toxicity, delirium is often seen on medical and surgical units. Delirium is often experienced by elderly clients, children with high fevers, postoperative clients, and clients with cerebrovascular disease and congestive heart failure. Delirium can occur in people with infections, metabolic disorders, drug intoxications and withdrawals, medication toxicity, neurologic diseases, tumors, and certain psychosocial stressors. Delirium is important to recognize because, if it continues without intervention, irreversible brain damage can occur.

## ASSESSMENT

### Presenting Signs and Symptoms

- Fluctuating levels of consciousness. The individual might be disoriented and severely confused at night and during early morning hours **(sundowning),** and remain lucid during the day.
- Impaired ability to reason and carry out goal-directed behavior

- Alternating patterns of *hyperactivity* to *hypoactivity* (slow down activity to stupor or coma)
- Behaviors seen when **hyperactive** include:
  - Hypervigilance
  - Restlessness
  - Incoherent, loud, or rapid speech
  - Irritability
  - Anger and/or combativeness
  - Profanity
  - Euphoria
  - Distractibility
  - Tangentiality
  - Nightmares
  - Persistent abnormal thoughts (delusions)
- Behaviors seen when **hypoactive** include:
  - Lethargy
  - Speaks and moves little or slowly
  - Has spells of staring
  - Reduced alertness
  - Generalized loss of awareness of the environment
- Impaired attention span
- Cognitive changes not accounted for by dementia:
  - Memory impairment
  - Disorientation to time and place
  - Language disturbance; might be incoherent
  - Perceptual disturbance (hallucinations and illusions)
- Alterations in sleep-wake patterns
- Fear and high levels of anxiety

## Assessment Tools

When assessing individuals with confusional states, it is helpful to use structured cognitive screening tests such as the Folstein Mini Mental State Exam or the Functional Dementia Scale. (The latter may be found in Appendix D-9.)

## Assessment Guidelines

*Delirium*

1. Assess for fluctuating levels of consciousness, which is key in delirium.
2. Interview family or other caregivers.

3. Assess for past confusional states (e.g., prior dementia diagnosis).
4. Identify other disturbances in medical status (e.g., dyspnea, edema, presence of jaundice).
5. Identify any electroencephalogram (EEG), neuroimaging, or lab abnormalities in client's record.
6. Assess vital signs, level of consciousness, and neurologic signs.
7. Ask the client (when lucid) or family what they think could be responsible for the delirium (e.g., medications, withdrawal of substance, other medical condition).
8. Assess potential for injury (is the client safe from falls, wandering).
9. Assess need for comfort measures (pain, cold, positioning).
10. Are immediate medical interventions available to help prevent irreversible brain damage?

# NURSING DIAGNOSES WITH INTERVENTIONS

## Discussion of Potential Nursing Diagnoses

Individuals experiencing delirium often misinterpret environmental cues **(illusions)** or imagine they see things **(hallucinations)** that they most likely believe are threatening or harmful. When clients act on these interpretations of their environment, they are likely to demonstrate a **Risk for Injury.** The symptoms of confusion usually fluctuate, and nighttime is the most severe (this is often called sundowning). Therefore, these clients often have **Disturbed Sleep Pattern.** During times of severe confusion, individuals are usually terrified, and cannot care for their needs or interact appropriately with others, so **Fear, Self-Care Deficit**, and **Impaired Social Interaction** are also potential diagnoses. This section on delirium concerns **Acute Confusion**, which covers many of the above problems.

**Please note that many of the interventions, especially those for communication with the client with delirium when confused, are also applicable to the client with dementia when confused.** Table 12-1 identifies potential nursing diagnoses useful for all confused clients (delirium or dementia).

Table 12-1 **Potential Nursing Diagnoses for the Confused Client**

| Symptoms | Nursing Diagnoses |
| --- | --- |
| Wandering, unsteady gait; acts out fear from hallucinations or illusions; forgets things (leaves stove on, doors open) | **Risk for Injury** |
| Awakes disoriented during the night (sundowning), frightened at night | **Disturbed Sleep Pattern** **Fear** **Acute Confusion** |
| Too confused to take care of basic needs | **Self-Care Deficit** **Ineffective Coping** **Urinary Incontinence** **Imbalanced Nutrition** **Deficient Fluid Volume** |
| Sees frightening things that are not there **(hallucinations)**, mistakes everyday objects for something sinister and frightening (illusions), might become paranoid, thinking that others are doing things to confuse them **(delusions)** | **Disturbed Sensory Perception** **Impaired Environmental Interpretation Syndrome** **Disturbed Thought Processes** |
| Does not recognize familiar people or places, has difficulty with short- and/or long-term memory, forgetful and confused | **Impaired Memory** **Impaired Environmental Interpretation Syndrome** **Acute Confusion** **Chronic Confusion** |
| Difficulty with communication, cannot find words, difficulty in recognizing objects and/or people, incoherence | **Impaired Verbal Communication** |
| Devastated over losing their place in life as they know it (during lucid moments); fearful and overwhelmed by what is happening to them | **Spiritual Distress** **Hopelessness** **Situational Low Self-Esteem** **Grieving** |
| Family and loved ones overburdened and overwhelmed; unable to care for client's needs | **Disabled Family Coping** **Compromised Family Coping** **Interrupted Family Processes** **Impaired Home Maintenance** **Caregiver Role Strain** |

## Overall Guidelines for Nursing Interventions

### Delirium

1. Delirium, unlike dementia, is transitory when interventions are instituted and if delirium does not last a prolonged period of time. Therefore, **immediate intervention** for the underlying cause of the delirium is needed to prevent irreversible damage to the brain. Medical interventions are the first priority.

2. When clients are confused and frightened and are having a difficult time interpreting reality, they might be prone to accidents. Therefore, **Safety** is a high priority.

3. Delirium is a terrifying experience for many clients. When some individuals recover to their premorbid cognitive function, they are left with frightening memories and images. Some clinicians advocate preventive counseling and education after recovery from acute brain failure (Borson, 1997).

4. Refrain from using restraints. Encourage one or two significant others to stay with client to provide orientation and comfort.

## Selected Nursing Diagnoses and Nursing Care Plans

### ACUTE CONFUSION

Abrupt onset of a cluster of global, transient changes and disturbances in attention, cognition, psychomotor activity, level of consciousness, and/or sleep/wake cycle

### Related To (Etiology)

- ▲ Age older than 60 years
- ▲ Dementia
- ▲ Alcohol abuse
- ▲ Drug abuse
- ▲ Delirium
- ● Metabolic disorder, neurologic disorder, chemicals, medications, infections, fluid and electrolyte imbalances

▲ NANDA International accepted; ● In addition to NANDA International

## As Evidenced By (Assessment Findings/Diagnostic Cues)

▲ Fluctuation in cognition
▲ Fluctuation in sleep-wake cycle
▲ Fluctuation in level of consciousness
▲ Agitation or restlessness
▲ Misperceptions of the environment (e.g., illusions, hallucinations)
▲ Lack of motivation to initiate and/or follow through with goal-directed or purposeful behavior

## Outcome Criteria

• Oriented to time, place, and person
• Resume usual cognitive and physical activities
• Absence of untoward effects from episode of delirium

## Long-Term Goals

• Client will correctly state time/place and person within a few days
• Client will remain free of injury (e.g., falls) throughout client's periods of confusion

## Short-Term Goals

• Client and others will remain safe during client's periods of agitation or aggressive behaviors
• Clients will respond positively to staff efforts to orient them to time/place and person throughout periods of confusion
• Clients will take medication as offered to help alleviate their condition

## Interventions and Rationales

| Intervention | Rationale |
|---|---|
| 1. Introduce self and call client by name at the beginning of each contact. | 1. With short-term memory impairment, person is often confused and needs frequent orienting to time, place, and person. |

▲ NANDA International accepted

| Intervention | Rationale |
|---|---|
| 2. Maintain face-to-face contact. | 2. If client is easily distracted, he or she needs help to focus on one stimulus at a time. |
| 3. Use short, simple, concrete phrases. | 3. Client might not be able to process complex information. |
| 4. Briefly explain everything you are going to do before doing it. | 4. Explanation prevents misinterpretation of action. |
| 5. Encourage the family and friends (one at a time) to take a quiet, supportive role. | 5. Familiar presence lowers anxiety and increases orientation. |
| 6. Keep room well lit. | 6. Lighting provides accurate environmental stimuli to maintain and increase orientation. |
| 7. Keep environment noise to a minimum (e.g., television, visitors). | 7. Noise can be misconstrued into something frightening or threatening. |
| 8. Keep head of bed elevated. | 8. Helps provide important environmental cues. |
| 9. Provide clocks and calendars. | 9. These cues help orient client to time. |
| 10. Encourage client to wear prescribed eye glasses or hearing aid. | 10. Helps increase accurate perceptions of visual, auditory stimuli. |
| 11. Make an effort to assign the same personnel on each shift to care for client. | 11. Familiar faces minimize confusion and enhance nurse-client relationships. |
| 12. When *hallucinations* are present, assure clients they are safe (e.g., "I know you are frightened. I'll sit with you a while and make sure you are safe."). | 12. Client feels reassured that he or she is safe, and fear and anxiety often decrease. |

| Intervention | Rationale |
|---|---|
| 13. When *illusions* are present, clarify reality (e.g., "This is a coat rack, not a man with a knife . . . see? You seem frightened. I'll stay with you for a while."). | 13. With illusion, misinterpreted objects or sounds can be clarified, once pointed out. |
| 14. Inform client of progress during lucid intervals. | 14. Consciousness fluctuates: client feels less anxious knowing where he or she is and who you are during lucid periods. |
| 15. Ignore insults and name calling, and acknowledge how upset the person might be feeling. For example: *Client:* You incompetent jerk! Get me a real nurse, someone who knows what they are doing. *Nurse:* What you are going through is very difficult. I'll stay with you. | 15. Terror and fear are often projected onto the environment. Arguing or becoming defensive only increases client's aggressive behaviors and defenses. |
| 16. If client behavior becomes physically abusive: <br> a. *First*, set limits on behavior (e.g., "Mr. Jones, you are not to hit me or anyone else. Tell me how you feel." *or* "Mr. Jones, if you have difficulty controlling your actions, we will help you gain control."). | 16. Clear limits need to be set to protect client, staff, and others. Often client can respond to verbal commands. Chemical and physical restraints are used as a last resort, if at all. |

| Intervention | Rationale |
|---|---|
| b. *Second*, check orders for use of chemical restraint. | |
| 17. After client returns to premorbid cognitive state, educate client and offer counseling for client's recollection of terrifying, frightening memories and images. | 17. Client can believe his or her illusions or hallucinations were real, and it may take time for client to come to terms with the experience. |

## DEMENTIA

Dementia is marked by progressive deterioration in intellectual function, memory, and ability to solve problems and learn new skills. Judgment and moral and ethical behaviors decline as personality is altered. Box 12-2 presents the DSM-IV-TR diagnostic criteria for dementia.

Unlike delirium, dementia can be of a primary nature and is usually *NOT* reversible. Dementia is usually a slow and insidious process progressing over months or years. Dementia affects memory and ability to learn new information, or to recall previously learned information. Dementia also compromises intellectual functioning and the ability to solve problems. Common causes of dementia are:

- Vascular dementia (multi-infarct)
- HIV disease
- Head trauma
- Parkinson's disease
- Huntington's disease
- Pick's disease
- Creutzfeldt-Jakob disease
- General medical condition (brain tumors, subdural hematoma, etc.)
- Substance use

However, the most prevalent primary dementia is **dementia of the Alzheimer's type (DAT)**. The second most common form of dementia is vascular dementia, which is caused by multiple strokes. As mentioned above, substances can also cause dementia (alcohol, inhalants, phencyclidine, piperidine), as can other medical conditions.

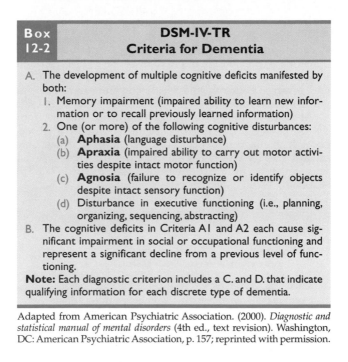

| Box 12-2 | **DSM-IV-TR**<br>**Criteria for Dementia** |
|---|---|

A. The development of multiple cognitive deficits manifested by both:

  1. Memory impairment (impaired ability to learn new information or to recall previously learned information)

  2. One (or more) of the following cognitive disturbances:

    (a) **Aphasia** (language disturbance)

    (b) **Apraxia** (impaired ability to carry out motor activities despite intact motor function)

    (c) **Agnosia** (failure to recognize or identify objects despite intact sensory function)

    (d) Disturbance in executive functioning (i.e., planning, organizing, sequencing, abstracting)

B. The cognitive deficits in Criteria A1 and A2 each cause significant impairment in social or occupational functioning and represent a significant decline from a previous level of functioning.

**Note:** Each diagnostic criterion includes a C. and D. that indicate qualifying information for each discrete type of dementia.

Adapted from American Psychiatric Association. (2000). *Diagnostic and statistical manual of mental disorders* (4th ed., text revision). Washington, DC: American Psychiatric Association, p. 157; reprinted with permission.

## ASSESSMENT

### Presenting Signs and Symptoms

- Memory impairment, usually short-term at first
- Cognitive impairment:
  - **Aphasia:** language disturbance, difficulty finding words, using words incorrectly
  - **Apraxia:** inability to carry out motor activities despite motor functions being intact (e.g., putting on one's pants, blouse, etc.)
  - **Agnosia:** loss of sensory ability; inability to recognize or identify familiar objects, such as a toothbrush, or sounds, such as the ringing of the phone; loses ability to problem-solve, plan, organize, or abstract
- A significant decline in previous level of functioning; poor judgment
- Mood disturbances, anxiety, hallucinations, delusions, and impaired sleep often accompany dementia

## Assessment Tools

A variety of other medical problems can masquerade as dementia. For example, depression in the elderly is often misdiagnosed as dementia. Table 12-2 highlights the difference between dementia and depression and can be a useful guide for assessment.

At times it is important to distinguish dementia from delirium. Table 12-3 helps the nurse identify differences in the symptoms between one and the other. One always has to keep in mind that delirium can coexist with dementia, and that often clouds the picture. Refer to Appendix D-9.

Table 12-2 **Dementia versus Depression**

| Dementia | Depression |
| --- | --- |
| 1. Recent memory is impaired. In early stages, patient attempts to hide cognitive losses; is skillful at covering up. | 1. Patient readily admits to memory loss; other cognitive disturbances might be present. |
| 2. Symptoms progress slowly and insidiously; difficult to pinpoint onset. | 2. Symptoms are of relatively rapid onset. |
| 3. Approximate or "near-miss" answers are typical; tries to answer. | 3. "Don't know" answers are common; client does not try to recall or answer. |
| 4. Client struggles to perform well but is frustrated. | 4. Little effort to perform; is apathetic; seems helpless and pessimistic. |
| 5. Affect is shallow or labile. | 5. Depressive mood is pervasive. |
| 6. Attention and concentration might be impaired. | 6. Attention and concentration are usually intact. |
| 7. Changes in personality (e.g., from cheerful and easygoing to angry and suspicious). | 7. Personality remains stable. |

From Varcarolis, E. (1998). *Foundations of psychiatric mental health nursing* (3rd ed.). Philadelphia, WB Saunders, p. 694; reprinted with permission.

Table 12-3 **Nursing Assessment: Delirium versus Dementia**

| | Delirium | Dementia |
|---|---|---|
| Onset | Acute impairment of orientation, memory, intellectual function, judgment, and affect. | Slow insidious deterioration in cognitive functioning. |
| Essential feature | Disturbance in consciousness, fluctuating levels of consciousness, and cognitive impairment. | Progressive deterioration in memory, orientation, calculation, and judgment; symptoms do not fluctuate. |
| Cause | The syndrome is secondary to many underlying disorders that cause temporary, diffuse disturbances of brain function. | The syndrome is either *primary* in etiology or *secondary* to other disease states or conditions. |
| Course | The clinical course is usually brief (hours to days); prolonged delirium may lead to dementia. | Progresses over months or years; often irreversible. |
| Speech | May be slurred; reflects disorganized thinking. | Generally normal in early stages; progressive aphasia; confabulation. |
| Memory | Short-term memory impaired. | Short-term, then long-term, memory destroyed. |
| Perception | Visual or tactile hallucinations; illusions. | Hallucinations not prominent. |
| Mood | Fear, anxiety, and irritability most prominent. | Mood labile; previous personality traits become accentuated (e.g., paranoid, depressed, withdrawn, and obsessive-compulsive). |
| Electroencephalogram | Pronounced diffuse slowing or fast cycles. | Normal or mildly slow. |

From Varcarolis, E. (2002). *Foundations of psychiatric mental health nursing* (4th ed.). Philadelphia: WB Saunders, p. 694; reprinted with permission.

## Assessment Guidelines

*Dementia*

1. Identify the underlying cause; for example, does the client have a history of
   - Depression
   - Substance abuse
   - Pernicious anemia

   See Box 12-3 for laboratory tests that might help root out possible causes.
2. How well is the family prepared and informed about the progress of the client's dementia (e.g., the phases and course of Alzheimer's disease [AD], vascular dementia, AIDS-related dementia, multiple sclerosis, lupus, brain injury)?
3. How is the family coping with the client? What are the main issues at this time?
4. What resources are available to the family? Does the family get help from other family members, friends, and community resources? Are the caregivers aware of community support groups and resources?
5. Obtain the data necessary to provide appropriate safety measures for the client.
6. How safe is the client's home environment (e.g., wandering, eating inedible objects, falls, provocative behaviors toward others)?
7. For what client behaviors could the family use teaching and guidance (e.g., catastrophic reaction, lability of mood, aggressive behaviors, nocturnal delirium [increased confusion and agitation at night; sundowning])?
8. Identify family supports in the community.

# NURSING DIAGNOSES WITH INTERVENTIONS

## Discussion of Potential Nursing Diagnoses

The care of a client with dementia requires a great deal of patience and creativity. These clients have enormous needs, and put enormous demands on staff caring for demented clients, and on families who carry the burden at home. As some of these diseases progress, most notably AD, so do the demands on the staff, caregivers, and family. Safety is

---

Box 12-3 **Basic Workup for Dementia**

- Chest and skull radiograph studies
- Electroencephalography
- Electrocardiography
- Urinalysis
- Sequential multiple analyzer: 12-test serum profile
- Thyroid function tests
- Folate levels
- Venereal Disease Research Laboratories (VDRL), HIV tests
- Serum creatine assay
- Electrolyte assessment
- Vitamin $B_{12}$ levels
- Vision and hearing evaluation
- Neuroimaging (when diagnostic issues are not clear)

---

always a major concern. **Risk for Injury** might be related to impaired mobility, sensory deficits, history of accidents, or lack of knowledge of safety precautions.

As time goes on, the person loses the ability to perform tasks that were once familiar and routine. The inability of the person to care for basic needs covers all areas (e.g., bathing, hygiene, grooming, feeding, and toileting). Therefore, **Self-Care Deficit** usually involves many functions. The goals are set up so that individuals can do as much for themselves as possible during each phase of the dementia.

**Impaired Verbal Communication** is often related to diminished comprehension, difficulty recognizing objects, aphasia, cerebral impairment, and severe memory impairment. Therefore, family and health care workers need to know ways to interact with a person with this nursing diagnosis.

The burden of caring for a family member with dementia can be enormous, especially over prolonged periods of time. Family members need a great deal of support, education, and guidance from community agencies and well-informed health care workers. Families might experience **Disabled Family Coping**, which should always be addressed when it is recognized. Therefore, **Risk for** and/or **Caregiver Role Strain** should be part of the initial assessment, and must be continuously assessed as the dementia progresses. Most families will need information, support, and periods of respite.

There are numerous nursing diagnoses that might be appropriate. Refer back to Table 12-1 for nursing diagnoses appropriate for confused clients.

## Overall Guidelines for Nursing Interventions

1. Educate family on safety features for impaired family member living at home—for example:
   a. Precautions for wandering (e.g., Medic-Alert bracelet, "Home Safe Program," effective locks)
   b. Home safety features (e.g., eliminating slippery rugs, labeling of rooms and drawers, installing complex locks on top of doors)
   c. Self-care guidelines on maintaining optimum nutrition, bowel and bladder training, optimum sleep patterns, and working to optimum ability in activities of daily living
2. Educate family (and staff) on effective communication strategies with a confused client, for example:
   a. Teaching alternative modes of communication when client is aphasic
   b. Teaching basic communication techniques with confused clients (for example: introduce self each time; use simple, short sentences; maintain eye contact; focus on one topic at a time; talk about familiar and simple topics)
3. **Family/caregiver support is a priority.** Provide names and telephone numbers of support groups, respite care, day care, protective services, recreational services, Meals on Wheels, hospice services, and so on that are within the family/caregivers community. Encourage the use of support groups for caregivers.
4. Provide family with information on all medications client is taking (use for each, potential side and toxic effects, any interactions that could occur) and name and number of whom to call with future questions.

## Selected Nursing Diagnoses and Nursing Care Plans

### RISK FOR INJURY

At risk of injury as a result of environmental conditions interacting with the individual's adaptive and defensive resources

## Related To (Etiology)

- ▲ Sensory dysfunction
- ▲ Cognitive or emotional difficulties
- ▲ Chemical (drugs, alcohol)
- ▲ Biochemical
- ● Confusion, disorientation
- ● Faulty judgment
- ● Loss of short-term memory
- ● Lack of knowledge of safety precautions
- ● Previous falls
- ● Unsteady gait
- ● Wandering
- ● Provocative behavior

## As Evidenced By (Assessment Findings/Diagnostic Cues)

- ● Getting into fights with others
- ● Choking on inedible object
- ● Wandering
- ● Burns
- ● Falls
- ● Getting lost
- ● Poisoning—wrong medication, wrong dose

## Outcome Criteria

- Highest level of functioning will be supported
- Optimum health is maintained (nutrition, sleep, elimination)
- Free of fractures, bruises, contusions, burns, and falls

## Long-Term Goals

- With guidance and environmental manipulation, client will not hurt himself/herself if falls occur
- With the aid of an identification bracelet, neighborhood or hospital alert, and enrollment in the Safe Return Program, client will be returned within 3 hours of wandering
- Client will ingest only correct doses of prescribed medication and appropriate food and fluids

▲NANDA International accepted; ● In addition to NANDA International

*Short-Term Goals*

- Client will remain injury free whether at home or in the hospital with the aid of environmental manipulation and family or nursing staff precautions and interventions

*Interventions and Rationales*

| Intervention | Rationale |
|---|---|
| **Safe Environment** | |
| 1. Restrict driving. | 1. Impaired judgment can lead to accidents. |
| 2. Remove throw rugs and other objects. | 2. Minimizes tripping and falling. |
| 3. Minimize sensory stimulation. | 3. Decreases sensory overload, which can increase anxiety and confusion. |
| 4. If clients become verbally upset, listen briefly, give support, then change the topic. | 4. When attention span is short, clients can be distracted to more productive topics and activities. |
| 5. Label all rooms and drawers with pictures. Label often-used objects (e.g., hairbrushes and toothbrushes). | 5. Might keep client from wandering into other client's rooms. Increases environmental clues to familiar objects. |
| 6. Install safety bars in bathroom. | 6. Prevents falls. |
| 7. Supervise clients when they smoke. | 7. Danger of burns is always present. |
| 8. If client wanders during the night, put mattress on the floor. | 8. Prevents falls when client is confused. |
| 9. Have client wear Medic-Alert bracelet that cannot be removed (with name, address, and telephone number). Provide police department with recent pictures. | 9. Client can easily be identified by police, neighbors, or hospital personnel. |

| Intervention | Rationale |
|---|---|
| 10. Alert local police and neighbors about wanderer. | 10. Can reduce time necessary to return client to home or hospital. |
| 11. Put complex locks on door. | 11. Reduces opportunity to wander. |
| 12. Place locks at top of door. | 12. In moderate and late DAT, ability to look up and reach upward is lost. |
| 13. Encourage physical activity during the day. | 13. Physical activity during the day might decrease wandering at night. |
| 14. Explore the feasibility of sensor devices. | 14. Provides warning if installing client wanders. |
| 15. Enroll the client in the Alzheimer's Association's Safe Return program *(www.alz.org)*. | 15. Helps track individuals with dementia who wander and are at risk of getting lost or injured. |

## SELF-CARE DEFICIT

Impaired ability to perform or complete feeding, bathing, toileting, dressing, and grooming activities for oneself

### *Related To (Etiology)*

▲ Perceptual or cognitive impairment
▲ Neuromuscular impairment
▲ Decreased strength and endurance
▲ Confusion
● Apraxia (inability to perform tasks that were once routine)
● Severe memory impairment

### *As Evidenced By (Assessment Findings/Diagnostic Cues)*

▲ Inability to wash properly
▲ Impaired ability to put on or take off necessary items of clothing

▲ NANDA International accepted; ● In addition to NANDA International

▲ Inability to maintain appearance at a satisfactory level
▲ Inability to get to toilet or commode
▲ Inability to carry out proper toilet hygiene

### Outcome Criteria

• Client's self-care needs will be met with optimal participation by client

### Long-Term Goals

• Client will participate in self-care at optimal level with supervision and guidance
• Client's skin will remain intact despite incontinence or prolonged pressure
• Client will maintain nutrition, hygiene, dress, and toileting activities with appropriate support from others (e.g., caregivers, family, staff)

### Short-Term Goals

Client will:
• Be able to follow step-by-step instructions for dressing, bathing, and grooming
• Put on own clothes appropriately with aid of fastening tape (Velcro) and supervision
• Participate in toilet training procedures daily
• Ingest adequate calories (1500 to 2200 calories/day)
• Maintain an adequate fluid intake (2400 to 3200 ml/day)

### Interventions and Rationales

| Intervention | Rationale |
|---|---|
| **Dressing and Bathing** | |
| 1. Always have clients perform all tasks that they are capable of. | 1. Maintains self-esteem, uses muscle groups, and minimizes further regression. |
| 2. Always have client wear own clothes, even if in the hospital. | 2. Helps maintain client's identity and dignity. |

▲ NANDA International accepted

| Intervention | Rationale |
|---|---|
| 3. Use clothing with elastic, and substitute fastening tape (Velcro) for buttons and zippers. | 3. Minimizes client's confusion, and increases independence of functioning. |
| 4. Label clothing items with name and name of item. | 4. Helps identify clients if they wander, and gives caregivers additional clues when aphasia or agnosia occurs. |
| 5. Give step-by-step instructions whenever necessary (e.g., "Take this blouse . . . put in one arm . . . now the next arm . . . pull it together in the front . . . now . . ."). | 5. Client can focus on small pieces of information more easily; allows client to perform at optimum level. |

**Nutrition**

| | |
|---|---|
| 1. Monitor food and fluid intake. | 1. Client might have anorexia or be too confused to eat. |
| 2. Offer finger food that client can walk around with. | 2. Increases input throughout the day; client might eat only small amounts at meals. |
| 3. During period of hyperorality, watch that client does not eat nonfood items (e.g., ceramic fruit or food-shaped soaps). | 3. Client puts everything into mouth; might be unable to differentiate inedible objects. |

**Bowel and Bladder Function**

| | |
|---|---|
| 1. Begin bowel and bladder program early; start with bladder control. | 1. Same time of day for bowel movements and toileting—in early morning, after meals and snacks, and before bedtime—can help prevent incontinence. |

2. Evaluate use of adult disposable undergarments.
3. Label bathroom door, as well as doors to other rooms, with a picture.

2. Prevents embarrassment if incontinent.
3. Additional environmental clues can maximize independent toileting. Pictures are more readily interpreted.

**Sleep**

1. Because client might awaken frightened and disoriented at night, keep area well lit.
2. Nonbarbiturates might be ordered (e.g., chloral hydrate).
3. Avoid the use of restraints.

1. Reinforces orientation, minimizes possible illusions.
2. Barbiturates can have a paradoxical reaction, causing agitation.
3. Can cause client to become more terrified and fight against restraints until exhausted to a dangerous degree.

---

## IMPAIRED VERBAL COMMUNICATION

Decreased, delayed, or absent ability to receive, process, transmit and use a system of symbols

---

*Related To (Etiology)*

▲ Decrease in circulation to the brain
▲ Physical barrier (e.g., brain tumor, subdural hematoma)
▲ Deterioration or damage to the neurologic centers in the brain that regulate speech and language
▲ Biochemical changes in the brain/physiologic conditions
● Severe memory impairment
● Escalating anxiety
● Delusions or illusions

---

▲ NANDA International accepted; ● In addition to NANDA International

## As Evidenced By
### (Assessment Findings/Diagnostic Cues)

- ▲ Difficulty forming words or sentences
- ▲ Difficulty expressing thoughts verbally
- ▲ Speaks or verbalizes with difficulty
- ▲ Does not or cannot speak
- ▲ Has difficulty finding the right word for objects (aphasia)
- ● Has difficulty identifying objects (agnosia)
- ● Inability to focus or concentrate on a train of thought
- ● Impaired comprehension
- ● Refers back to first language

## Outcome Criteria

- Communicates with aid of variety of verbal and nonverbal techniques for optimum period of time

## Long-Term Goals

- Client will communicate basic needs with the use of visual and verbal clues when needed
- Client will communicate important thoughts with the use of visual and verbal clues when needed
- Client's family and caregivers demonstrate ability to minimize client's agitation and fear when client is delusional or having illusions

## Short-Term Goals

- Client's basic needs will be met when in the hospital (hydration and nutrition, hygiene, dress, bowel and bladder function)
- Client will learn to adopt alternative modes of communication with the use of nonverbal techniques (e.g., writing, pointing, demonstrating an action [pantomime])
- Client's anxiety and fear will be decreased when delusions or illusions occur through the use of appropriate nursing techniques

---

▲ NANDA International accepted;  ● In addition to NANDA International

*Interventions and Rationales*

**Follow the guidelines for intervention with a confused client in the first half of this chapter. Communication techniques specific for dementia follow.**

| Intervention | Rationale |
|---|---|
| 1. Use a variety of nonverbal techniques to enhance communication:<br>a. Point, touch, or demonstrate an action while talking about it.<br>b. Ask clients to point to parts of their body or things that they want to communicate about.<br>c. When client is searching for a particular word, guess at what is being said and ask if you are correct (e.g., "You are pointing to your mouth, saying pain. Is it your dentures? No. Is your mouth sore? Yes. OK, let me take a look to see if I can tell what is hurting you."). Always ask client to confirm whether your guess is correct. | 1. Both delirium and dementia can pose huge communication problems, and often alternative nonverbal or verbal methods have to be used. |

| Intervention | Rationale |
|---|---|
| d. Use of cue cards, flash cards, alphabet letters, signs, and pictures on doors to various rooms is often helpful for many clients and their families (e.g., bathroom, "Charles' bedroom"). Use of pictures is helpful when ability to read decreases. | |
| 2. Encourage reminiscing about happy times in life. | 2. Remembering accomplishments and shared joys helps distract client from deficit and gives meaning to existence. |
| 3. If a client gets into an argument with another client, stop the argument and get them out of each other's way. After a short while (5 minutes), explain to each client matter-of-factly why you had to intervene. | 3. Prevents escalation to physical acting out. Shows respect for client's right to know. Explaining in an adult manner helps maintain self-esteem. |
| 4. Reinforce client's speech through pictures, nonverbal gestures, X's on calendars, and other methods used to anchor client in reality. | 4. When aphasia starts to hinder communication, alternate methods of communication need to be instituted. |

Burnside (1988) suggests useful guidelines for implementing nursing interventions or teaching a severely cognitively impaired person (Box 12–4).

> Box 12-4 **Guidelines for Caring for the Cognitively Impaired**
>
> 1. Provide only one visual clue (object) at a time.
> 2. Know that the client might not understand the task assigned.
> 3. Remember that relevant information is remembered longer than irrelevant information.
> 4. Break tasks into very small steps.
> 5. Give only one instruction at a time.
> 6. Report, record, and document all data.

## CAREGIVER ROLE STRAIN

A caregiver's felt or exhibited difficulty in performing the family caregiver role

### Related To (Etiology)

▲ Severity of the care receiver's illness
▲ 24-hour care responsibility
▲ Duration of caregiving
▲ Lack of support from significant others
▲ Lack of respite and recreation for the caregiver
▲ Inadequate physical environment for providing care
▲ Family's and/or caregiver's isolation

### As Evidenced By (Assessment Findings/Diagnostic Cues)

▲ Difficulty in performing required activities
▲ Altered caregiver health status (hypertension, cardiovascular disease, etc.)
▲ Inability to complete caregiving tasks
● Expressions by caregiver of:
  • Feelings of stress in relationship with client
  • Feelings of anger and/or depression
  • Family conflict regarding issues of providing care
  • Feelings that caregiving interferes with other important roles in his/her life

---

▲ NANDA International accepted; ● In addition to NANDA International

## *Outcome Criteria*

- Satisfaction with physical health
- Satisfaction with social support
- Satisfaction with professional support

## *Long-Term Goals*

Caregivers will:
- State that they have help from family and/or friends, and/or the community, that has helped stabilize their situation
- Demonstrate adaptive coping strategies for dealing with the stress of the caregiver role
- Demonstrate effective problem-solving techniques they can use to deal with issues of caring for their family member
- Identify resources they can use when new situations arise that appear to need new coping strategies
- State that they now maintain social relationships with other individuals and families as evidenced by involvement in community groups, with extended family members, and with friends

## *Short-Term Goals*

Caregivers will:
- State they understand and have written information on their family member's/friend's type of dementia (e.g., AD, multi-infarct dementia) and appropriate caregiving techniques by (date)
- Know and discuss the available resources in their community, national resources, and sites on the Internet that will provide information, support, and how to arrange respite by (date)
- Identify at least three steps they can take to relieve some of the family stress and enhance well-being to all members of the family unit by (date)
- Learn at least three new coping strategies and coping mechanisms to diffuse the tension and strain on caregiver and family by (date)
- Care for their own needs through diet, exercise, and plenty of rest and give five examples of healthy changes by (date)

- Be aware of where to go to get legal and financial planning advice early in the disease process by (date)
- Acknowledge realistic goals of treatment for their family member by (date)

## Interventions and Rationales

| Intervention | Rationale |
|---|---|
| 1. Assess what caregivers and family know about client's dementia, and educate regarding the client's specific illness. | 1. Point out areas that will benefit from planning and preparation (e.g., legal issues, financial issues, additional caregiving techniques, and knowing what they can and what they cannot change or accomplish). |
| 2. Provide a list of community agencies and support groups where family and primary caregiver can receive support, further education, and information regarding how to arrange respite. | 2. Help diminish a sense of hopelessness and increase a sense of empowerment. |
| 3. Help the caregiver and family to identify areas that need intervention, and those areas that are presently stable. | 3. Identify specific areas needing assistance, and those that will need assistance in the future. |
| 4. Teach the caregiver and family specific interventions to use in response to behavioral or social problems brought on by the dementia. | 4. Caregivers need to learn many new ways to intervene in situations that are common with demented clients (agitation, catastrophic reactions, sleep-wake disturbances, wandering). |

| Intervention | Rationale |
|---|---|
| 5. Safety is a major concern. Box 12-5 identifies some steps that caregivers and family can take to make the home a safer place. | 5. These steps, prepared by the Alzheimer's Association, can help make the home safe for the person with dementia. |
| 6. Encourage spending nonstressful time with the client at client's present level of functioning (e.g., watching a favorite movie together, reading with client a simple book with pictures, performing simple tasks like setting the table, washing dishes, washing the car). | 6. Encourages the client to participate as much as possible in family life. Helps diminish feelings of isolation and alienation temporarily. |
| 7. Encourage caregiver/ family members to follow family traditions (church activities, holidays, and vacations). | 7. Helps family maintain their family rituals and helps client's sense of belonging. |
| 8. Encourage caregivers/ family members to use respite care during regular intervals (e.g., vacations). | 8. Regular periods of respite can help caregivers/family prevent burnout, can allow caregivers to continue participating in their life, and can help minimize feelings of resentment. |
| 9. Identify financial burdens placed on caregiver/family. Refer to community, national associations, or other resources that might help. | 9. Any kind of long-term illness within a family can place devastating financial burdens on all members. |

## Box 12-5 Home Safety

### Make Potentially Dangerous Places Less Accessible
- Install door locks out of sight.
- Use special safety devices, such as child-proof locks and door knobs, to limit access to places where knives, appliances, equipment, and cleaning fluids are stored.

### Accommodate Visual Changes
- Add extra lighting in entries, outside landings, areas between rooms, stairways, and bathrooms because changes in level of light can be disorienting.
- Place contrasting colored rugs in front of doors or steps to help the individual anticipate staircases and room entrances.

### Avoid Injury during Daily Activities
- Monitor the temperature of water faucets and food because the person might have a decreased sensitivity to temperature.
- Install walk-in showers, grab bars, and decals on slippery surfaces in the bathroom to prevent falls.
- Supervise the person in taking prescription and over the-counter medications.

### Beware of Hazardous Objects and Substances
- Limit the use of certain appliances and equipment such as mixers, grills, knives, and lawnmowers.
- Supervise smoking and alcohol consumption.
- Remove objects, such as coffee tables, floor lamps, to create safe wandering areas and reduce the possibility of injury.

### Be Prepared for Emergencies
- Keep a list of emergency phone numbers and addresses for the local police departments, hospitals, and poison control help lines.
- Check fire extinguishers and smoke alarms, and conduct fire drills regularly.
- If the person with AD tends to wander, enroll him or her in the Safe Return program.

# MEDICAL TREATMENTS

## Psychopharmacology for Dementia

**Alzheimer's disease (AD)** is the most common dementia, accounting for 70% of all dementias, and is the fourth most prevalent cause of death in the adult population. Cholinesterase inhibitors can help in Alzheimer's dementia. Unfortunately, they do not affect ongoing neural destruction (Maxmen & Ward, 2002). The result of the action is to prevent the metabolism of acetylcholine. Acetylcholine is the neurotransmitter associated with memory and learning. Since acetylcholine is often lower in people with AD, these drugs may temporarily reduce, and later delay, cognitive and behavioral symptoms of dementia.

**Tacrine (Cognex)** was the first anticholinesterase approved for the treatment of Alzheimer's disease. Because of liver toxicity, it is rarely used today. Other cholinesterase inhibitors have been useful for many AD clients.

**Donepezil (Aricept)**, another cholinesterase inhibitor, also appears to slow down deterioration in cognitive functions in individuals with mild-to-moderate dementia, without the serious liver toxicity that is attributed to tacrine. **Rivastigmine (Exelon)** and *Galantamine* (**razadyne**) are two others in use today.

**Memantine (Namenda)** is the most recent drug approved at this writing. This drug is the first in a new class of drugs. Memantine is an $N$-methyl-D-aspartate (NMDA) receptor antagonist that has demonstrated significant effectiveness in clients with moderate-to-severe AD.

## *Other Agents Used for Targeting Specific Symptoms in Dementia*

**Agitation and Aggression** (Maxmen & Ward, 2002)
- **Hypoanxiolytics (lorazepam 0.5 mg PO)** have less drug accumulation and induce less confusion than do longer-acting anxiolytics. Watch for sedation/falls.
- **Trazodone (Desyrel; doses between 25 and 500 mg/day),** and **buspirone (Buspar; doses between 10 and 60 mg/day)** can decrease agitation and aggression without decreasing cognitive performance.
- **Atypical antipsychotics (risperidone 800-1000 mg bid)**

  **Anxiety Buspirone** is not a sedative and does not produce many unwanted side effects, such as psychomotor impairment, drowsiness, or cognitive impairment. For this reason, many prefer this drug to the benzodiazepines. **Lorazepam** is also used.

**Depression** The **selective serotonin-uptake inhibitors (SSRIs)** are effective and are tolerated better than drugs with high anticholinergic side effects, such as the tricyclic antidepressants (TCAs). Tricyclics also produce orthostasis (leading to falls or fractures) and cardiac conduction delays. Useful medications included in this group are fluoxetine (Prozac), paroxetine (Paxil), and sertraline (Zoloft).

**Psychotic Features (Hallucinations and Delusions)** The newer atypical antipsychotics have been found to help clear client's thinking but do not have the more troubling and potentially serious side-effect profile of the standard (phenothiazine-like) drugs. Appropriate atypical drugs include: olanzapine (Zyprexa), quetiapine (Seroquel), and risperidone (Risperdal).

## Integrative Approaches (CAM)

There are some drugs currently under investigation for the use in AD.

**Estrogens:** Some studies have indicated that hormone replacement therapy (HRT) appears to reduce the risk of AD by 30% to 40%. The principal concern with HRT is that recent studies seem to point to an increase in breast cancer, along with other risk factors.

**Nonsteroidal Antiinflammatory Drugs (NSAIDs):** It seems that there is mounting evidence that the use of nonsteroidal antiinflammatory drugs (e.g., ibuprofen) might reduce the risk of AD.

**Ginkgo Biloba:** At present, there is little evidence that, Ginko Biloba provides significant benefit (Stern et al, 2004).

**Vitamin E:** Early in disease, vitamin E may slow down or prevent neural destruction and declines in dementia; however, it does not directly reduce cognitive or behavioral symptoms (Maxmen & Ward, 2002; Stern et al, 2004).

# NURSE, CLIENT, AND FAMILY RESOURCES

## ASSOCIATIONS

**Alzheimer's Disease and Related Disorders Association**
225 North Michigan Avenue, Suite 1700
Chicago, IL 60601-7633
(312) 335-8700; (800) 272-3900
For caregivers of Alzheimer's clients

**Alzheimer's Disease Education and Referral
    Center Hotline**
(800) 438-4380
Information, referrals, and publications regarding
    clinical trials

## INTERNET SITES

**Alzheimer's Association**
http://www.alz.org

**Alzheimer Society of Canada**
http://www.alzheimer.ca

# PART III

# PSYCHIATRIC EMERGENCIES AND FORENSIC ISSUES

# CHAPTER 13

# Crisis Intervention and Rehabilitation

## OVERVIEW

A **crisis** is an acute, time-limited phenomenon experienced as an overwhelming emotional reaction to a:
- Stressful situational event
- Developmental event
- Societal event
- Cultural event, or to the perception of that event

A crisis is not a pathologic state, and being in crisis is not pathologic. It is a struggle for equilibrium and adjustment when problems are perceived as insolvable.

Nurses intervene through a variety of crisis-intervention modalities, such as disaster nursing, mobile crisis units, group work, health education and crisis prevention, victim outreach programs, and telephone hotlines.

It is important to keep in mind that, in crisis work, particularly, the client might be an individual, a group, or a community:
- **Individual client** (as in physical abuse)
- **Group** (as in students in a classmate's suicide event or shootings)
- **Community** (as in disaster nursing—tornadoes, hurricanes, shootings, airplane crashes)

It is difficult to predict what one person will perceive as a disastrous event constituting a crisis. A pregnancy, a breakup of a relationship, failing a test, or being given an adverse medical diagnosis can be catastrophic for one person but not to another. Some crises are more universal, such as the death of a child or spouse; these events are experienced as crises to almost everyone.

Crisis by definition is self-limiting and is resolved within 4 to 6 weeks. The goal of crisis intervention is to maintain the precrisis level of functioning. However, a person can emerge from the crisis at a higher level of functioning, at the same level, or at a lower level of functioning. Crisis intervention deals with the present (here-and-now) only, and nurses take a much more active and directive role with their clients in crisis.

## Types of Crises

There are basically three types of crises: maturational, situational, and adventitious crises.

### Maturational

Erikson identified eight stages of growth and development that must be completed to reach maturity. Each stage identifies a specific task that must be successfully mastered to progress through the growth process. When a person arrives at a new stage, former coping styles might no longer be age appropriate, and new coping mechanisms have yet to be developed. During this period of transition, psychological disequilibrium might occur. This temporary disequilibrium might affect interpersonal relationships, body image, and social and work roles (Hoff, 1995).

### Situational

A situational crisis arises from an external rather than an internal source. Examples of internal situations that could precipitate a crisis include loss of job, the death of a loved one, witnessing a crime, abortion, a change of job, a change in financial status, "coming out" as to homosexual orientation, divorce, and school problems. These external situations are often referred to as "life events" or "crucial life problems" because most people encounter some of these problems during the course of their lives.

### Adventitious

An adventitious crisis is a crisis of disaster, and is not a part of everyday life; it is unplanned and accidental. Adventitious crises can be divided into three subcategories:

1. Natural disaster (floods, earthquakes, fires, tornadoes)
2. National disasters (wars, riots, airplane crashes, terror attacks)
3. Crimes of violence (assault or murder in the workplace, bombing in crowded places, spousal or child abuse, sexual assault)

## Phases of Crisis

1. A problem arises that contributes to increased anxiety levels. The anxiety stimulates the use of usual problem-solving techniques.
2. If the usual problem-solving techniques do not work, anxiety continues to rise, and trial-and-error attempts at restoring balance are tried.
3. If trial-and-error attempts fail, anxiety escalates to severe or panic levels, and the person adopts automatic relief behaviors.
4. If these measures do not reduce anxiety, anxiety can overwhelm the person and lead to serious personality disorganization, which signals the person is in crisis.

## Levels of Crisis Intervention

There are three levels of crisis intervention: (1) preventive, (2) crisis intervention, and (3) rehabilitation. Psychotherapeutic nursing interventions are directed toward these three levels of care.

### Preventive (Primary Care)

Primary preventions are interventions that promote mental health and reduce the incidence of mental illness in an individual, group, or community. Interventions are aimed at altering causative factors before they can do harm—for example, anticipating and preparing people for stressful events, such as parenting classes, premarital counseling, preoperative teaching, respite care, or child-birth classes. Environmental manipulation can also help allay a crisis by providing support or removing the client from the stressor. Examples include finding shelter for an abused woman and her children, offering sick leave to an individual, or obtaining shelter for a homeless individual.

## Crisis Intervention (Secondary Care)

Intervention during an acute crisis aims to prevent prolonged anxiety from diminishing personal effectiveness and personality organization.

## Rehabilitation (Tertiary Care)

Rehabilitation provides support for those who have experienced and are now recovered from a disabling mental state and are, as a result, psychologically disabled. There are notably different aspects of response between a mentally healthy person and a severe and persistently mentally ill person in crisis. The mentally healthy person can make good use of crisis intervention (secondary care). The severely mentally ill or psychologically disabled person, in contrast, will fare much better with rehabilitation (tertiary care). Table 13-1 gives the reader an idea of some of the basic differences.

# ASSESSMENT

## Assessing History

A positive history for potential crises might include:
- Overwhelming life event (situational, maturational, or adventitious)
- A history of violent behavior
- A history of suicidal behavior
- A history of a psychiatric disorder (e.g., depression, personality disorder, bipolar disorder, schizophrenia, or an anxiety disorder)
- A history of or concurrent serious medical condition (cancer, ongoing cardiac problems, uncontrolled diabetes, lupus, multiple sclerosis)
- Religious or cultural beliefs that can affect the way the person experiences the crisis event

## Presenting Signs and Symptoms

People in crisis present with a variety of behaviors. Some of these behaviors are:
- Confusion; disorganized thinking
- Immobilization; social withdrawal
- Violence against others; suicidal thoughts or attempts

Table 13-1 **Mentally Healthy versus Severe and Persistently Mentally Ill Person in Crisis**

| Mentally Healthy Person | Long-Term Mentally Ill Person |
| --- | --- |
| 1. Has realistic perception of potential crisis event. | 1. Because of severe biologically based mental illness or psychologically disabling illness, potential crisis event is usually distorted by minimizing or maximizing the event. |
| 2. Has healthy sense of self, place, and purpose in life. Good problem-solving abilities. | 2. Inadequate sense of self and purpose or abilities. Inadequate problem-solving abilities. Nurse becomes more active in assisting the person in crisis. |
| 3. Usually has adequate situational supports. | 3. Person often has no family or friends and might be living an isolated existence, or even homeless. |
| 4. Usually has adequate coping skills. Has a number of techniques that can be used to lower anxiety and adapt to the situation. | 4. Because coping ability for the severely and persistently mentally ill is poor, coping mechanisms are usually inadequate or poorly utilized. |

- Running about aimlessly; agitated, increased psychomotor activity
- Crying; sadness
- Flashbacks; intrusive thoughts; nightmares
- Forgetfulness; poor concentration

## Sample Questions

*The nurse uses a variety of therapeutic techniques to obtain the answers to the following questions. Use your discretion and decide which questions are appropriate to complete your assessment.*

The nurse assesses three main areas during a crisis: (1) the meaning of the precipitating event, (2) support system, and (3) coping skills.

### Determine the Meaning of the Precipitating Event

1. "What happened in your life before you started to feel this way?"
2. If this is an ongoing problem, ask the person, "What is different today than it was yesterday about the problem? Be specific."
3. "What does this event/problem mean to you?"
4. "How does this event/problem affect your life?"
5. "How do you see this event/problem as affecting your future?"

### Evaluate the Client's Support System

1. "To whom do you talk when you feel overwhelmed?"
2. "Whom can you trust?"
3. "Who is available to help you?"
4. "Are these people available now?"
5. "Where do you worship (talk to God)? Go to school? Are there community-based activities that you are involved in?"

### Identify Personal Coping Skills

1. "What do you usually do when you feel stressed or overwhelmed?"
2. "What has helped you get through difficult times in the past?"
3. "When these things have not helped, why do you think your previous coping skills are not working now?"
4. "What have you done so far to cope with this situation?"
5. "Have you thought of killing yourself or someone else?"

## Assessment Tools

There are many factors that can influence how a person responds to a potential crisis situation. Some factors that can limit a person's ability to cope with stressful life events are:

- The number of other stressful life events with which the person is currently coping
- The presence of other unresolved losses the person is dealing with
- The presence of concurrent medical problems
- The experiencing of excessive fatigue or pain

Assessing for stressful life events can be a very useful tool (see Appendix D-10 for the Life-Changing Events Questionnaire).

## Assessment Guidelines

### Crisis

1. Identify if the client's response to the crisis warrants psychiatric treatment or hospitalization to minimize decompensation (suicidal behavior, psychotic thinking, violent behavior).
2. Do the nurse and client have a clear understanding of the *precipitating event*?
3. Assess client's understanding of his or her present *situational supports*.
4. What *coping styles* does the client usually use? What coping mechanisms might help the situation in the present?
5. Are there certain religious or cultural beliefs that need to be considered in assessing and intervening in this person's crisis?
6. Is this situation one in which the client needs primary (education, environmental manipulation, or new coping skills), secondary (crisis intervention), or tertiary (rehabilitation) intervention?

# NURSING DIAGNOSES WITH INTERVENTIONS

## Discussion of Potential Nursing Diagnoses

During a crisis, a person might exhibit a variety of behaviors that indicate a number of human problems. When anxiety levels escalate to high-moderate, severe, or panic levels, the ability to problem solve is impaired, if present at all. Essentially, in an acute crisis, what happens is that a person's usual coping skills are not effective in meeting the crisis situation. In a person with already compromised coping skills, this situation is compounded. **Ineffective Coping** is evidenced by inability to meet basic needs, use of inappropriate defense mechanisms, and/or alteration in social participation.

**Anxiety** (moderate, severe, panic) is always present, and lowering of anxiety so that clients can start problem solving on their own is key in crisis management.

**Compromised Family Coping** or **Disabled Family Coping** can be related to a situational or maturational event within the family, or two or more events going on simultaneously. Family members might have difficulty responding to each other in a helping manner. Communications become confused, and an inability to express feelings is evident.

## Overall Guidelines for Nursing Interventions

### Acute Crisis

1. Safety first: Assess for any suicidal or homicidal thoughts or plans.
2. Initial steps focus on increasing feelings of safety and decreasing anxiety.
3. Initially, nurse can take an active approach (make phone calls, set up and mobilize social supports, etc.).
4. Plan with client interventions acceptable to both nurse and client.
5. Crisis intervention calls for creative directive approaches.
6. Plan follow-up on client's progress.

### Crisis Stabilization and Rehabilitation

1. People with severe and long-term mental health problems are readily susceptible to crisis.
2. Adapting the crisis model to this group includes focusing on client's strengths, modifying and setting realistic goals, and taking a more active role.

### After Crisis Stabilization

1. Assess and provide for client's and family's psychoeducational needs.
2. Assess and provide for needed social skills training.

3. Assess and refer to a vocational rehabilitation program, when appropriate.
4. Evaluate and refer to supportive group therapy.
5. Teach or refer clients to cognitive-behavioral therapy programs, where they can learn to manage their psychotic symptoms.

## Selected Nursing Diagnoses and Nursing Care Plans

The following sections thread **Ineffective Coping** through **Acute Crisis Intervention** and then to **Rehabilitation**.

*ACUTE CRISIS INTERVENTION*

### INEFFECTIVE COPING

Inability to form a valid appraisal of the stressors, inadequate choices of practiced responses, and/or inability to use available resources

*Related To (Etiology)*

- ▲ Inadequate level of confidence in ability to cope
- ▲ Inadequate social support created by characteristics of relationships
- ▲ Inadequate level of perception of control
- ▲ Inadequate resources available
- ▲ High degree of threat; situational or maturational crises
- ▲ Inadequate opportunity to prepare for stressors
- ▲ Disturbance in pattern of appraisal of threat
- ▲ Disturbance in pattern of tension release
- ▲ Situational or maturational crisis
- ● Mass disaster (bombing, tornado, flood, hostage situation)
- ● Act of terrorism/threat or actual attack
- ● Crime of violence (rape, witnessing robbery or murder, spouse/child abuse)

---

▲ NANDA International accepted; ● In addition to NANDA International

## As Evidenced By
## (Assessment Findings/Diagnostic Cues)

- ▲ Inability to meet basic needs
- ▲ Destructive behavior toward self or others
- ▲ Inability to meet role expectations
- ▲ Use of forms of coping that impede adaptive behavior
- ▲ Abuse of chemical agents
- ▲ Change in usual communication patterns
- ▲ Risk taking
- ▲ Decreased use of social support
- ▲ Inadequate problem solving
- ▲ Verbalization of inability to cope or inability to ask for help

## Outcome Criteria

- ■ Uses effective coping strategies
- • Reports increase in psychologic comfort
- • Verbalizes sense of control
- • Functions well in precrisis level or higher

## Long-Term Goals

Client will:
- • Return to precrisis level of functioning within 4 to 6 weeks
- • Identify skills and information that can help prevent future crises
- • State that he/she has learned more adaptive ways to cope with stress
- • State that he/she has a stronger existing support system

## Short-Term Goals

- • Client's anxiety level will go from severe to moderate or moderate to mild by end of first encounter (a person in mild-to-moderate levels of anxiety can still problem solve)
- • Client and nurse will clarify the problem in solvable terms by end of first session

---

▲ NANDA International accepted; ■ NOC Outcome, Anxiety Self-Control

- Client and nurse will identify existing supports and identify other needed supports by end of first session
- Client and nurse will set realistic goals to deal with problem situations by end of first session
- Client and nurse will identify a clear step-by-step plan of action by end of first session, revised throughout
- Client will remain safe throughout crisis situation

## *Interventions and Rationales*

| Intervention | Rationale |
|---|---|
| 1. Provide liaison to social agencies to take care of emergency needs. | 1. Physical needs such as shelter, food, protection from abuser need to be handled immediately. |
| 2. Make appointments for needed medical or other health-care providers. Write out time of appointment and directions for client. | 2. For example, child or elder might have acute physical problems that need emergency attention. |
| 3. Assess for client's safety, for example: Are there suicidal thoughts? Is there child or spouse abuse? Are there unsafe living conditions? | 3. Client safety is first consideration. |
| 4. Identify client's perception of the event. Reframe perception of the event if event is seen as overwhelming or hopeless, and/or client views self as helpless. | 4. Distorted perception raises anxiety. Help client experience event as a problem that can be solved. |
| 5. Assess stressors and precipitating cause of the crisis. | 5. Identify areas for change and intervention. |

| Intervention | Rationale |
|---|---|
| 6. Identify client's current skills, resources, and knowledge to deal with problems. | 6. Encourage client to use strengths and usual coping skills. |
| 7. Identify other skills client might need to develop (e.g., decision-making skills, problem-solving skills, communication skills, relaxation techniques). | 7. Additional skills can help minimize crisis situations in the future and help clients regain more control over their present situation. |
| 8. Assess client's support systems. Rally existing supports *(with client's permission)* if client is overwhelmed at present. | 8. Client might be immobilized initially. Nurses often need to take an active role during crisis intervention. |
| 9. Identify and arrange for extra supports if current support system is either not available or insufficient. | 9. Client might have lost important supports (death, divorce, distance) or simply not have sufficient supports in place. |
| 10. Nurse often needs to take an active role in crisis intervention (e.g., make telephone calls; arrange temporary child care; arrange for shelters, emergency food, first aid, etc.). | 10. Clients in crisis are often temporarily immobilized by anxiety and unable to problem solve. Nurse organizes situation so that it is seen as solvable and controllable. |
| 11. Give only small amounts of information at a time. | 11. Only small pieces of information can be understood when a person's anxiety level is high. |

| Intervention | Rationale |
|---|---|
| 12. Encourage client to stay in the "here-and-now" to deal with the immediate situation only. | 12. Crisis intervention deals with the immediate problem disrupting client's present situation. |
| 13. Listen to client's story. Refrain from interrupting. | 13. Telling of the story can in itself be healing. |
| 14. Help client to set achievable goals. | 14. Working in small, achievable steps helps client gain sense of control and mastery. |
| 15. Work with client on devising a plan to meet goals. | 15. A realistic and specific plan helps decrease anxiety and promote hopefulness. |
| 16. Identify and contact other members of the health team who can work with client to solve crisis event. | 16. Provides a broad base of support to intervene with problem, and enlarges client's network for future problems. |
| 17. In some situations, **debriefing** is a valuable technique for use with a group of people. Examples of debriefing: with staff on a unit when a client attempts suicide; in a disaster situation (e.g., plane crashes, bombings, natural disasters). | 17. Survivors, family members, and staff all need to discuss the impact of a disaster, and debriefing provides a structure in which to do so (Weeks, 1999). |

## *REHABILITATION*

### INEFFECTIVE COPING

Inability to form a valid appraisal of the stressors, inadequate choices of practiced responses, and/or inability to use available resources

## Related To (Etiology)

- ▲ Inadequate social supports
- ▲ Disturbance in pattern of tension release
- ▲ Disturbance in pattern of appraisal of threat
- ● Poor coping skills
- ● Inability to problem solve
- ● Inadequate level of personal resources

## As Evidenced By
## (Assessment Findings/Diagnostic Cues)

- ▲ Inability to meet role expectations
- ▲ High illness rate
- ▲ Inability to meet basic needs
- ▲ Abuse of chemical agents
- ▲ Destructive behavior toward self and others
- ▲ Risk taking
- ▲ Verbalization of inability to cope or inability to ask for help
- ● Lack of ability to function at precrisis level
- ● Altered thought processes or inappropriate mood states
- ● Prolonged confusion

## Outcome Criteria

Maintenance of optimum level of functioning in:
- Work
- Home
- Community

## Long-Term Goals

Client will:
- Function in the community with minimal use of inpatient services
- Increase life skills and available supports to use during times of stress
- Maintain stable functioning between episodes of exacerbation

---

▲ NANDA International accepted; ● In addition to NANDA International

## Short-Term Goals

Client will:

- Retain positive coping strategies during times of stress with aid of nurse/family/friends
- Work with nurse to find needed supports (e.g., residential, financial, employment/education, medical, social, recreational)

## Interventions and Rationales

| Intervention | Rationale |
|---|---|
| 1. Nurse works with client and family to assess the variety of needs that the client has. | 1. Client with psychiatric disabilities has a wide range of needs. |
| 2. Identify client's highest level of functioning in terms of: <br> a. Living skills <br> b. Learning skills <br> c. Working skills <br> See Table 13-2. | 2. Identifies client's potential so that arrangements can incorporate the client's potential. |
| 3. Identify the social supports available to the family: <br> a. Education about the disease, treatment, prognosis, and medications <br> b. Community supports to help client function optimally <br> c. Community supports that offer family support/ groups/ongoing psychoeducation | 3. Family members need a variety of supports to prevent family deterioration. |

| Intervention | Rationale |
|---|---|
| 4. Identify specific community supports that can provide client and family with continuity of care, for example (Public Policy Committee, 1999): | 4. The National Alliance for the Mentally Ill (NAMI) (Public Policy Committee, 1999) contends that a comprehensive array of community support services must be available for individuals to help people function at optimum levels and slow down relapse rate. |
| a. Residential support individuals to help services | |
| b. Transportation support services | |
| c. Intensive case management | |
| d. Psychosocial rehabilitation | |
| e. Peer support | |
| f. Consumer-run services | |
| g. Around-the-clock crisis services | |
| h. Outpatient services with mobile capabilities | |
| 5. Provide *social skills training*, especially if client is living with family. | 5. Some studies have shown that social skills training lowers relapse over time, especially for those living with families (Public Policy Committee, 1999). |
| 6. Work with family and client to identify client's prodromal (early) signs of impending relapse. | 6. Client and family can secure medical help before exacerbation of illness occurs. |
| 7. Work with client and family to identify an appropriate vocational rehabilitation service for client. Box 13-1 describes types of vocational rehabilitation services available. | 7. Employment makes a significant contribution to relapse prevention, improved clinical outcomes, and improved self-image. |

Intervention

8. Teach client and family about psycho-active medications:
   a. Side effects
   b. Toxic effects
   c. What medication can do
   d. What medication cannot do
   e. Whom/where to call with questions, or in emergencies

Rationale

8. Medication teaching can do a lot to reduce relapse rate and prolong time between relapses.

Table 13-2 **Living, Learning, and Working Skills for Psychiatrically Disabled Clients**

Potential skilled activities needed to achieve goal of psychiatric rehabilitation:

| Physical | Emotional | Intellectual |
| --- | --- | --- |
| **Living Skills** | | |
| Personal hygiene | Human relations | Money management |
| Physical fitness resources | Self-control | Use of community resources |
| Use of public transportation | Selective reward | Goal setting |
| Cooking | Stigma reduction | Problem development |
| Shopping | Problem solving | |
| Cleaning | Conversational skills | |
| Participating in sports | | |
| Using recreational facilities | | |
| **Learning Skills** | | |
| Being quiet | Making speeches | Reading |
| Paying attention | Asking questions | Writing |
| Staying seated | Volunteering answers | Arithmetic |
| Observing | Following directions | Study skills |
| Being punctual | Asking for directions | Hobby activities |
| | Listening | Typing |

Data from Anthony, W.A. (1980). *Principles of psychiatric rehabilitation.* Baltimore, MD: University Park Press.

*Continued*

Table 13-2 **Living, Learning, and Working Skills for Psychiatrically Disabled Clients—cont'd**

Potential skilled activities needed to achieve goal of psychiatric rehabilitation:

| Physical | Emotional | Intellectual |
|---|---|---|
| **Working Skills** | | |
| Punctuality | Job interviewing | Job qualifying |
| Use of job tools | Job decision making | Job seeking |
| Job strength | Human relations | Specific job tasks |
| Job transportation | Self-control | |
| Specific job tasks | Job keeping | |
| | Specific job tasks | |

---

**Box 13-1 Some Vocational Rehabilitation Models**

**Supported Employment (SE) Programs**
This model has proven to be most successful in assisting persons with the most serious disabilities to attain and maintain an attachment to the work force. It is individualized and provides on-site, one-on-one supports and job-coaching services, and occurs in competitive, "real work" settings; job coach services are gradually reduced and removed.

**Transitional Employment (TE) Programs**
This model offers a temporary work experience to individuals offering the same supports and services as SE. TE positions are contracted to a service program that fills openings and staffs positions to meet contractual obligations. No individual participants receive permanent TE positions; they must move on to competitive employment within an agreed-upon length of time. Staff often cover contract positions, working on the job for a day in cases of illness or with changes in participants' schedules.

Box 13-1  **Some Vocational Rehabilitation Models—cont'd**

### Clubhouses

Programs are "member directed," with members defined as individuals with serious mental illness. Clubhouse services and supports are provided to members according to the structure of the "work-ordered day." Members have individual daily responsibilities and schedules to fulfill as preparation for entry or re-entry into the world of work. Membership in a clubhouse is lifelong, and members provide each other ongoing support.

### Job Clubs

There are two main types: in-house clubs and postprogram graduate clubs. Members discuss issues, uncertainties, and problems that they face while seeking employment or maintaining employment gains. In-house clubs can provide practical guidelines in résumé writing, guidelines for work exploration, opportunities to practice interviewing skills, and, in some cases, vocational assessment and interest identification. Postprogram graduate clubs provide essential off-site support services, such as working with new coworkers, adjusting to job requirements, handling issues of stigma and disclosure, and feelings of isolation.

### Peer and Natural Supports

These circles of support are central to the continued success of individuals with serious psychiatric conditions who are attaining and maintaining employment. Circles expand connections beyond the usual family and friends to include wider community links to religious organizations, recreational/activity groups, public libraries, volunteer activities, and peer support activities (such as job clubs; support groups that meet regularly; one-on-one relationships; "warm lines" for crisis intervention and supports; and Internet chat rooms).

Adapted from Donegan, K.R., & Palmer-Erbs, V.K. (1998). Promoting the importance of work for persons with psychiatric disabilities. *Journal of Psychosocial Nursing, 36,* 13–23; reprinted with permission.

# NURSE, CLIENT, AND FAMILY RESOURCES

## ASSOCIATIONS

**Emotions Anonymous**
PO Box 4245
St. Paul, MN 55104-0245
(612) 647-9712
12-Step program of recovery from emotional difficulties

**Workaholics Anonymous**
PO Box 289
Menlo Park, CA 94026-0289
(510) 273-9253
12-Step program of recovery from compulsive
    overworking

**Red Cross Disaster Mental Health Services (DMHS)**
Contact local Red Cross for information

## INTERNET SITES

**Alliance for Psychosocial Nursing**
http://www.psychnurse.org

**NAMI (National Alliance for the Mentally Ill)**
http://www.nami.org

**Mental Help Net**
http://mentalhelp.net

# CHAPTER 14

# Family Violence

## OVERVIEW

Physical and psychological trauma causes long-lasting and devastating damage to people's lives, their children's lives, and lives of generations to come. Violence has moved from the home into schools, the workplace, and neighborhoods, onto the road, and into the air, and touches every corner of community life. This chapter deals with child, spouse, and elder abuse.

### Child, Spouse, and Elder Abuse

One of the most disturbing aspects of family violence or victimization is the horrifying legacy of violence:

> I and the public know
> what all school children learn
> Those to whom evil is done
> do evil in return (W.H. Auden)

Victims of abuse are often debilitated when their ability to cope is overwhelmed. Zerbe (1999) states that, during a course of a lifetime, few escape traumatic events, but the victims are often left to deal with the devastating consequences by themselves.

The nurse is often the first point of contact for people experiencing family violence, and is in the ideal position to contribute to prevention, detection, and effective intervention. All forms of interpersonal abuse can be devastating. Abuse can take the form of emotional, physical, and/or sexual abuse and neglect. Emotional abuse kills the spirit and the ability to succeed later in life, to feel deeply, or to make emotional contact with others. Physical abuse includes emotional abuse in addition to the potential for long-term physical deformity, internal damage, and acute painful tissue damage, bone damage, and/or, in some cases, death. The consequences of being sexually abused as a child are devastating and often neverending. Survivors of sexual abuse experience low self-esteem, self-hatred, affective instability, poor control of aggressive impulses, and disturbed interpersonal relationships compounded by an inability to trust and difficulty in protecting themselves. Sexual abuse occurs all too often in conjunction with spouse abuse and elder abuse.

## ASSESSMENT

### Assessing History

Sensitivity is required on the part of the nurse who suspects family violence. Interview guidelines are suggested in Box 14-1. A person who feels judged or accused of

---

**Box 14-1 Interview Guidelines**

**Do's**
- Conduct the interview in private.
- Be direct, honest, and professional.
- Use language the client understands.
- Ask client to clarify words not understood.
- Be understanding.
- Be attentive.
- Inform the client if you must make a referral to child/adult protective services, and explain the process.
- Assess safety, and help reduce danger (at discharge).

**Don'ts**
- Do *not* try to "prove" abuse by accusations or demands.
- Do *not* display horror, anger, shock, or disapproval of the perpetrator or situation.
- Do *not* place blame or make judgments.
- Do *not* allow the client to feel "at fault" or "in trouble."
- Do *not* probe or press for responses or answers the client is not willing to give.
- Do *not* conduct the interview with a group of interviewers.
- Do *not* force a child to remove clothing.

wrongdoing is most likely to become defensive, and any attempts at changing coping strategies in the family will be thwarted. It is better for the nurse to ask about ways of solving disagreements or methods of disciplining children, rather than use the word *abuse* or *violence*, which appear judgmental and, therefore, are threatening to the family (Smith-DiJulio, 2002).

1. **Child:** Is there a history of unexplained "accidents" and physical injuries?
2. **Child:** Does the child appear well nourished, appropriately dressed, clean, and appropriately groomed?
3. **Adult woman:** Does she have a history of abuse as a child?
4. **Adult man:** Does he have a history of abuse as a child?
5. **Elder:** Is there a history of unexplained "accidents" or physical injuries?
6. **Elder:** Does the elder have a history of being abused as a child, or abusing his or her children?
7. Does there seem to be a history of drug or alcohol abuse within the family system?
8. Does the client reexperience the abuse through flashbacks, dreams or nightmares, or intrusive thoughts?
9. Does the client or other family member state that he or she has had suicidal or homicidal thoughts in the past?

## Presenting Signs and Symptoms

- Feelings of helplessness or powerlessness
- Repeated emergency room or hospital visits
- Vague complaints, including insomnia, abdominal pain, hyperventilation, headache, or menstrual problems
- Poorly explained bruises in various stages of healing
- Injuries (bruises, fractures, scrapes, lacerations) that do not seem to fit the description of the "accident"
- Frightened, withdrawn, depressed, and/or despondent appearance

## Assessment Questions

*The nurse uses a variety of therapeutic techniques to obtain the answers to the following questions. Use your discretion and decide which questions are appropriate to complete your assessment.*

## For All Clients

1. "Tell me about what happened to you?"
2. "Who takes care of you?" (for children or dependent elderly)
3. "What happens when you do something wrong?" (for children)
4. "How do you and your partner/caregiver resolve disagreements?" (for women and elderly)
5. "What do you do for fun?"
6. "Who helps you with your children? Parents?"
7. "What time do you have for yourself?"

## For Spouse

1. "Have you been hit, kicked, or otherwise hurt by someone in the past year? By whom?"
2. "Do you feel safe in your current relationship?"
3. "Is there a partner from a previous relationship who is making you feel unsafe now?"

## For Parents

1. "What arrangement do you make when you have to leave your child alone?"
2. "How do you discipline your child?"
3. "When your infant cries for a long time, how do you get him or her to stop?"
4. "What about your child's behavior bothers you the most?"

## Assessment Tools

The Abuse Assessment Screen developed by the Nursing Research Consortium on Violence and Abuse is a helpful tool for nurses in the clinical area and is found in Appendix D-11.

## Assessment Guidelines

### Family Abuse

**During your assessment and counseling, maintain an interested and empathetic manner. Refrain from displaying**

**horror, anger, shock, or disapproval of the perpetrator or the situation. Assess for:**

1. Presenting signs and symptoms of victims of family violence
2. Potential problems in vulnerable families. For example, some indicators of vulnerable parents who might benefit from education and effective coping techniques are listed in Box 14-2.
3. Physical, sexual, and/or emotional abuse and neglect and economic maltreatment in the case of elders
4. Family coping patterns
5. Client's support system
6. Drug or alcohol use
7. Suicidal or homicidal ideas
8. Posttrauma syndrome
9. If the client is a child or an elder, identify the protection agency in your state that will have to be notified

## NURSING DIAGNOSES WITH INTERVENTIONS

### Discussion of Potential Nursing Diagnoses

Violence brings with it pain; psychological and physical injury and anguish; the potential for disfigurement; and the potential for death. Therefore, **Risk for Injury** is a

---

**Box 14-2  Assessing for Parents Who Are Vulnerable for Child Abuse**

1. New parents whose behavior toward the infant is rejecting, hostile, or indifferent.
2. Teenage parents, most of whom are children themselves, require special help and guidance in handling the baby and discussing their expectations of the baby and their support systems.
3. Retarded parents, for whom careful, explicit, and repeated instructions on caring for the child and recognizing the infant's needs are indicated.
4. People who grew up in abusive homes. This is the biggest risk factor for perpetuation of family violence.

major concern for nurses and other members of the health care team.

Within all families where violence occurs, severe communication problems are evident. Coping skills are not adequate to handle the emotional and environmental events that trigger the crisis situation. Inadequate coping skills among family members result in family members not getting their needs met, including the need for safety, security, and sense of self. Therefore, there exists **Ineffective Role Performance** within the family.

There are many other nursing diagnoses that the nurse can use in caring for children and adults who are suffering from abuse at the hands of others. Some include **Anxiety, Fear, Disabled Family Coping, Posttrauma Syndrome, Powerlessness, Caregiver Role Strain, Disturbed Body Image, Chronic Low Self-Esteem, Impaired Parenting,** and **Acute/Chronic Pain.**

This chapter discusses **Risk for Injury** for the child, adult, and elder and **Ineffective Role Performance** geared toward the abuser.

## Overall Guidelines for Nursing Interventions

*Child, Adult, and Elder*

1. Establish rapport before focusing in on the details of the violent experience.
2. Reassure client that he or she did nothing wrong.
3. Allow client to tell his or her story without interruptions.
4. If client is an **adult,** assure client of confidentiality, and that any changes are his or hers to make.
5. If client is a **child,** report abuse to appropriate authorities designated in your state.
6. If client is an **elder,** check with state laws for reporting information.
7. Establish a safety plan in situations of **spouse abuse.** (Refer to Box 14-4 for a full, personalized plan.)
8. **Keep your charting detailed, accurate, and up-to-date.**
   - Verbatim statements of who caused the injury and when it occurred
   - A body map to indicate size, color, shape, areas, and types of injuries with explanation
   - Physical evidence, when possible, of sexual abuse
   - Ask for permission to take photos

9. Be aware of your own feelings of anger, frustration, and need to rescue.
10. Use peer supervision for validation, support, and guidance.

## Selected Nursing Diagnoses and Nursing Care Plans

### RISK FOR INJURY

At risk of injury as a result of environmental conditions interacting with the individual's adaptive and defensive resources

*Related To (Etiology): Perpetrator's*

- Rage reaction (parents, partner, caregiver)
- Poor coping skills
- History of violence, neglect, or emotional deprivation as a child
- History of drug or alcohol abuse
- Poor impulse control
- Decline in mental status or has a mental illness
- Pathologic family dynamics

*As Evidenced By*
*(Assessment Findings/Diagnostic Cues): Abused's*

- Recurrent emergency department (ED) visits for injuries attributed to being "accident prone"
- Presenting problems reflecting signs of high anxiety and chronic stress:
  - ▲ Hyperventilation
  - ▲ Panic attacks
  - ▲ Gastrointestinal disturbances
  - ▲ Hypertension
  - ▲ Physical injuries
- Depression
- Stress-related conditions:

---

▲ NANDA International accepted; ● In addition to NANDA International

▲ Insomnia
▲ Violent nightmares
▲ Anxiety
▲ Extreme fatigue
▲ Eczema, loss of hair
● Inability to concentrate as seen in poor school or work performance
● Poor hygiene and disheveled appearance at school or work or in the home
● Bruises of various ages and specific shapes (fingers, belts)

## CHILD-ABUSE CLIENT

### Outcome Criteria

• Physical abuse, sexual abuse, and/or neglect has ceased
■ Have plans to maintain safety of child

### Long-Term Goals

Child will:
• Know what plans are made for the child's protection and state them to nurse after decision is made by health care team
• Demonstrate renewed confidence and feelings of safety during follow-up visits

### Short-Term Goals

Child will:
• Be safe until adequate home and family assessment is made by (date)
• Be treated by nurse practitioner or physician and receive medical care for injuries within 1 hour
• Participate with therapists (nurse, social worker, counselor) for purpose of ongoing therapy and emotional support (art, play, group, or other) within 24 to 48 hours

---

▲ NANDA International accepted; ● In addition to NANDA International

## Interventions and Rationales

| Intervention | Rationale |
|---|---|
| 1. Adopt a nonthreatening, nonjudgmental relationship with parents. | 1. If parents feel judged or blamed or become defensive, they may take the child and either seek help elsewhere or seek no help at all. |
| 2. Understand that children do not want to betray their parents. | 2. Even in an intolerable situation, the parents are the only security that child knows. |
| 3. Provide (or have physician provide) a complete physical assessment of child. | 3. To provide competent care and to substantiate reporting to child welfare agency, if required. |
| 4. Use of dolls might help child tell his or her story of how "accident" happened. | 4. Child might not know how to articulate what happened or might be afraid of punishment. Dolls can be an easier way for child to act out what happened. |

**Forensic Issues**

| Intervention | Rationale |
|---|---|
| 5. **Be aware of your agency's and state's policy on reporting child abuse.** Contact supervisor and/or social worker to implement appropriate reporting. | 5. Health care workers are mandated to report any cases of suspected or actual child abuse. |
| 6. Ensure that proper procedures are followed, and evidence is collected. | 6. If child is temporarily taken to a safe environment, appropriate evidence helps protect the child's future welfare. |
| 7. Keep accurate and detailed records of incident:<br>• Verbatim statements of who caused the injury and when it occurred | 7. Accurate records could help ensure child's future safety and court presentation. |

| Intervention | Rationale |
|---|---|
| • A body map to indicate size, color, shape, areas, and types of injuries with explanation | |
| • Physical evidence, when possible, of sexual abuse | |
| • Use of photos can be helpful. Check hospital policy. | |
| 8. Forensic examination of the sexually assaulted child should be conducted according to specific protocols: | 8. Proper collection, handling, and storage of forensic specimens are crucial to court presentation. |
| • Provided by law enforcement agencies | |
| • Particular medical facilities | |

## SPOUSE-ABUSE CLIENT

### Outcome Criteria

• Physical, emotional, sexual, financial abuse has ceased
■ Have plans to maintain safety of spouse and children

### Long-Term Goals

Client will:
• Within 3 weeks, state that they believe that they do not deserve to be beaten
• Within 3 weeks, state they have joined a support group or are receiving counseling (families, couples, individual)
• State that their living conditions are now safe from spouse abuse or potential abuse; or
• Within 2 months, state that they have found safe housing for self and children

---

■ NOC Outcome, Anxiety Self-Control

## *Short-Term Goals*

Client will:
- Have timely access to medical care for fractures, wounds, burns, and other injuries
- After initial interview, name four community resources they can contact (hotlines, shelters, support groups, neighbor, crisis center, or spiritual advisors who do not support violence)
- After initial interview, describe a safety plan to be used in future violent situations
- State their right to live in a safe environment by (date)

## *Interventions and Rationales*

| Intervention | Rationale |
|---|---|
| 1. Ensure that medical attention is provided to client. Ask permission to take photos. | 1. If client wants to file charges, photos boost victim's confidence to press charges now or in the future. |
| 2. Set up interview in private and ensure confidentiality. | 2. Client might be terrified of retribution and further attacks from partner if she tells. |
| 3. Assess in a non-threatening manner information concerning:<br>a. Sexual abuse<br>b. Chemical abuse<br><br>c. Thoughts of suicide or homicide | 3. These are all vital issues in determining appropriate interventions:<br>a. Increases risk for posttrauma syndrome.<br>b. Many victims self-medicate.<br>c. Might seem the only way out of an intolerable, catastrophic situation. |
| 4. Encourage client to talk about the battering incident without interruptions. | 4. When you ask clients to share their story, you understand that you are there to listen. |

| Intervention | Rationale |
|---|---|
| 5. Assess for level of violence in the home (Box 14-3). | 5. Each cycle of violence can become more intense. Danger for life of victim and children increases during escalation. |
| 6. Ask how client is faring with the children in the home. | 6. In homes in which the mother is abused, children also tend to be abused. |
| 7. Assess if clients have a safe place to go when violence is escalating. If no, include a list of shelters or safe houses with other written information. | 7. When abused clients are ready to go, they will need to go quickly. |

**Forensic Issues**

| | |
|---|---|
| 8. Identify if client is interested in pressing charges. If yes, give information on:<br>a. Local attorneys who handle spouse abuse cases<br>b. Legal clinics<br>c. Battered women's advocates | 8. Often clients are afraid of spouse or partner retaliation, but when they are ready to seek legal advice, an appropriate list of lawyers well trained in this area is needed. |
| 9. **Know the requirement in your state about reporting suspected spouse abuse.** | 9. Many states have or are developing laws and/or guidelines for protecting battered women. |
| 10. Discuss with client an escape plan during escalation of anxiety, before actual violence erupts. (Box 14-4 is an example of a personalized safety plan.) | 10. Write out plan, and include shelter and referral numbers. This can prevent further abuse to children and client. |

| Intervention | Rationale |
|---|---|
| 11. Throughout work with battered spouses emphasize:<br>a. *"No one* deserves to be beaten."<br>b. *"You cannot make anyone hurt you."*<br>c. "It is *not* your fault." | 11. When self-esteem is eroded, people often buy into the myth that they deserved the beatings because they did something "wrong," and if they had not done X, then it would not have happened. |
| 12. Encourage clients to reach out to family and friends whom they might have been avoiding. | 12. Old friends and relatives can make helpful allies and validate that client does not deserve to be beaten. |
| 13. Know the psychotherapists in your community who have experience working with battered spouses/partners. | 13. Psychotherapy with victims of trauma requires special skills on the part of even an experienced therapist. |
| 14. If client is not ready to take action at this time, give her a list of community resources available:<br>a. Hotlines<br>b. Shelters<br>c. Battered women's groups<br>d. Battered women's advocates<br>e. Social services<br>f. Medical assistance/Aid to Families with Dependent Children (AFDC) | 14. It can take time for clients to make decisions to change their life situation. People need appropriate information. |

---

### Box 14-3 Spouse Abuse—Assessing the Level of Violence in the Home

1. Does the client feel safe?
2. Has there been a recent increase in violence?
3. Has the client been choked?
4. Is there a weapon in the house?
5. Has the abuser used/threatened to use a weapon?
6. Has the abuser threatened to harm the children?
7. Has the abuser threatened to kill the client?

---

Adapted from Jezierski, M. (1994). Abuse of women by male partners: Basic knowledge for emergency nurses. *Journal of Emergency Nursing, 20,* 361; reprinted with permission.

Box 14-4 provides a personalized safety plan for when the client is in the relationship and when the relationship is over.

---

### Box 14-4 Personalized Safety Plan

**Suggestions for Increasing Safety—In the Relationship**
- I will have important phone numbers available to my children and myself.
- I can tell _____ and _____ about the violence and ask them to call the police if they hear suspicious noises coming from my home.
- If I leave my home, I can go (list four places) _____, _____, _____, or _____.
- I can leave extra money, car keys, clothes, and copies of documents with _____.
- If I leave, I will bring _____ (see checklist next page).
- To ensure safety and independence, I can: keep change for phone calls with me at all times; open my own savings account; rehearse my escape route with a support person; and review my safety plan on _____ (date).

**Suggestions for Increasing Safety—When the Relationship Is Over**
- I can: change the locks; install steel/metal doors, a security system, smoke detectors, and an outside lighting system.

## Box 14-4 Personalized Safety Plan—cont'd

- I will inform _____ and _____ that my partner no longer lives with me and ask them to call the police if he or she is observed near my home or my children.
- I will tell people who take care of my children the names of those who have permission to pick them up. The people who have permission are: _____, _____, and _____.
- I can tell _____ at work about my situation and ask _____ to screen my calls.
- I can avoid stores, banks, and _____ that I used when living with my battering partner.
- I can obtain a protective order from _____. I can keep it on or near me at all times as well as have a copy with _____.
- If I feel down and ready to return to a potentially abusive situation, I can call _____ for support or attend workshops and support groups to gain support and strengthen my relationships with other people.

### Important Phone Numbers
Police _____
Hotline _____
Friends _____
Shelter _____

### Items To Take Checklist
Identification
Birth certificates for me and my children
Social Security cards
School and medical records
Money, bankbooks, credit cards
Keys (house/car/office)
Driver's license and registration
Medications
Change of clothes
Welfare identification
Passports, Green Cards, work permits
Divorce papers
Lease/rental agreement, house deed
Mortgage payment book, current unpaid bills
Insurance papers
Address book
Pictures, jewelry, items of sentimental value
Children's favorite toys and/or blankets

*ELDER-ABUSE CLIENT*

## Outcome Criteria

- Physical, emotional, sexual abuse has ceased
- Neglect and/or financial exploitation has ceased
- Have plans to maintain safety of elderly client

## Long-Term Goals

Client will:
- State that caregiver has provided adequate food, clothing, housing, and medical care by (date)
- Be free of physical signs of abuse by (date)

## Short-Term Goals

Client will:
- State that they feel safer and more comfortable by (date) using a scale of 1 to 5 (1 being the safest); *or*
- Ask to be removed from violent situation by (date)
- Name two people who can be called for help by (date)

## Interventions and Rationales

| Intervention | Rationale |
|---|---|
| 1. Assess severity of signs and symptoms of abuse and potential for further abuse on a weekly level. | 1. Determines need for further intervention. |
| 2. Assess environmental conditions as factors in abuse or neglect (Box 14-5). | 2. Identifies areas in need of intervention and degree of abuse or neglect. |
| 3. If abuse is suspected, talk with client and caregiver separately. | 3. Helps attain a better understanding of what is happening, and minimizes friction among parties involved. |
| 4. Discuss with client factors leading to abuse. | 4. Identifies triggers to abusive behaviors and areas for teaching for abuser. |
| 5. Stress concern for physical safety. | 5. Validates situation is serious. |

| Intervention | Rationale |
|---|---|
| **Forensic Issues** | |
| 6. Know your state laws regarding elder abuse. Notify supervisor, physicians, and social services when a suspected abuse is reported. | 6. Keeps channels of communication open. Emphasizes the need for accurate and detailed records. |
| 7. If **undue influence** is suspected, an expert in geriatric or forensic psychiatry who has experience should be called in. | 7. Determine if the elder is making medical, legal, or financial decisions based on coercion and manipulations of others to gain control of the elder's finances, home, and/or decision making. |
| 8. Stress that no one has the right to abuse another person. | 8. Often people who have been abused begin to believe that they "deserve" the abuse. |
| 9. Discuss with client: <br> a. Hotlines <br> b. Crisis units <br> c. Emergency numbers | 9. Maximizes client safety through use of support systems. |
| 10. Explore with client ways to make changes. | 10. Directs assessment to positive areas. |
| 11. Assist client in making decisions for future action. | 11. Helps lower feelings of helplessness and identifies realistic options to an abusive situation. |
| 12. Involve community supports to help monitor and support elder. | 12. Involve as many agencies as can take a legitimate role in maintaining client safety. |

> ### Box 14-5  Elder Abuse/Neglect—Home Assessment
>
> **Environmental Conditions**
> - House in poor repair
> - Inadequate heat, lighting, furniture, cooking utensils
> - Presence of garbage or vermin
> - Old food in kitchen
> - Lack of assistive devices
> - Locks on refrigerator
> - Blocked stairways
> - Elder lying in urine, feces, or food
> - Unpleasant odors
>
> **Medication**
> - Medication not being taken as prescribed

## FOR THE ABUSER

### INEFFECTIVE ROLE PERFORMANCE

Patterns of behavior and self-expression that do not match the environmental context, norms, and expectations

### Related To (Etiology)

- ▲ Domestic violence
- ▲ Inadequate support system
- ▲ Family conflict
- ▲ Young age, developmental level
- ▲ Low socioeconomic status
- ▲ Substance abuse
- ▲ Mental-health disorder
- ▲ Lack of resources
- ▲ Lack of knowledge about role skills

### As Evidenced By
### (Assessment Findings/Diagnostic Cues)

- ▲ Inadequate external support for role enactment
- ▲ System conflict

---

▲ NANDA International accepted

▲ Change in usual patterns of responsibility
▲ Domestic violence
▲ Inadequate role competency and skills
▲ Role overload
▲ Inadequate coping
● Anxiety or depression

## PARENTS OF ABUSED CHILDREN

### Outcome Criteria

■ Uses alternative coping mechanisms for stress rather than abusive strategies
● Use of emotional, physical, sexual, and neglectful abusive behaviors has ceased

### Long-Term Goals

Parent will:
● State that group meetings with other parents who have battered are useful
● Demonstrate at least four new parenting skills that they find effective
● Share in two planned pleasurable activities twice a day with child when child returns home
● Attend workshops/group classes for effective parenting on an ongoing basis
● Attend an anger management training (AMT) course within 2 weeks

### Short-Term Goals

Parent will:
● Be able to name and call three agencies that can help financially during the crisis within 24 hours
● Name two places they can contact to discuss feeling of rage and helplessness by end of first interview
● Be able to name three alternative actions to take when feelings of helplessness and rage start to surface within 1 week

---

▲ NANDA International accepted; ● In addition to NANDA International; ■ NOC Outcome, Abusive Behavior Self-Restraint

*Interventions and Rationales*

| Intervention | Rationale |
| --- | --- |

**Abusive Parents**

1. Identify if the child needs:
   a. Hospitalization for treatment and observation, *and/or*
   b. Referral to child protective services

1. Immediate safety of the child is foremost. Temporary removal of the child in volatile situations gives the nurse/counselor time to assess the family situation and coping skills, and rally community resources to lower family stress.

2. Discuss with parents stresses the family unit is currently facing. Contact appropriate agencies to help reduce stress:
   *Economic*
   a. Job opportunities
   b. Social services
   c. Family-service agencies
   *Social supports*
   a. Public health nurse
   b. Day care teacher
   c. Schoolteacher
   d. Social worker
   e. Respite worker
   f. AMT
   Encourage and provide family therapy.

2. With the help of outside resources, family stress can be lowered, leading to improved ability to problem solve.

3. Reinforce parents' strengths, and acknowledge the importance of continued medical care for the child (Gorman et al., 1996).

3. Gives parents credit and support for positive parenting skills.

| Intervention | Rationale |
|---|---|
| 4. Work with parents to try out safe methods to effectively discipline the child. | 4. Gives parents alternatives, and can help minimize feelings of frustration and helplessness. |
| 5. Strongly encourage parents to join a self-help group (e.g., Parents Anonymous, family counseling, group counseling). | 5. Learning new ways of dealing with stress takes time, and support from others acts as an important incentive to change. |
| 6. Provide written information on hotlines, community supports, and agencies. | 6. Have resources available for immediate use. |

*PERPETRATOR AND CLIENT IN SPOUSE ABUSE*

*Outcome Criteria*

- Physical, emotional, sexual, and financial abuse of partner has ceased.
- Uses alternative coping mechanisms for stress rather than abuse

*Long-Term Goals*

Abuser will:
- State he must change in order to stay with family
- Join and attend a group for spouses who batter
- Recognize inner states of anger
- Attend a structured AMT program
- Demonstrate at least four alternative ways to deal with anger and frustration
- Within 6 months, couple will state that violence has ceased altogether

---

■ NOC Outcome, Abusive Behavior Self-Restraint

## Short-Term Goals

Client will:
- State that they are interested in knowing about family treatment modalities
- State that they no longer choose to live in a situation with violence
- Name three places they can call to receive counseling for self and family
- Obtain a restraining order
- Have information on safe houses, or name people they can stay with

## Interventions and Rationales

| Intervention | Rationale |
|---|---|
| **Spouse Abuser** | |
| 1. If abuser is motivated, make arrangements for abuser to participate in an AMT program. | 1. Empirical results show a 6- to 8-week structural program trains clients to deactivate angry emotional state (Suinn, 1998). |
| 2. Work with abuser to recognize signs of escalating anger. | 2. Often abuser is unaware of process of what leads up to rage reaction. |
| 3. Work with abuser to learn ways of channeling anger nonviolently. | 3. Violence is often a learned coping skill. Adaptive skills for dealing with anger must be learned. |
| 4. Encourages abuser to discuss thoughts and feelings with others who have similar problems. | 4. Minimizes isolation, and encourages problem solving. |
| 5. Refer to self-help groups in the community for abusive men, such as Batterers Anonymous. | 5. Self-help groups help clients look at own behaviors among those who have similar problems. |

*PERPETRATOR AND CLIENT OF ELDER ABUSE*

### Outcome Criteria

- Physical, emotional, and sexual abuse and neglect have ceased
- Use of **undue influence** for monetary/financial control or all other control of elder has ceased
- ■ Uses alternative coping strategies for stress rather than abuse

### Long-Term Goals

- Client will state the abuse has stopped, or state that he or she is now in a safe place
- Family members will state that they will meet the nurse/counselor on a weekly basis for counseling starting by (date)
- Abuser will meet with other family members and discuss feelings on care of elderly by (date)
- Family members will meet together and discuss alternatives for care of elder by (date)
- Client and family will meet together and discuss resources and supports they feel are important to them by (date)
- Abuser will demonstrate, instead of violence, two appropriate methods of dealing with frustration by (date)

### Short-Term Goals

- Family members will meet together with nurse/counselor and discuss alternative approaches toward their elderly family member within 1 week
- Family members will role play two strategies for avoiding physical or emotional violence toward elder (relaxation, assertive behaviors, anger management techniques) by (date)
- Family members will demonstrate two safe alternative methods of dealing with their emotions in "hot" situations by (date)
- Family members will name two support services to whom they can turn for help within 2 days
- One other family member or support person will spend time with elder and relieve abuser of caregiving duties for stated periods of time within 1 week

---

■ NOC Outcome, Abusive Behavior Self-Restraint

*Interventions and Rationales*

| Intervention | Rationale |
|---|---|
| **Elder Abuser** | |
| 1. **Check your state for laws regarding elder abuse.** | 1. Many states have adopted laws to help protect elders and support their needs for safety. |
| 2. Encourage abuser to verbalize feelings about elder and the abusive situation. | 2. The abused might feel overwhelmed, isolated, and unsupported. |
| 3. Encourage problem solving when identifying stressful areas. | 3. Assesses abuser's approach to problem-solving skills, and explores alternatives. |
| 4. Meet with entire family, and identify stressors and problem areas. | 4. Other family members might not be aware of the strain the abuser is under or the lack of safety to the abused family member. |
| 5. If there are no other family members, notify other community agencies that might help abuser and elder stabilize situation, for example: <br> a. Support group for elder <br> b. Support group for abuser <br> c. Meals on Wheels <br> d. Day care for seniors <br> e. Respite services <br> f. Visiting nurse service | 5. Minimizes family stress and isolation, and increases safety. |
| 6. Initiate referrals for available support services. | 6. Rallies needed support for abusive situation. |

| Intervention | Rationale |
|---|---|
| 7. Encourage abuser's use of counseling. | 7. Increases coping skills and social supports. |
| 8. Suggest that family members meet together on a regular basis for problem solving and support. | 8. Encourages family to learn to solve problems together. |
| 9. Act as a facilitator in the beginning to assess and teach problem-solving skills and offer referral information. | 9. Families increase their communication skills, effectiveness in inter-actions, and self-esteem. |

# NURSE, CLIENT, AND FAMILY RESOURCES

## ASSOCIATIONS

**Family Violence and Sexual Assault Institute (FVSAI)**
6160 Cornerstone Court East
San Diego, CA 92121
(858) 623-2777
http://www.fvsai.org

**National Domestic Violence Hotline (NDV Hotline)**
3616 Far West Boulevard, Suite 101-297
Austin, TX 78731-3074
(800) 799-SAFE (hotline)

**Rape, Abuse, and Incest National Network (RAINN)**
(800) 656-HOPE
http://www.feminist.com/rainn.htm

**Batterers Anonymous**
8485 Tamarinal #D
Fontana, CA 92335
(909) 355-1100
For men who wish to control their anger and eliminate their abusive behavior

**Sexual Abuse Survivors Anonymous (SASA)**
PO Box 241046
Detroit, MI 48224
(313) 882-6446
12-Step program for survivors of rape, incest, or sexual
   abuse

**Survivors of Incest Anonymous (SIA)**
PO Box 190
Benson, MD 21018-9998
(410) 893-3322
12-Step program for survivors of incest

**Child Abuse Prevention—KidsPeace**
(800) 334-4KID
http://www.kidspeace.org

**Childhelp USA Hotline**
(800) 422-4453 (24 hours)

**Youth Crisis Hotline**
(800) HIT-HOME

**Runaway Hotline**
(800) 231-6946

## INTERNET SITES

**National Coalition Against Domestic Violence**
http://www.ncadv.org

**Prevent Child Abuse America Home Page**
http://www.childabuse.org

**Child Abuse Prevention Network**
http://child-abuse.com

**Victim Services Domestic Violence Shelter Tour**
http://www.dvsheltertour.org

**David Baldwin's Trauma Information Pages**
http://www.trauma-pages.com/
Site focuses on emotional trauma and traumatic stress

**MaleSurvivor**
http://www.malesurvivor.org/

**Men Can Stop Rape**
http://www.mencanstoprape.org
Helping men who rape

# CHAPTER 15

# Sexual Assault

## OVERVIEW

Rape is a violent crime with an increasing prevalence (Stern et al, 2004), an act of violence, and sex is the weapon used by the perpetrator. **Rape is a nonconsensual vaginal, anal, or oral penetration, obtained by force or threat of bodily harm, or when a person is incapable of giving consent**. It is usually men who rape, and most of those raped are women. A male who is sexually assaulted is more likely to have physical trauma and to have been victimized by several assailants than is a female. Males experience the same devastating severe and long-lasting trauma as do females. Long-term psychological effects of sexual assault might include the development of depression, dysfunction, and somatic complaints in many survivors. Incest victims might experience a negative self-image, self-destructive behavior, and substance abuse. All catastrophic events can result in a post-trauma syndrome. **Rape-trauma syndrome** is a variant of posttraumatic stress disorder (PTSD) and consists of two phases: (1) the acute phase, and (2) the long-term reorganization phase. Nurses might encounter clients right after the sexual assault or weeks, months, or even years after the sexual assault. In either case, the individual will benefit from compassionate and effective nursing interventions.

## ASSESSMENT

### Assessing History

A positive history includes:
1. A history of a previous sexual assault
2. A history of incest within the family

3. The individual suffers from any of the signs and symptoms of PTSD

## Presenting Signs and Symptoms

### Acute Phase of Rape-Trauma Syndrome (0 to 2 Weeks after the Rape)

*Typical reactions to crisis reflecting cognitive, affective, and behavioral disruptions:*
- Shock, numbness, and disbelief
- Might appear calm and self-contained
- Might appear hysterical, restless
- Might cry a lot; *or*
- Might smile or laugh a lot
- Complains of disorganization in his or her life
- Complains of somatic symptoms

### Long-Term Reorganization Phase (2 Weeks or More)

- Intrusive thought of the rape throughout day and night
- Flashbacks of the incident (reexperiencing the traumatic event)
- Dreams with violent content
- Insomnia
- Increased motor activity (moving, taking trips, changing phone numbers, staying with friends)
- Mood swings, crying spells, depression
- Fears and phobias can develop:
  - Fear of indoors (if rape occurred indoors)
  - Fear of outdoors (if rape occurred outdoors)
  - Fear of being alone
  - Fear of crowds
  - Fear of sexual encounters

Questioning should be done in a very nonthreatening manner using open-ended types of questions (e.g., "It must have been very frightening to know you had no control over what was happening").

## Assessment Guidelines

### Sexual Assault

1. Assess physical trauma—use a body map and ask permission to take photos.
2. Assess psychological trauma—write down verbatim statements of client.

3. Assess available support system. Often partners or family members do not understand about rape, and might not be the best supports to rally at this time.
4. Assess level of anxiety. If clients are in severe to panic levels of anxiety, they will not be able to problem-solve or process information.
5. Identify community supports (e.g., attorneys, support groups, therapists) who work in the area of sexual assault.
6. Encourage clients to tell their story. **Do not** press them to.

# NURSING DIAGNOSES WITH INTERVENTIONS

## Discussion of Potential Nursing Diagnoses

**Rape-Trauma Syndrome** is the nursing diagnosis that applies to the physical and psychological effects resulting from a sexual assault. The diagnosis includes the acute phase of disorganization of the survivor's lifestyle and the long-term phase reorganization.

**Rape-Trauma Syndrome: Compound Reaction** includes the above diagnosis with:
- Reliance on alcohol or other drugs
- Reactivated symptoms of previous conditions, such as physical or psychiatric illness

**Rape-Trauma Syndrome: Silent Reaction** is a complex stress reaction to rape. The individual is usually unable to describe or discuss the rape. Some of the symptoms are:
- Abrupt changes in relationships with men
- Nightmares
- Increasing anxiety during the interview, silence, blocking, stuttering
- Marked change in sexual behavior
- Sudden onset of phobic reactions
- No verbalization of the occurrence of rape

FORENSIC NOTE: Each emergency department (ED) or crisis center needs to have its own protocol for the forensic examination of the sexual assault survivor. Most EDs and crisis centers also have rape kits that facilitate collection of specimens, such as blood, semen, hair, and fingernail scrapings.

## Overall Guidelines for Nursing Interventions

*Survivor of Sexual Assault*

1. Follow your institution's protocol for sexual assault.
2. Do not leave the person alone.
3. Maintain a nonjudgmental attitude.
4. Ensure confidentiality.
5. Encourage the person to talk; listen empathetically.
6. Emphasize that the person did the right thing to save his or her life.
7. **Forensic issues:**
   - Physical trauma—size, color, distribution of trauma with a body map.
   - Ask permission to take photos.
   - Take verbatim statements as to client's reaction to rape.
   - Document emotional status.
8. Explain everything that you are going to do beforehand.
9. Ascertain forensic examination is done, and specimens are obtained with client's written permission.
10. Alert client as to what he or she might experience during the long-term reorganization phase.
11. Arrange for support follow-up, for example:
    - Support groups
    - Group therapy
    - Individual therapy
    - Crisis counseling

## Selected Nursing Diagnoses and Nursing Care Plans

### RAPE-TRAUMA SYNDROME

Sustained maladaptive response to a forced, violent, sexual penetration against the victim's will and consent

*Related To (Etiology)*

▲ Sexual assault

---

▲NANDA International accepted

## As Evidenced By
### (Assessment Findings/Diagnostic Cues)

- ▲ Disorganization
- ▲ Change in relationships
- ▲ Physical trauma (e.g., bruising, tissue irritation)
- ▲ Suicide attempts
- ▲ Denial
- ▲ Guilt, humiliation, embarrassment
- ▲ Aggression; muscle tension
- ▲ Mood swings
- ▲ Nightmare and sleep disturbances
- ▲ Sexual dysfunction
- ▲ Feelings for revenge
- ▲ Phobias
- ▲ Loss of self-esteem
- ▲ Inability to make decisions
- ▲ Vulnerability, helplessness
- ▲ Substance abuse
- ▲ Depression, anxiety
- ▲ Shame, shock, fear
- ▲ Self-blame
- ▲ Dissociative disorders
- ▲ Hyperalertness

## Outcome Criteria

- ■ Acknowledgment of right to disclose and discuss abusive situations
- • Resolution of anger, guilt, hurt, fear, depression, low self-esteem
- • Experiences hopefulness and confidence in going ahead with life plans

## Long-Term Goals

Survivor will:
- • Discuss the need for follow-up crisis counseling and other supports by (date)
- • State that the acuteness of the memory of the rape subsides with time and is less vivid and less frightening within 3 to 5 months

---

▲ NANDA International accepted; ■ NOC Outcome, Abuse Recovery: Sexual; ● In addition to NANDA International

- Verbalization of details of abuse
- State that the physical symptoms (e.g., sleep disturbances, poor appetite, and physical trauma) have subsided within 3 to 5 months

## Short-Term Goals

Survivor will:

- Begin to express reactions and feelings about the assault
  before leaving the ED or crisis center
- Have a short-term plan for handling immediate situational needs before leaving the ED or crisis center
- List common physical, social, and emotional reactions
  that often follow a sexual assault before leaving the ED or
  crisis center
- Speak to a community-based rape victim advocate in the
  ED or crisis center
- State the results of the physical examination completed
  in the ED or crisis center
- Have access to information on obtaining competent legal
  council

## Interventions and Rationales

| Intervention | Rationale |
|---|---|
| 1. Have someone stay with the client (friend, neighbor, or staff member) while he or she is waiting to be treated in the ED. | 1. People in high levels of anxiety need some-one with them until anxiety level is down to moderate. |
| 2. **Very important:** Approach client in a nonjudgmental manner. | 2. Nurses' attitudes can have an important therapeutic impact. Displays of shock, horror, disgust, or disbelief are not appropriate. |
| 3. Confidentiality is crucial. | 3. The client's situation is not to be discussed with anyone other than medical personnel involved unless client gives consent. |

| Intervention | Rationale |
|---|---|
| 4. Explain to client the signs and symptoms that many people experience during the long-term phase, for example:<br>  a. Nightmares<br>  b. Phobias<br>  c. Anxiety, depression<br>  d. Insomnia<br>  e. Somatic symptoms | 4. Many individuals think they are going crazy as time goes on and are not aware that this is a process that many people in their situation have experienced. |
| 5. Listen and let the client talk. **Do not** press client to talk. | 5. When people feel understood, they feel more in control of their situation. |
| 6. Stress that they did the right thing to save their life. | 6. Rape victims might feel guilt or shame. Reinforcing that they did what they had to do to stay alive can reduce guilt and maintain self-esteem. |
| 7. Do *not* use judgemental language. | 7. Use (Stern et al, 2004)<br>  • Reported *not* alleged<br>  • Declined *not* refused<br>  • Penetration *not* intercourse |

### Forensic Examination and Issues

| | |
|---|---|
| 8. Assess the signs and symptoms of physical trauma. | 8. Most common injuries are to face, head, neck, extremities. |
| 9. Make a body map to identify size, color, and location of injuries. Ask permission to take photos. | 9. Accurate records and photos can be used as medicolegal evidence for the future. |

| Intervention | Rationale |
|---|---|
| 10. Carefully explain all procedures before doing them (e.g., "We would like to do a vaginal examination and do a swab. Have you had a vaginal examination before?" [rectal examination in case of male who has been raped]). | 10. The individual is experiencing high levels of anxiety. Matter-of-factly explaining what you plan to do and why you are doing it can help reduce fear and anxiety. |
| 11. Explain the forensic specimens you plan to collect; inform client that they can be used for identification and prosecution of the rapist, for example: <br> a. Combing pubic hairs <br> b. Skin from underneath nails <br> c. Semen samples <br> d. Blood | 11. Collecting body fluids and swabs is essential (DNA) for identifying the rapist. |
| 12. Encourage client to consider treatment and evaluation for sexually transmitted diseases before leaving the ED. | 12. Many survivors are lost to follow-up after being seen in the ED or crisis center and will not otherwise get protection. |
| 13. Many clinics offer prophylaxis to pregnancy with norgestrel (Ovral). | 13. Approximately 3% to 5% of women who are raped become pregnant. |

| Intervention | Rationale |
|---|---|
| 14. All data must be carefully documented:<br>  a. Verbatim statements<br>  b. Detailed observations of physical trauma<br>  c. Detailed observations of emotional status<br>  d. Results from the physical examination<br>  e. All lab tests should be noted | 14. Accurate and detailed documentation is crucial legal evidence. |
| 15. Arrange for support follow-up:<br>  a. Rape counselor<br>  b. Support group<br>  c. Group therapy<br>  d. Individual therapy<br>  e. Crisis counseling | 15. Many individuals carry with them constant emotional trauma. Depression and suicidal ideation are frequent sequelae of rape.<br>The sooner the intervention, the less complicated the recovery may be. |

# NURSE, CLIENT, AND FAMILY RESOURCES

## ASSOCIATIONS

**Family Violence and Sexual Assault Institute (FVSAI)**
6160 Cornerstone Court East
San Diego, CA 92121
(858) 623–2777
http://www.fvsai.org

**Rape, Abuse, and Incest National Network (RAINN)**
(800) 656-HOPE
http://www.feminist.com/rainn.htm

**Sexual Abuse Survivors Anonymous (SASA)**
PO Box 241046
Detroit, MI 48224
(313) 882–6446
12-Step program for survivors of rape, incest, or sexual
  abuse

**Survivors of Incest Anonymous (SIA)**
PO Box 190
Benson, MD 21018-9998
(410) 893–3322
12-Step program for survivors of incest

**Child Abuse Prevention—Kids Peace**
(800) 334-4KID
http://www.kidspeace.org

**Childhelp USA Hotline**
(800) 422–4453 (24 hours)

**Youth Crisis Hotline**
(800) HIT-HOME

**Runaway Hotline**
(800) 231–6946

## INTERNET SITES

**Victim Services Domestic Violence Shelter Tour**
http://www.dvsheltertour.org

**David Baldwin's Trauma Information Pages**
http://www.trauma-pages.com
Site focuses on emotional trauma and traumatic stress

**MaleSurvivor**
http://www.malesurvivor.org

**Men Can Stop Rape**
htt://www.mencanstoprape.org
Helping men who rape

# CHAPTER 16

# Suicide Behaviors

## OVERVIEW

Suicide is the eighth leading cause of death in the United States (Stern and colleagues, 2004). Although suicide is a behavior that needs careful assessment in depression, alcoholism/substance abuse, schizophrenia, and personality disorders (borderline, paranoid, and antisocial), suicide is not necessarily synonymous with mental disorders.

Physical illness can play a role in suicide behavior (pain, recent surgery, chronic physical illness). Suicide seems to be most prevalent among clients with diseases that result in suffering and dependency, such as AIDS and cancer. Therefore, nurses might encounter suicidal individuals in outpatient settings, intensive care units, nursing homes, or medical/surgical units; during home visits; or even among one's own circle of family and friends. People who are taking medications that contribute to depression and psychotic symptoms could also be at risk.

Suicide seems to cluster in some families; therefore, family history is pertinent. This could be the result of inherited markers for depression, learned problem-solving behavior within the family, inherited low cerebrospinal fluid (CSF) levels of 5-hydroxyindole-acetic acid (low CSF levels are associated with higher risk of attempted suicide), or some other genetic factor associated with suicide.

Suicidal people share other commonalties. They are often poor problem solvers, have troubled emotional lives (depression, anger, anxiety, guilt, and/or boredom), have a low threshold for emotional pain, are often impulsive, and might engage in extreme solutions sooner than non–suicide-prone individuals (Chiles & Strosahl, 1997). People who are isolated (have poor social supports) and people who are experiencing severe life stress at any age might also be at risk. Risk factors for age were compiled by the National Institute of Mental Health (1995) as follows:

- The strongest risk factors for *youth* are alcohol or other drug use disorders and aggressive or disruptive behaviors. Depression and social isolation are also risk factors. Suicide in youths is the second leading cause of death following accidents.
- The strongest risk factors for *adults* are depression, alcohol abuse, cocaine use, and separation or divorce.
- Most *elderly* people who commit suicide have visited their primary care physician in the month before suicide. Recognition and treatment of depression in the medical setting is a promising way to prevent suicide in the elderly. Other risk factors include social isolation, solitary living arrangements, widowhood, lack of financial resources, and poor health. The elderly commit suicide more than any other group in the United States.

## ASSESSMENT

### Assessing History

- Past history of suicidal attempts or self-mutilation
- Family history of suicide attempts or completion
- History of a mood disorder, drug or alcohol abuse, or schizophrenia
- History of chronic pain, recent surgery, or chronic physical illness
- Client has a history of personality disorder (borderline, paranoid, antisocial)
- Client is bereaved or experiencing other significant loss (divorce, job, home)

### Presenting Signs and Symptoms

- Presents with:
  - Suicidal ideation—thoughts of harming self
  - Suicidal threat—communicates desire to harm/kill self
  - Suicide attempt, failed—attempted to kill self
  - Deliberate self-harm syndrome—clients who mutilate their bodies

○ A high degree of hopelessness, helplessness, and anhedonia, which are crucial factors in suicide
○ Client states they have a plan for how they will kill
themselves.

## Assessment Tools

There are a number of tools one can use to ascertain risk
factors when assessing for potential suicidal behaviors. An
acronym can facilitate the health care worker's recall when
in the midst of crisis situations. One such acronym, the
SAD PERSONS Scale (Patterson et al., 1983), is presented in
Appendix D-12.

## Assessment Guidelines

*Suicide*

1. Assess risk factors, including history of suicide (family,
   client, friends); degree of hopelessness, helplessness,
   and anhedonia; and lethality of plan.
2. Determine the appropriate level of suicide precautions
   for the client (physician or nurse clinician), even in the
   emergency room. If client is at a high risk, hospitalization might be necessary. For example: If individuals
   state they do have a *plan* of how to kill themselves, it is
   important to ascertain concrete behavioral information
   in order to assess the measure of lethality. Shea (1998)
   suggests the following steps:
   a. Find out what plans have been contemplated.
   b. Determine how far the person took actions or plans to
      take action on these plans.
   c. Determine how much of the person's time is spent on
      these plans and accompanying ruminations about
      suicide.
   d. Determine how accessible and lethal the mode of
      action is.
3. A red flag goes up if the client suddenly goes from
   sad/depressed to happy and seemingly peaceful. Often
   a decision to commit suicide "gives a way out of severe
   emotional pain."
4. If the client is to be managed on an outpatient basis,
   then:

- Assess social supports.
- Assess friends' and family's knowledge of signs and symptoms of potential suicidal behavior (e.g., increasing withdrawal, preoccupation, silence, and remorse).
- Identify community supports and groups the client and family could use for support.

# NURSING DIAGNOSES WITH INTERVENTIONS

## Discussion of Potential Nursing Diagnoses

A sound assessment provides the framework for determining the level of protection the client warrants at that time. Therefore, **Risk for Suicide** is the first area of concern.

Believing that one's situation or problem is intolerable, inescapable, and interminable leads to feelings of hopelessness. Therefore, **Hopelessness** is most often a crucial phenomenon requiring intervention.

A third area of intervention is to tackle the phenomenon of "tunnel vision" that suicidal clients have during times of acute stress and pain. That is, problem-solving skills are poor, and suicidal people have difficulty in performing flexible cognitive operations. Therefore, teaching the client, or reinforcing the client's own, effective problem-solving skills and helping him or her reframe life difficulties as events that can be controlled is a strategic part of the counseling process with suicidal clients. Therefore, **Ineffective Coping** can be viewed as the third leg of intervention. Other potential nursing diagnoses include **Risk for Loneliness, Situational/Chronic Low Self-Esteem, Deficient Knowledge, Social Isolation, Disabled Family Coping,** and **Spiritual Distress**.

## Overall Guidelines for Nursing Interventions

### Suicide

#### Hospitalized: Put on Suicide Precautions

- Suicide precautions range from arm's-length constraint (one-on-one with staff member at arm's length at all times), to one-on-one contact with staff at all times but may attend activities off the unit maintaining one-on-one contact, to knowing the client's whereabouts at all times on the unit and accompanied by staff while off the unit.

- If there is fear of imminent harm, restraints might be required.
- **Follow unit protocols and keep detailed records in client chart.**

## Outside the Hospital

- If a client is to be managed outside the hospital, the family, significant other, or friends should be alerted to the risk and treatment plan and informed of signs of deepening depression, such as a return or worsening of hopelessness.
- When the client is to be managed on an outpatient basis (Slaby, 1994), then:
  - Social support should be rallied.
  - Appropriate psychopharmacotherapy, psychotherapy, or sociotherapy should be initiated.
  - Clients and their family and friends should be given the psychiatric clinician's telephone number as well as that of a backup clinician or emergency room where they can go if the clinician is unavailable.
  - A return visit (as early as the next day, if decisions concerning hospitalization need to be reconsidered) should be scheduled.
  - Friends and family should be alerted to signs such as increasing withdrawal, preoccupation, silence, remorse, and sudden change from sad to happy and "worry-free."
  - Careful records should be kept in all instances documenting specific reasons why a client was or was not hospitalized.
- If the client is to be managed on an outpatient basis, then medication should be given in a limited amount (e.g., 1- to 3-day supply with no refill).

## If an Accepted Procedure at Your Facility/Clinic:

- Form a written no-suicide contract with the client, such as "I will not kill myself for any reason, and if I should feel suicidal, I will (a) talk to a staff member, or (b) talk to my therapist."
- List support people and agencies to use as outpatient and crisis hotline numbers for clients/family/friends.

## Selected Nursing Diagnoses and Nursing Care Plans

### RISK FOR SUICIDE

At risk for self-inflicted, life-threatening injury

*Related To (Etiology)*

- ▲ History of prior suicide attempt
- ▲ Family history of suicide
- ▲ Alcohol and substance use/abuse
- ▲ Abuse in childhood
- ▲ Fits demographics (elderly, young adult male, adolescent, widowed, Caucasian, Native American)
- ▲ Physical illness, chronic pain, terminal illness
- ▲ Grief, bereavement/loss of important relationship
- ▲ Legal or disciplinary problems
- ▲ Poor support system, loneliness
- ▲ Hopelessness/helplessness
- ▲ Psychiatric illness (e.g., depression, schizophrenia, bipolar disorder)

*As Evidenced By*
*(Assessment Findings/Diagnostic Cues)*

- ▲ Suicidal behavior (attempt, talk, ideation, plan, available means)
- ▲ Suicide plan (clear and specific, lethal method and available means)
- ● Suicidal cues
  - ● **Overt**—"No one will miss me"; "Nothing left to live for"; "I'd be better off dead"
  - ● **Covert**—Making out a will, giving valuables away, writing forlorn love notes, taking out large life insurance policy
- ● Statements of despair, hopelessness, helplessness, and nothing left to live for

*Outcome Criteria*

- ■ Refrains from attempting suicide
- ● Behavior manifestation of depression absent

---

▲ NANDA International accepted; ● In addition to NANDA International; ■ NOC Outcome, Suicide Self-Restraint

- Satisfaction with quality of life
- Satisfaction with coping ability
- Verbalizes control of impulses

## Long-Term Goals

Client will:
- State he/she wants to live
- Name two people he/she can call if thoughts of suicide recur before discharge
- Name at least one acceptable alternative to his/her situation by (date)
- Uphold a suicide contract
- Identify at least one goal for the future

## Short-Term Goals

Client will:
- Remain safe while in the hospital, with the aid of nursing intervention and support (if in the hospital)
- Make a no-suicide contract with the nurse covering the next 24 hours, then renegotiate the terms at that time (if in hospital and accepted at your institution)
- Stay with a friend or family if person still has potential for suicide (if in the community)
- Keep an appointment for the next day with a crisis counselor (if in the community)
- Join family in crisis family counseling
- Have links to self-help groups in the community

## Interventions and Rationales

| Intervention | Rationale |
|---|---|
| **In the Hospital** | |
| 1. During the crisis period, health care workers will continue to emphasize the following four points:<br>a. The crisis is temporary.<br>b. Unbearable pain can be survived.<br>c. Help is available.<br>d. You are not alone. | 1. Because of "tunnel vision," clients do not have perspective on their lives. These statements give perspective to the client and help offer hope for the future. |

| Intervention | Rationale |
|---|---|
| **Forensic Issues** | |
| 2. **Follow unit protocol** for suicide regarding creating a safe environment (taking away potential weapons—belts, sharp objects, items, and so on. See Box 16-1 about ensuring hospital safety.). | 2. Provide safe environment during time client is actively suicidal and impulsive; self-destructive acts are perceived as ties, the only way out of an intolerable situation. |
| 3. Keep accurate and thorough records of client's behaviors (verbal and physical) and all nursing/physician actions. | 3. These might become court documents. If client checks and attention to client's needs or requests are not documented, they do not exist in a court of law. |
| 4. Put on either *suicide precaution* (one-on-one monitoring at one arm's length away) or *suicide observation* (15-minute visual check of mood, behavior, and verbatim statements), depending on level of suicide potential. | 4. Protection and preservation of the client's life at all costs during crisis is part of medical and nursing staff responsibility. **Follow hospital protocol**. |
| 5. Keep accurate and timely records, document client's activity, usually every 15 minutes (what client is doing, with whom, and so on). **Follow unit protocols**. | 5. Accurate documentation is vital. The chart is a legal document as to client's "ongoing status," interventions taken, and by whom. |

| Intervention | Rationale |
|---|---|
| 6. Construct a *no-suicide contract* between the suicidal client and nurse. Use clear, simple language. When contract is up, it is renegotiated (if this is accepted procedure at your institution). | 6. The no-suicide contract helps clients know what to do when they begin to feel overwhelmed by pain (e.g., "I will speak to my nurse/ counselor/support group/family member when I first begin to feel the wish to harm myself"). |
| 7. Encourage clients to talk about their feelings and problem-solve alternatives. | 7. Talking about feelings and looking at alternatives can minimize suicidal acting out. |

**In the Community**

| | |
|---|---|
| 1. Arrange for client to stay with family or friends. If no one is available and the person is highly suicidal, hospitalization must be considered. | 1. Relieve isolation and provide safety and comfort. |
| 2. Weapons and pills are removed by friends, relatives, or the nurse. | 2. To help ensure safety. |
| 3. Encourage clients to talk freely about feelings (anger, disappointments) and help plan alternative ways of handling anger and frustration. | 3. Gives clients alternative ways of dealing with overwhelming emotions and gaining a sense of control over their lives. |
| 4. Encourage client to avoid decisions during the time of crisis until alternatives can be considered. | 4. During crisis situations, people are unable to think clearly or evaluate their options. |

| Intervention | Rationale |
|---|---|
| 5. Contact family members, arrange for individual and/or family crisis counseling. Activate links to self-help groups. | 5. Reestablishes social ties. Diminishes sense of isolation, and provides contact from individuals who care about the suicidal person. |
| 6. If anxiety is extremely high, or client has not slept in days, a tranquilizer might be prescribed. **Only a 1- to 3-day supply of medication should be given. Family member or significant other should monitor pills for safety.** | 6. Relief of anxiety and restoration of sleep loss can help the client think more clearly and might help restore some sense of well-being. |

## HOPELESSNESS

Subjective state in which an individual sees limited or no alternatives or personal choices available and is unable to mobilize energy on his/her own behalf

---

### Box 16-1 Guidelines for a Safe Hospital Environment

1. Use plastic utensils.
2. Do not allow clients to spend too much time alone in their rooms. Do not assign to a private room.
3. Jump-proof and hang-proof the bathrooms by installing break-away shower rods and recessed shower nozzles.
4. Keep electrical cords to minimal length.
5. Install unbreakable glass in windows. Install tamper-proof screens or partitions too small to pass through. Keep all windows locked.
6. Lock all utility rooms, kitchens, adjacent stairwells, and offices. All nonclinical staff (e.g., housekeepers and maintenance workers) should receive instructions to keep doors locked.

*Continued*

---

**Box 16-1  Guidelines for a Safe Hospital Environment—cont'd**

7. Take all potentia1lly harmful gifts (e.g., flowers in glass vases) from visitors before allowing them to see clients.
8. Go through client's belongings with client and remove all potentially harmful objects (e.g., belts, shoelaces, metal nail files, tweezers, matches, and razors).
9. Take care that client does not hoard medical supplies (e.g., intravenous [IV] tubing) or, if on an IV, client is carefully observed.
10. Ensure that visitors do not leave potentially harmful objects in client's room (e.g., matches and nail files).
11. Search clients for harmful objects (e.g., drugs, sharp objects, and cords) on return from pass.

---

Data from Schultz, B.M. (1982). *Legal liability in psychotherapy*. San Francisco: Jossey-Bass Publishing.

## Related To (Etiology)

▲ Failing or deteriorating physiologic conditions (AIDS, cancer)
▲ Prolonged isolation
▲ Long-term stress
▲ Abandonment
▲ Lost belief in transcendent values/God
● Chronic pain
● Perceived helplessness, powerlessness
● Loss of significant support systems
● Severe stressful events (financial reversals, relationship turmoil, loss of job)
● Perceiving the future as bleak and wasted

## As Evidenced By
## (Assessment Findings/Diagnostic Cues)

▲ Passivity, decreased verbalization
▲ Decreased affect
▲ Verbal cues (despondent content: "I can't," "Life is hopeless," "What's the use?", "There is no way out")

---

▲ NANDA International accepted; ● In addition to NANDA International

- ▲ Lack of involvement in care
- ▲ Turning away from speaker
- ▲ Lack of initiative
- ● Decreased judgment
- ● Decreased problem solving
- ● Lack of motivation
- ● Loss of interest in life
- ● Impaired decision making

## *Outcome Criteria*

- Connectedness with others to share thoughts, feelings, and beliefs
- Expression of positive future orientation
- Expression of meaning in life
- ■ Expresses will to live

## *Long-Term Goals*

Client will:
- State three optimistic expectations for the future by (date)
- Demonstrate reframing skills when viewing aspects of client's life that appear all negative by (date)
- Demonstrate two new problem-solving skills that client finds effective in making life decisions by (date)
- Describe and plan for at least two future-orientated goals by (date)

## *Short-Term Goals*

Client will:
- Identify two alternatives for one life problem area by (date)
- Identify three things that he/she is doing right by (date)
- Reframe two problem areas in his/her life that encourage problem-solving alternative solutions
- Make two decisions related to his/her care by (date)
- Name one community resource (support group, counseling, social service, family counseling) that he/she has attended at least twice

---

▲ NANDA International accepted; ● In addition to NANDA International; ■ NOC Outcome, Hope

*Interventions and Rationales*

| Intervention | Rationale |
|---|---|
| 1. Teach client steps in the problem-solving process. | 1. Stress that it is not so much *people* who are ineffective, but rather it is often the coping strategies they are using that are not effective. |
| 2. Encourage clients to look into their negative thinking, and reframe negative thinking into neutral objective thinking. | 2. Cognitive reframing helps people look at situations in ways that allow for alternative approaches. |
| 3. Point out unrealistic and perfectionistic thinking. | 3. Constructive interpretations of events and behavior open up more realistic and satisfying options for the future. |
| 4. Work with client to identify strengths. | 4. When people are feeling overwhelmed, they no longer view their lives or behavior objectively. |
| 5. Spend time discussing client's dreams and wishes for the future. Identify short-term goals they can set for the future. | 5. Renewing realistic dreams and hopes can give promise to the future and meaning to life. |
| 6. Identify things that have given meaning and joy to life in the past. Discuss how these things can be reincorporated into their present lifestyle (e.g., religious or spiritual beliefs, group activities, creative endeavors). | 6. Reawakens in client abilities and experiences that tapped areas of strength and creativity. Creative activities give people intrinsic pleasure and joy, and a great deal of life satisfaction. |

CHAPTER 16 Suicide Behaviors **491**

| Intervention | Rationale |
|---|---|
| 7. Encourage contact with religious or spiritual persons or groups that have supplied comfort and support in client's past. | 7. During times of hopelessness people might feel abandoned and too paralyzed to reach out to caring people or groups. |

## INEFFECTIVE COPING

Inability to form a valid appraisal of the stressors, inadequate choices of practiced responses, and/or inability to use available resources

### Related To (Etiology)

- ▲ Situational or maturational crises
- ▲ Disturbance in pattern of tension release
- ▲ Inadequate opportunity to prepare for stressor
- ▲ Inadequate resources available
- ▲ Inadequate social support created by characteristics of relationship
- ● Inadequate coping skills
- ● Poorly developed social skills
- ● Personal loss or threat of rejection
- ● Impulsive use of extreme solutions

### As Evidenced By
### (Assessment Findings/Diagnostic Cues)

- ▲ Lack of goal-directed behavior
- ▲ Verbalization of inability to cope or inability to ask for help
- ▲ Abuse of chemical agents
- ▲ Inability to meet basic needs
- ▲ Decreased use of social supports
- ▲ Inability to problem solve
- ▲ Poor problem solving
- ▲ Destructive behavior toward self or others

---

▲ NANDA International accepted; ● In addition to NANDA International

▲ Inability to meet role expectations
▲ Use of forms of coping that might impede adaptive behavior
▲ Change in usual communication pattern
▲ Expression of anxiety, depression, fear, impatience, frustration, and/or discouragement

## Outcome Criteria

- Refrains from using or abusing chemical agents
- Reports adequate supportive social contacts
- Identifies multiple coping strategies
- Uses effective coping strategies

## Long-Term Goals

Client will:

- Demonstrate a reduction of self-destructive behaviors by (date)
- Demonstrate two new behaviors in dealing with emotional pain by (date)
- Name two persons to whom he/she can talk if suicidal thoughts recur in the future by (date)
- State that he/she believes his/her life has value and that they have an important role to play (mother, son, husband, father, provider, friend, job-related position, etc.)
- State willingness to learn new coping strategies (through group, individual, therapy, coping skills training, cognitive-behavior skills, and so on) by (date)

## Short-Term Goals

Client will:

- Discuss with the nurse/counselor at least three situations that trigger suicidal thoughts, as well as feelings about these situations by (date)
- Name two effective ways to handle difficult situations in the future by (date)
- State that he/she feels comfortable with one new coping technique after three sessions of role playing by (date)

---

▲ NANDA International accepted

*Interventions and Rationales*

| Intervention | Rationale |
|---|---|
| 1. Identify situations that trigger suicidal thoughts. | 1. Identify targets for learning more adaptive coping skills. |
| 2. Assess client's strengths and positive coping skills (talking to others, creative outlets, social activities, problem-solving abilities). | 2. Use these to build upon and draw from in planning alternatives to self-defeating behaviors. |
| 3. Assess client's coping behaviors that are not effective and that result in negative emotional sequelae: drinking, angry outbursts, withdrawal, denial, procrastination. | 3. Identify areas to target for teaching and planning strategies for supplanting more effective and self-enhancing behaviors. |
| 4. Role play with client adaptive coping strategies that client can use when situations that lead to suicidal thinking begin to emerge. | 4. Not all new coping strategies are effective. *The idea is that the nurse and client work together to find what does work, and that there is no one right way to behave.* |
| 5. Assess need for assertiveness training. Assertiveness skills can help client develop a sense of control and balance. | 5. When people have difficulty getting their needs met or asking for what they need, frustration and anger can build up, leading to, in some cases, ineffective outlets for stress. |
| 6. Clarify those things that are not under the person's control. One *cannot* control another's actions, likes, choices, or health status. | 6. Recognizing one's limitations in controlling others is, paradoxically, a beginning to finding one's strength. |

| Intervention | Rationale |
|---|---|
| 7. Assess client's social supports. | 7. Have client experiment with attending at least two chosen possibilities. |

# NURSE, CLIENT, AND FAMILY RESOURCES

## ASSOCIATIONS

**American Foundation for Suicide Prevention**
120 Wall Street, 22nd Floor
New York, NY 10005
(888) 333-2377; (212) 363-3500
http://www.afsp.org

**American Suicide Foundation**
1045 Park Avenue, Suite 3C
New York, NY 10028
(800) ASF-4042; (212) 410-1111
Provides referrals to national support groups for suicide survivors

**American Association of Suicidology**
4201 Connecticut Avenue NW, Suite 408
Washington, DC 20008
(202) 237-2280
http://www.suicidology.org

**Friends for Survival, Inc.**
PO Box 214463
Sacramento, CA 95821
(916) 392-0664
For family, friends, and professionals after a suicide death

**Ray of Hope**
PO Box 2323
Iowa City, IA 52244
(319) 337-9890

**Save Our Sons and Daughters (SOSAD)**
2241 West General Boulevard
Detroit, MI 48208
(313) 361-5200
http://sosad.com
For family and friends of survivors of homicide and
    suicide

## INTERNET SITES

**Suicide Awareness Voices of Education**
http://www.save.org

**Samaritans**
http://www.samaritans.org.uk

**(If You Are Thinking About) Suicide . . . Read This First**
http://www.metanoia.org/suicide

**Suicide@rochford.org**
http://www.rochford.org/suicide

# CHAPTER 17

# Anger and Aggression

## OVERVIEW

People who are prone to acting out anger and assaultive behavior are becoming an increasing public health concern. An increase in such behaviors has become a national concern, and anger is now being recognized as a crucial problem area. One example is the phenomenon of "road rage." Another example is the need to develop programs to train flight attendants to deal with aggression and assaultive behavior by passengers in flight. Child/family abuse, community property damage, dysfunctional work performance, and physical or verbal assaults are the result of inappropriate and destructive acting out of anger.

Anger is a universal emotion, perhaps one of the most difficult for people to deal with, whether it is one's own or someone else's angry or aggressive impulses. Anger and aggression are the last stages of a response that begins with feelings of vulnerability and then uneasiness (Alvarez, 2002). Ideally, the most useful nursing interventions would be instituted during these **initial phases,** before a client's anger starts to escalate out of control. An understanding of the kinds of situations and client attributes that might make a client predisposed to angry and aggressive behaviors is important for nurses. Assessment skills guiding the nurse to signals of escalating anger and aggression are vital. Accurate assessment and intervention during the early stages of escalating anger are the best prevention of violent or aggressive behavior, which, in most instances, is the physical attempt to take control (Alvarez, 2002).

However, there are times when anger has already escalated, and the threat of violence is imminent. At this time, different intervention strategies are needed. Therefore, an entirely different set of guidelines is needed when a client threatens to become physically violent.

Nurses encounter angry and aggressive clients in various settings. Clients in emergency rooms or medical units, in community health settings, and even during a home visit might feel anxious, overwhelmed, and/or threatened and lash out verbally or threaten aggressive physical behavior toward health care personnel. Some clients are more prone toward angry and aggressive behaviors than others. For example, clients who abuse substances; have poor coping skills; are psychotic; have antisocial, borderline, or narcissistic traits; and have cognitive disorders, paranoia, or mania might at times be at risk for violent behaviors.

**No nurse need ever accept or tolerate anger or aggression. Preventive measures are required for the safety of the nurse as well as the client's safety.**

The following sections offer nursing guidelines for assessing anger and potential aggression for when a client is angry and verbally abusive, and interventions for when a client's anger has escalated to physical abuse.

In the hospital, specific protocols that follow legal and ethical guidelines should be followed when restraining or secluding clients.

There are psychopharmacologic agents that have been found useful for angry and aggressive clients as well. Guidelines for working with angry and aggressive clients follow the least restrictive means of helping a client in gaining control. Least restrictive usually starts with verbal restraints, then chemical restraints, and finally physical restraints/seclusion.

# ASSESSMENT

## Assessing History

- Any past history of violence **(The best predictor of future behavior is past behavior.)**
- Paranoia
- Alcohol/drug ingestion

- Certain clients with mania or agitated depression
- Personality disorder clients prone to rage, violence, or impulse dyscontrol (antisocial, borderline, and narcissistic)
- Oppositional defiant disorder or conduct disorder
- Clients experiencing command hallucinations
- Any client with psychotic features (hallucinations, delusions, illusions)
- Clients with a cognitive disorder (e.g., dementia or delirium)
- Clients known to have intermittent explosive disorder (e.g., domestic violence)
- Certain medical conditions (e.g., chronic illness or loss of body function) can strain a person's coping abilities and lead to uncharacteristic anger

## Presenting Signs and Symptoms

- Violence is usually (but not always) preceded by:
  - Hyperactivity: most important predictor of imminent violence (e.g., pacing, restlessness)
  - Increasing anxiety and tension: clenched jaw or fist, rigid posture, fixed or tense facial expression, mumbling to self—also, shortness of breath, sweating, and rapid pulse
  - Verbal abuse (e.g., uses profanity, is argumentative)
  - Loud voice, change of pitch, or very soft voice, forcing others to strain to hear
  - Intense eye contact or avoidance of eye contact
- Recent acts of violence, including property violence
- Stone silence
- Alcohol or drug intoxication
- Carrying a weapon or object that might be used as a weapon (e.g., fork, knife, rock)
- Milieu conducive to violence:
  - Overcrowding
  - Staff inexperience
  - Staff provocative/controlling
  - Poor limit setting
  - Arbitrarily taking away privileges

## Assessment Tools

Refer to Appendix D-13 for an overt aggression scale.

## Assessment Guidelines

*Violence and Aggression*

1. History of violence is the single best predictor of violence.
2. *Assess client for risk of violence:*
   - Has violent wish or intention to harm another?
   - Has a plan?
   - Has availability or means to carry out plan?
   - Consider demographics: sex (male), age (14 to 24), socioeconomic status (low), and support systems (few).
3. Assess situational characteristics (Box 17-1).
4. Assess self for defensive response or taking client's anger personally, which may accelerate the anger cycle. For example, are you:
   - Responding aggressively toward client?
   - Avoiding client?
   - Suppressing or denying either your own or client's anger?
5. Assess your level of comfort in the situation and the prudence of enlisting other staff to work with you to deal with a potentially explosive situation.

---

### Box 17-1 Assessing Situational Characteristics for Violence

- **Availability of Potential Victims:** Most violent crimes occur between people who know each other.
- **Access to Weapons:** People with martial arts training or combat experience and those who possess great physical strength are capable of inflicting great harm.
- **Substance Use**
- **Stressors:** Daily stressor, such as relationship and financial problems, can reduce a person's frustration tolerance.

Data from Vandercreek, L. (1998). Models for clinical decision making with dangerous patients. In G.P. Koocher, S.C. Norcross, & S.S. Hill (Eds.). *Psychologists' desk reference*. New York: Oxford University Press, pp. 496–499.

# NURSING DIAGNOSES WITH INTERVENTIONS

## Discussion of Potential Nursing Diagnoses

People who commit acts of violence often lack conflict resolution skills, and resort to more primitive and physical ways of acting and responding. Many believe that a lack of assertiveness or problem-solving skills is an area of dysfunction in violent people (Mairo, 1997). Therefore, teaching clients new coping skills and effective behavioral alternatives to manage their anger is helpful for many clients and is a primary prevention intervention. Many practitioners use psychoeducational and cognitive-behavioral approaches for people with anger, violence, and abuse control problems. Some of the focus in therapy is directed toward (Mairo, 1997):

- Increasing client's awareness, appreciation, and accountability for his or her acts
- Enhancing the client's ability to identify and manage the attitudes and emotions that are associated with violent behaviors
- Decreasing social isolation and providing a supportive milieu for change
- Decreasing hostile-dependent relationships when they exist
- Developing nonviolent and constructive conflict resolution skills

**Ineffective Coping** is an appropriate nursing diagnosis for clients who have angry and aggressive responses to stressful, frustrating, or threatening situations. When a client's anxiety and anger escalate to levels at which there is a threat of harm to self or others, **Risk for Other-Directed Violence** is more appropriate and necessitates an entirely different set of interventions. During this time, talking-down skills are employed. If psychopharmacology or chemical restraints are not effective, restraint or seclusion of an aggressive client might be warranted.

Nurses are better prepared when they are familiar with the medications that can be effective during an episode of acute aggression or violence. Again, the least restrictive intervention is usually used first: (1) interpersonal (verbal), then (2) chemical (psychopharmacology), and finally, (3) physical restraint or seclusion.

The following text discusses two nursing diagnoses: one for intervention with **clients who are angry and hostile**, and a second for intervention with those whose anger has escalated to **threat of violence toward self or others**. Guidelines are given for restraint procedures, and appropriate pharmacologic agents for acute anger and aggression are noted.

## Overall Guidelines for Nursing Interventions

*Anger and Violence*

1. Always minimize personal risks; stay at least one arm's length away from client. Give client lots of space.
2. Set limits at the outset:
   - Use *direct approach* (e.g., "Violence is unacceptable."). Describe the consequences (restraints, seclusion). Best for confused or psychotic clients.
   - Use *indirect approach* if client is **not** confused or psychotic (e.g., "You have a choice. You can take this medication and go into the interview room [or hallway] and talk, or you can sit in the seclusion room until you feel less anxious.").
3. Follow guidelines for setting limits as identified in Box 17-2.

## Selected Nursing Diagnoses and Nursing Care Plans

*CLIENTS WHO ARE ANGRY AND HOSTILE*

### INEFFECTIVE COPING

Inability to form a valid appraisal of the stressors, inadequate choices of practiced responses, and/or inability to use available resources

*Related To (Etiology)*

- ▲ Inadequate level of perception of control
- ▲ High degree of threat
- ▲ Disturbance in pattern of tension release

---

▲NANDA International accepted

---

#### Box 17-2 Setting Limits

1. Set limits only in those areas in which a clear need to protect the client or others exists.
2. Establish realistic and enforceable consequences of exceeding limits.
3. Make the client aware of the limits and the consequences of not adhering to the limits before incidents occur. The client should be told in a clear, polite, and firm manner what the limits and consequences are and should be given the opportunity to discuss any feelings or reactions to them.
4. All limits should be supported by the entire staff. The limits should be written in the care plan, if the client is hospitalized, and should also be communicated verbally to all those involved.
5. When the limits are consistently adhered to, a decision to discontinue the limits should be made by the staff and should be noted on the nursing care plan. The decision should be based on consistent behavior, not on promises or sporadic efforts.
6. The staff should formulate a plan to address their own difficulty in maintaining consistent limits.

---

From Chitty, K.K., & Maynard, C.K. (1986). Managing manipulation. *Journal of Psychosocial Nursing and Mental Health Services, 24,* 9; reprinted with permission.

▲ Inadequate opportunity to prepare for stressors
▲ Disturbance in pattern of appraisal of threat
● Ineffective problem-solving strategies/skills
● Inappropriate/ineffective use of defense mechanisms
● Personal vulnerability
● Knowledge deficit
● Overwhelming crisis situations
● Impaired reality testing
● Excessive anxiety
● Intoxication or withdrawal of substances of chemical abuse
● Chemical or biologic brain changes

---

▲ NANDA International accepted; ● In addition to NANDA International

## As Evidenced By
### (Assessment Findings/Diagnostic Cues)

▲ Inappropriate/ineffective use of defense mechanisms
▲ Inability to meet role expectations
▲ Use of forms of coping that impede adaptive behavior
▲ Abuse of chemical agents
▲ Destructive behavior toward self and others
▲ Change in usual communication patterns
● Verbal manipulations
● Expresses inability to cope
● Perceptual distortions
● Aggressive rather than assertive behaviors
● Immature maladaptive behaviors
● Reports feeling anxious, apprehensive, fearful, and/or depressed, angry

## Outcome Criteria

● Client and others will remain free from injury
● Destructive behavior toward others, property, animals, and so on will cease
● Use of assertive and healthy behaviors to get needs met is in constant evidence

## Long-Term Goals

Client will:
● Identify two new safe and appropriate behaviors that will reduce anxiety, frustration, and anger by (date)
● Discuss alternative ways of meeting demands of current situation by (date)
● Recognize when anger and aggressive tendencies begin to escalate and employ tension-reducing behaviors at that time (time outs, deep breathing, talking to a previously designated person, employing an exercise, such as jogging) by (date)
● Verbalize an understanding of aggressive behavior, associated disorders, and medications, if any, by (date)

---

▲ NANDA International accepted; ● In addition to NANDA International

- Identify own strengths and skills to cope with problems, and work with nurse to build upon these skills (e.g., problem solving) (ongoing)
- Practice stress-management techniques (exercising, talking, relaxation, journal writing) as evidenced by staff observations and family report (ongoing)

## Short-Term Goals

Client will:
- Refrain from harming others or destroying property
- Be free of self-inflicted harm
- Be rule-compliant during hospitalization
- Begin to implement at least two new coping techniques when angry and aggressive feelings begin to escalate
- Experience a decrease of anxiety and anger using a self-reported scale of 1 to 10 (1 feeling least anger and 10 feeling the most anger) after trying new coping techniques

## Interventions and Rationales

| Intervention | Rationale |
|---|---|
| 1. Assess your own feelings in the situation, guard against taking client's abusive statements personally or becoming defensive. | 1. Although clients are often skillful at making personal and pointed statements, they do not know nurses personally, and have no basis on which they can make accurate judgments. |
| 2. Refrain from responding with sarcasm or ridicule, no matter how threatened or angry you feel. | 2. An angry or sarcastic remark by an authority figure will serve as an attack on the client's self-esteem, and encourage more defensive behaviors (e.g., increased hostility). |
| 3. Pay attention to angry and aggressive behavior; do not minimize such behavior in the hope that it will go away. | 3. *Minimization of angry behaviors* and *ineffective limit setting* are the **most frequent factors contributing to the escalation of violence.** |

| Intervention | Rationale |
|---|---|
| 4. Set clear, consistent, and enforceable limits on behavior (see Box 17-2 for guidelines). | 4. Clear limits give client understanding of expectations for acceptable behaviors and stress the consequences of not adhering to those behaviors. |
| 5. Emphasize to clients that they are responsible for all consequences of their aggressive behavior, including legal charges. | 5. Focusing on the "here and now" rules, and that client is responsible for the consequences of any and all aggressive behaviors, can help decrease the chronically angry client's need to "test limits." |
| 6. Emphasize to the client that you are setting limits on specific behaviors, not feelings (e.g., "It is OK to be angry at Tom, but it is not OK to threaten him or verbally abuse him."). | 6. Underlines that behavioral limits are not punitive, while communicating expectation for positive behaviors. |
| 7. Use a matter-of-fact, neutral approach. Remain calm and use a moderate, firm voice and calming hand gestures. | 7. Fear, indignation, and arguing are gratifying to many verbally abusive clients. A matter-of-fact approach can help interrupt the cycle of escalating anger. |
| 8. When a client starts to become abusive, and anger threatens to escalate, inform the client that the nurse will leave the room for a period of time (20 minutes) and will be back when the situation is calmer. Return when time is up. | 8. When this response is given in a neutral, matter-of-fact manner, the client's abusive behavior does not get rewarded. Always return in the time specified, and focus communication on neutral topics. |

| Intervention | Rationale |
|---|---|
| 9. Attend positively to nonabusive communication, such as non-illness-related topics, by responding to requests and by providing emotional support. | 9. Reinforces appropriate communication and behaviors. This gives the client and nurse time to share healthier communication and build up a sounder working relationship. |
| 10. Avoid power struggles and control battles. | 10. Power struggles and control battles are perceived as a challenge, and generally lead to escalation of the conflict. |
| 11. Respond to client anxiety or anger with active listening and validation of client distress. Apologize when appropriate. | 11. Allows the client to feel heard and understood; builds trust. |
| 12. Work with client to identify the internal and interpersonal factors that provoke violence or that strengthen a relationship against anger and aggression. | 12. Helps both nurse and client identify triggers for aggression, and factors that can mitigate or reduce the escalation of anger and aggression. **This is the first step in a structured violence prevention strategy** (Goodwin, 1985). |
| 13. Identify serious risk factors for further violence (family chaos, other mental or environmental risk factors). | 13. Whenever possible, reduce the possibility of continued violence by treating the risk factors (e.g., getting family counseling, finding a job). **This is the second step in a structured violence-prevention strategy** (Goodwin, 1985). |

| Intervention | Rationale |
|---|---|
| 14. Work with client to identify what supports are lacking, and problem-solve ways to achieve needed support. | 14. Advocacy with support is **the third step in intervention for violence** (Goodwin, 1985). |
| 15. Teach the client (and family) the steps in the problem-solving process. | 15. Many people have never learned a systematic and effective approach to dealing with and mastering tough life situations/problems. |
| 16. Role play alternative behaviors with clients that they can use in stressful and overwhelming situations when anger threatens. | 16. Role playing allows client to rehearse alternative ways of handling stressful and angry feelings in a safe environment. |
| 17. Work with clients to set goals for their behavior. Give positive feedback when clients reach their goals. | 17. Gives client a sense of control while learning goal-setting skills. Achieving self-set goals might enhance a person's sense of self, and can foster new and more effective approaches to frustrating feelings. |
| 18. Provide the client with other outlets for stress and anxiety (exercising, listening to music, reading, talking to a friend, attending support groups, participating in a sport). | 18. Alternative means of channeling aggression and angry feelings can help clients decrease their anxiety and stress, and allow for more cognitive approaches to their situation (e.g., using a problem-solving approach). |

| Intervention | Rationale |
|---|---|
| 19. Provide the client and family with community resources that teach assertiveness training, anger management, and stress reduction techniques. These might take a while to master, but will give the client more satisfying experiences in life. | 19. When clients are motivated, there are a number of techniques they can learn that can aid in helping them get what they want through acceptable and rewarding means. |

*CLIENTS WHO THREATEN HARM TO SELF OR OTHERS*

## RISK FOR OTHER-DIRECTED VIOLENCE

At risk for behaviors in which an individual demonstrates that he/she can be physically, emotionally, and/or sexually harmful to others

*Related To (Etiology)*

▲ History of violent, antisocial behavior
▲ History of violence against others (hitting, biting, kicking, spitting, rape, and so on)
▲ Panic states
▲ Stamping feet, running in corridors
▲ Rage reactions
▲ Neurologic impairment (positive electroencephalogram, computed tomography scan, or magnetic resonance image; head trauma, positive neurologic findings, seizure disorders)
▲ Manic excitement
▲ Cognitive impairment
▲ Substance abuse or withdrawal
▲ Psychotic symptoms (auditory, visual, common hallucinations, paranoid delusions, illogical thought processes)
▲ Poor impulse control

---

▲ NANDA International accepted

## *As Evidenced By*
## *(Assessment Findings/Diagnostic Cues)*

- ▲ Increased motor activity, pacing, excitement, irritability, agitation
- ▲ Provocative behavior (argumentative, overactive, complaining, demanding behaviors)
- ▲ Hostile, threatening verbalizations (loud, threatening, profane speech)
- ▲ Overt and aggressive acts; goal-directed destruction of objects in the environment
- ▲ Possession of destructive means (gun, knife, other weapon)
- ▲ Verbal threats against property/person, threatening notes/letters
- ▲ Body language: angry facial expressions, rigid posture, clenched fists, threatening posture
- ▲ History of assaultive behavior

## *Outcome Criteria*

- • Refrains from abusive behaviors (in all forms) toward others
- ■ Controls impulse

## *Long-Term Goals*

Client will:
- • Display nonviolent behaviors toward self and others
- • Demonstrate three new ways to deal with tension and aggression in a nondestructive manner
- • Make plans to continue with long-term therapy (individual, family, group) to work on violence-prevention strategies and increasing coping skills
- • Identify factors contributing to abusive behaviors

---

▲ NANDA International accepted; ■ NOC Outcome, Controls Impulse

## Short-Term Goals

- Client's behavior will not escalate to aggressive acts toward self, others, or property while in hospital.
- Client will demonstrate increased self-control while in hospital.
- Client will participate in time outs, moving to a less stimulating environment, and verbal limits set by staff during hospital stay.
- Client will refrain from hurting self or others with the aid of verbal, chemical, or physical restraints.
- Client will identify available community resources for help.

## Interventions and Rationales

| Intervention | Rationale |
|---|---|
| 1. Keep environmental stimulation at a minimum (e.g., lower lights, keep stereos down, ask clients and visitors to leave the area or have staff take client to another area). | 1. Increased stimulation can increase client's anxiety level, leading to increased agitation or aggressive behaviors. |
| 2. Keep voice calm, speak in a low tone. | 2. High-pitched rapid voice can increase anxiety levels in others; the opposite is true when the tone of voice is low and calm, and the words are spoken slowly. |
| 3. Call client by name, introduce yourself, orient the client when necessary, tell the client beforehand what you are going to do. | 3. Calling client by name helps to establish contact. Orienting and giving information can minimize misrepresentation of nurses' intentions. |

| Intervention | Rationale |
|---|---|
| 4. Always use personal safety precautions:<br>  a. Either leave the door open in the interview room or use a hallway.<br>  b. If you feel uncertain of client's potential for violence, other staff should be nearby.<br>  c. Never turn your back on an angry client.<br>  d. Have a quick exit available.<br>  e. If on home visit, go with a colleague if there is concern regarding aggression.<br>**Leave the home immediately if there are any signs that the client's behavior is escalating out of control.** | 4. **Your safety is first always.** Always call in colleagues or other staff if you feel threatened or in physical danger. Nursing and security staff should have received frequent training in dealing with angry and hostile clients, including frequent training in steps in anger de-escalation and seclusion and restraint procedures. Ask for training, and learn from more experienced colleagues about unit precautions for staff as well as client safety. |

**Forensic Issues**

| Intervention | Rationale |
|---|---|
| 5. Always document client's behaviors and staff interventions during each level of restrictive intervention. | 5. Staff can demonstrate the appropriate use for each level of restraint in court of law, if necessary. |
| 6. When interventions are needed to reduce escalating anger, always use the least restrictive first, when possible:<br>  a. Interpersonal—verbal interventions | 6. Seclusion or restraints should never be used as punishment or substitute for staff. Restraints should be used only when there is no less restrictive alternative. |

| Intervention | Rationale |
|---|---|
| b. Chemical—appropriate medications | |
| c. Physical—restraints or seclusion | |
| 7. *Verbal interventions:* Encourage the client to talk about angry feelings and find ways to tolerate or reduce angry and aggressive feelings. | 7. When client feels heard and understood and has help with problem-solving alternative options, de-escalation of anger and aggression is often possible. |
| 8. Use empathetic *verbal interventions* (e.g., "It must be frightening to be here and to be feeling out of control."). | 8. Empathetic verbal intervention is the most effective method of calming an agitated, fearful, panicky client. |
| 9. When interpersonal interventions fail to decrease the client's anger, consider the need for *chemical* or *physical restraints.* Assessment includes determination if aggression is acute or chronic. (See Table 17-1 in the next section for medications used for clients with acute anger and Table 17-2 for clients with chronic aggression.) | 9. Often psychopharmacologic interventions can help clients gain control of their behavior, and prevent continued escalation of anger and hostile impulses. Appropriate medications for acute aggression differ from those appropriate for chronic aggression. |

| Intervention | Rationale |
|---|---|
| 10. Alert hospital security and other staff in a quiet and unobtrusive manner *before* violent behavior escalates so that they are prepared to intervene in a safe and knowledgeable manner if needed. | 10. **Hospital staff and security should have frequent training in restraining or secluding clients**. Alerting staff and security beforehand best ensures that the restraint or seclusion process will be handled safely for client, staff, and other clients on the unit. |
| 11. When interpersonal and pharmacologic interventions fail to control the angry client, *physical intervention (restraints or seclusion)* is the final resort. **Always follow hospital protocols, which should reflect HICFA standards**. Refer to Box 17-3 for some guidelines for use of restraints. | 11. Hospital protocols that are clear and well written tell staff when to restrain, how to restrain, how long before a physician's order is needed, nursing interventions for client during period of restraints or seclusion, how often to check restraints or client in seclusion, whom to call, and how often the need for restraints/seclusion needs to be reevaluated by physician. |
| 12. As mentioned, specific interventions should be documented, including times, types of intervention, and behavioral responses before restraints/seclusion was employed. | 12. Record what works with client, so that client-specific intervention information can be gleaned from careful documentation in the future. |

| Intervention | Rationale |
|---|---|
| 13. If restraints or seclusion has been used, check on client every 15 minutes, check restraints and circulation (color, temperature, pulses on extremities), need for toileting, nutrition, and hydration. **Use unit protocol as a guide.** | 13. Client safety is an important part of our care. Checking client frequently helps ensure client safety **(use unit protocol as a guide)**, and written records are kept in client's permanent record. |

---

**Box 17-3 Guidelines for Restraining a Client**

1. The specific indications should be clearly documented.
2. Anyone impaired enough to require restraints should have continuous staff observation.
3. Restraints are used when there is not a less restrictive alternative.
4. Restraints should be properly used and designed.
5. Five staff members are necessary to restrain a resistant client.
6. Security should be called to assist.
7. During the procedure, the client should be told in calm, simple terms, what is happening.
   *"You are in a hospital . . . these people are nurses and security staff . . . no one is going to hurt you . . . we are trying to make things safe for you."*
8. Nursing and security staff should receive training in this procedure on a regular basis.
9. Unit protocol should meet HICFA regulations, which are usually more stringent than any state or JCAHO regulations.

Adapted from Goldberg, R.J. (1998). *Practical guide to the care of the psychiatric patient.* St. Louis, Mosby, p. 168; reprinted with permission.

# MEDICAL TREATMENTS

## Psychopharmacology

### Acute Aggression

Distinctions need to be made as to whether the presenting behavior is acute aggression or chronic aggression. Acute aggression can be medically managed best with short-term use of medication with rapid onset of action. Table 17-1 helps identify some medications useful for acute aggression.

### Chronic Aggression

Chronic aggression is a more common problem, and aggression can diminish only after a therapeutic dose of the appropriate medication is used for 4 to 8 weeks. Table 17-2 lists drugs used to treat chronic aggression.

Table 17-1 **Medication Useful for Acute Aggression**

| Medication | Comments |
| --- | --- |
| Atypical antipsychotics (e.g., risperidone, olanzapine) or high-potency traditional neuroleptics (e.g., haloperidol) | Should be limited to psychosis-induced violence. Not to be used for aggression alone for more than 6 weeks. |
| **Benzodiazepines (Short-acting):** | Effective in episodic dyscontrol and rage reactions. |
| Lorazepam (Ativan) | Initially 1 to 2 mg orally or intramuscularly every hour until calm, Taper at 10% per day from highest dose to avoid withdrawal symptoms unless drug is used less than 1 week. Not to be used for aggression alone for more than 6 weeks. |
| Trazodone (Desyrel) | Acutely lowers aggression and agitation in demented or mentally retarded clients without impairing cognition. Doses up to 500 mg have been used. |

Data from Maxmen, J.S., & Ward, N.G. (2002). *Psychotropic drugs: Fast facts* (3rd ed.). New York: WW Norton & Co.

Table 17-2 **Medication Useful for Chronic Aggression**

| Generic Group | Indications |
|---|---|
| Beta blockers (e.g., propranolol) | Recurrent or chronic aggression in organically based violence; for example: Alzheimer's disease Stroke Huntington's disease Psychosis in which aggression is unrelated to psychotic thought |
| Anticonvulsants | Bipolar disorder Borderline personality disorder (BPD) Conduct disorder Episodic dyscontrol Posttraumatic stress disorder (PTSD) Central nervous system (CNS) disorder |
| Lithium | Mania-associated violence Uncontrolled rage triggered by nothing or minor stimuli (e.g., BPD, PTSD, variety of other situations) |
| Buspirone (BuSpar) | Cognitively impaired, developmentally disabled, head injuries, and dementia |
| Nadolol | Diminishes assaultiveness in chronic paranoid schizophrenia, CNS disorders, and developmentally disabled |
| Carbamazepine | Intermittent explosive disorder and BPD, as well as PTSD and schizophrenia |

Adapted from Maxmen, J.S., & Ward, N.G. (2002). *Psychotropic drugs: Fast facts* (3rd ed.). New York: WW Norton & Co.

# NURSE, CLIENT, AND FAMILY RESOURCES

## INTERNET SITES

**Focus Adolescent Service**
http://www.focusas.com
Search for "anger" to find relevant articles

**SIUC Mental Health Web**
http://www.siu.edu/office/counsel/
Managing anger and understanding the dynamics of violence, abuse, and control

**Anger Management Institute**
http://www.manageanger.com/guidelines.htm
Guidelines for understanding and managing anger

**Centers for Disease Control and Prevention**
http://www.cdc.gov
Search for "anger" to find multiple articles

**About Anger and Raging**
http://www.recovery-man.com/abusive/
   rage_vs_anger.htm

**Anger Management**
http://mentalhelp.net

# CHAPTER 18

# Grieving and Dysfunctional Grieving

## OVERVIEW

Loss is part of the human experience, and grief is the normal response to loss. There can be loss of a relationship (divorce, separation, death, abortion); of health (a body function or part, mental or physical capacity); of status or prestige; of security (occupational, financial, social); of self-confidence; of self-concept; or of a dream; or loss can be of a symbolic nature.

Even though grief and loss are universal experiences, loss through death is a major life crisis for most people. Grief is not a mood disorder, although a depressive syndrome is often part of the grieving process.

**Grief** is the characteristic painful feelings precipitated by the death of a loved one or by some other significant loss. **Bereavement** is the state of being deprived of a loved one by death. **Mourning** is the process (grief work) by which the grief is resolved, and includes various phenomena, which are discussed later.

Although grief is a normal phenomenon, it can be the focus of treatment. Most bereaved persons resolve their loss with help and support from family and friends. However, more than 30% require professional support (Lloyd-Williams, 1995). Acute grief can trigger an exacerbation of any pre-existing medical or psychological problems. A history of depression, substance abuse, or posttraumatic stress disorder can complicate grief and require treatment (Prigerson, 1995). Unresolved grief reactions account for many of the physical symptoms seen in medical clinics and hospital units. Suicide is higher among people who have had a significant loss, especially if losses are multiple and grieving mechanisms are limited (Gregory, 1994). The death of a child and multiple deaths are regarded as the most severe types of loss. Nurses are not immune to grief reactions. As health care workers, as nurses, as friends, as people who will experience grief and loss throughout our own lifetimes, it is helpful to know what happens during the process of mourning, what might help others through this process, and how to identify a person who is having difficulty resolving his or her pain and sorrow (dysfunctional grieving).

Dr. Elisabeth Kübler-Ross began listening to the terminally ill, and out of her groundbreaking work came a construct of the human response to death that has entered the mainstream (Kramer-Howe, 2005). Most nurses and clinicians are familiar with Kübler-Ross's (1969) classic review of the stages of death and dying (denial, isolation, anger, bargaining, depression, and acceptance).

The resolution of the loss usually occurs through these stages, and a person might demonstrate a different clinical picture at each stage of mourning. Each stage has its own characteristics, and the duration and form of each stage varies considerably from person to person. People react within their own cultural patterns and their own value and personality structure, as well as within their own social environment. Most of us are programmed in our response to death. Distinct characteristics, however, can be identified throughout the grieving process. It is important to keep in mind that these stages do not necessarily progress in an orderly fashion, and might overlap during the grief process.

**What we are not often taught is what to say or do to facilitate the healing of those who must learn to live with their anguish.**

Normal grief reaction includes depressed mood, insomnia, anxiety, poor appetite, loss of interest, guilt feelings, dreams about the deceased, and poor concentration. Psychological states include shock, denial, and yearning and searching for the deceased. The acute grief reaction lasts from 4 to 8 weeks; the active symptoms of grief usually last from 3 to 6 months; and the complete work of mourning can take from 1 to 2 years or more to complete. However, acute grief can be a time of exacerbation of any medical or psychiatric problems, as mentioned on the previous page.

Nurses can care for the bereaved through listening, assisting in communication, teaching families about the process of dying, or facilitating bereavement with opportunities to prevent ill health and to help families find new directions for growth.

# ASSESSMENT

## Assessing History

- Does the bereaved exhibit some of the factors that can complicate the successful completion of mourning?
  - ○ Was the bereaved heavily dependent on the deceased?
  - ○ Were there persistent, unresolved conflicts with the deceased?
  - ○ Was the deceased a child (often the most profound loss)?
  - ○ Does the bereaved have a meaningful relationship/support system?
  - ○ Has the bereaved experienced a number of previous losses?
  - ○ Does the bereaved have sound coping skills?
- Was the deceased's death associated with a cultural stigma (e.g., AIDS, suicide)?
- Was the death unexpected or associated with violence (murder, suicide)?
- Has the bereaved had difficulty resolving past significant losses?
- Does the bereaved have a history of depression, drug or alcohol abuse, or other psychiatric illness?
- If the bereaved is young, are there indications for special interventions?

## Presenting Signs and Symptoms of Dysfunctional Grief

- Prolonged, severe symptoms lasting for 2 or more months
- Limited response to support
- Profound and persistent feelings of hopelessness
- Completely withdrawn, or fears being alone
- Inability to work, to create, or to feel emotion and positive states of mind
- Maladaptive behaviors in response to the death, for example:

- ○ Drug or alcohol abuse
- ○ Promiscuity
- ○ Fugue states
- ○ Feeling dead or unreal
- ○ Suicidal ideation
- ○ Aggressive behaviors
- ○ Compulsive spending
- Recurrent nightmares, night terrors, compulsive reenactments
- Exhaustion from lack of sleep and hyperarousal
- Prolonged depression, panic attacks
- Self neglect

## Assessment Tools

Table 18-1 presents a comparison of the symptoms seen in a "normal" mourning process contrasting those seen in a dysfunctional grief reaction. This can be used as a helpful guide in your assessment.

Table 18-1 **Common Experiences during Grief and their Pathologic Intensification**

| Phase | Typical Response | Pathologic Intensification |
|---|---|---|
| Dying | Emotional expression and immediate coping with the dying process. | Avoidant; overwhelmed, dazed, confused; self-punitive; inappropriately hostile. |
| Death and outcry | Outcry of emotions with news of the death and turning to others for help or isolating self with self-succoring. | Panic; dissociative reactions, reactive psychoses. |
| Warding off (denial) | Avoidance of reminders, social withdrawal, focusing elsewhere, emotional numbing, not thinking of implications to self or certain themes. | Maladaptive avoidances confronting the implications of death. Drug or alcohol abuse, counterphobic frenzy, promiscuity, fugue states, phobic avoidance, feeling dead or unreal. |

*Continued*

Table 18-1 **Common Experiences during Grief and their Pathologic Intensification—cont'd**

| Phase | Typical Response | Pathologic Intensification |
|-------|------------------|---------------------------|
| Re-experience (intrusion) | Intrusive experiences, including recollections of negative relationship experiences with the deceased, bad dreams, reduced concentration, compulsive re-enactments. | Flooding with negative images and emotions, uncontrolled ideation, self-impairing compulsive reenactments, night terrors, recurrent nightmares, distraught from intrusion of anger, anxiety, despair, shame, or guilt themes; physiologic exhaustion from hyperarousal. |
| Working through | Recollection of the deceased and contemplation of self with reduced intrusiveness of memories and fantasies, increased rational acceptance, reduced numbness and avoidance, more "dosing" of recollections, and a sense of working through it. | Sense that one cannot integrate the death with a sense of self and continued life. Persistent, warded-off themes can manifest as anxious, depressed, enraged, shame-filled, or guilty moods, and psychophysiologic syndromes. |
| Completion | Reduction in emotional swings with a sense of self-coherence and readiness for new relationships. | Failure to complete mourning might be associated with inability to work, to create, to feel emotion, or to experience positive states of mind. |

From Horowitz, M.J. (1990). A model of mourning: Change in schemas of self and others. *Journal of the American Psychoanalytic Association, 38,* 297-324; reprinted with permission.

Assessment Guidelines

*Grieving and Dysfunctional Grieving*

1. Identify if the individual is at risk for complicated dysfunctional grieving (see Assessing History).
2. Evaluate for psychotic symptoms, agitation, increased activity, alcohol/drug abuse, and extreme vegetative symptoms (anorexia, weight loss, not sleeping).
3. Do not overlook people who do not express significant grief in the context of a major loss. Those individuals might have an increased risk of subsequent complicated or unresolved grief reaction (Kaplan & Sadock, 1999).
4. Complicated grief reactions require significant interventions. Suicidal or severely depressed people might require hospitalization. **Always assess for suicide** with signs of depression or other dysfunctional signs.
5. Assess support systems. If support systems are limited, find bereavement groups in the bereaved's community.
6. When grieving is stalled or dysfunctional, a variety of therapeutic approaches have proved extremely beneficial (e.g., cognitive-behavioral interventions). Provide referrals.
7. Grieving can bring with it severe spiritual anguish. Would spiritual counseling or a specific counselor be useful for the bereaved at this time?

# NURSING DIAGNOSES WITH INTERVENTIONS

## Discussion of Potential Nursing Diagnoses

The North American Nursing Diagnosis Association (NANDA, International, 2005-2006) identifies three nursing diagnoses for nursing actions: **Dysfunctional Grieving, Risk for Dysfunctional Grieving,** and **Anticipatory Grieving.** However, because nurses are in constant contact with people and their families experiencing painful losses, **Acute Grief Reaction** (not a NANDA International nursing diagnosis) can also be the focus of treatment. During this time, the nurse might need to intervene for **Ineffective Coping** or **Compromised Family Coping, Disturbed Sleep Pattern, Risk for Spiritual Distress** or **Spiritual Distress, Disturbed Thought Processes,** or other problems.

## Overall Guidelines for Nursing Interventions
### Grieving and Dysfunctional Grieving

1. Employ methods that can facilitate the grieving process and give support to a grieving person: (Robinson, 1997)
   - Be there for the bereaved; give your full presence.
   - Offer physical touch suited to the moment and your relationship. Do not use touch if it will presume an intimacy that does not exist or as a tool to coerce a person to mourn.
   - Identify family or friends to assist with practical concerns.
   - Try to provide beauty or nourishment in some suitable form.
   - Encourage the individual and family to mourn on their own schedule.
2. Identify and treat/refer an individual with a pathologic process.
3. Assess for suicide if there is persistent, severe depression and deep, enduring feelings of hopelessness.
4. Know, share, and support with the bereaved the normal phenomena that occur during the normal mourning process, which might concern some people (intense anger at the deceased, guilt, symptoms the deceased had before death, unbidden flood of memories). Give bereaved a written handout to refer to.
5. Apply appropriate measures when the family member dies in the hospital that can help facilitate grieving for families (Table 18-2).

   Remember, we each grieve differently depending upon age, culture, and spiritual levels. Make an effort to identify the special/specific needs of the bereaved.

## Selected Nursing Diagnoses and Nursing Care Plans

### ACUTE GRIEF REACTION

Focuses on the devastating and often overwhelming pain people experience upon the death of someone they care about and who was an integral part of their lives; the acute phase lasts from 4 to 8 weeks after the death or a significant loss (The *long-term phase* follows the acute phase and constitutes the main work of mourning; it might last for 1 to 2 years or more)

## Related To (Etiology)

- Recent loss of loved one (e.g., person, pet) or forced change (e.g., loss of job, home, or body part; disaster; divorce)

## As Evidenced By
## (Assessment Findings/Diagnostic Cues)

Signs of grief:
- Anguish and pain
- Anger at deceased or health care professionals
- Guilt

Table 18-2 **Nursing Interventions for Grieving Families in a Hospital Setting**

| Intervention | Rationale |
| --- | --- |
| 1. At the death or imminent death of a family member: | |
| • Communicate the news to the family in an area of privacy. | • Family members can support each other in an atmosphere in which they can behave naturally. |
| • If only one family member is available, stay with that member until clergy, a family member, or a friend arrives. | • The presence and comfort of the nurse during the initial stage of shock can help minimize feelings of acute isolation and anxiety. |
| • If the nurse feels unable to handle the situation, the aid of another who can support the family should be enlisted. | • The individual or family will need support, answers to questions, and guidance as to immediate tasks and information. |
| 2. If the family requests to see and take leave of the dying or dead person: | |
| • Grant this request. | • The need to take leave can be of overwhelming importance for some—to kiss good-bye, ask for forgiveness, or take a lock of hair. This helps people face the reality of death. |

*Continued*

● In addition to NANDA International

Table 18-2 **Nursing Interventions for Grieving Families in a Hospital Setting—cont'd**

| Intervention | Rationale |
|---|---|
| 3. If angry family members accuse the nurse or doctor of abusing or mismanaging the care of the deceased: | |
| • Continue to provide the best care for the dying or final care to the dead. Avoid becoming involved in angry and painful arguments and power struggles. | • Complaints are not directed toward the nurse personally. The anger may serve the purpose of keeping grieving relatives from falling apart. Projected anger may be an attempt to deal with aggression and guilt toward the dying person. |
| 4. If relatives behave in a grossly disturbed manner (e.g., refuse to acknowledge the truth, collapse, or lose control): | |
| • Show patience and tact, and offer sympathy and warmth. | • Shock and disbelief are the first responses to the news of death, and people need ways to protect themselves from the overwhelming reality of loss. |
| • Encourage the person to cry. | • Crying helps provide relief from feelings of acute pain and tension. |
| • Provide a place of privacy for grieving. | • Privacy facilitates the natural expression of grief. |
| 5. If the family requests specific religious, cultural, or social customs strange or unknown to the nurse: | |
| • Help facilitate steps necessary for the family to carry out the desired arrangements. | • Institutional mourning rituals of various cultures provide important external supports for the grief-stricken person. |

Data from Engel, G.L. (1964). Grief and grieving. *American Journal of Nursing, 64*(9), 93.

- Crying
- Vegetative signs (anorexia, insomnia, bowel dysfunction, immobility)
- Withdrawal from usual activities and preoccupation with the deceased

## Outcome Criteria

- Expresses positive expectations about the future
- The family will engage in life and pursue other activities

## Long-Term Goals

- The bereaved will seek support during the grieving process.
- The bereaved will demonstrate behaviors that signify the individual is completing the process of mourning (Box 18-1).
- The bereaved will participate in planning the funeral.
- The bereaved will state they find comfort and support through their religious/spiritual practices.

---

### Box 18-1 Behaviors Signaling Successful Mourning

The person:
1. Can tolerate intense emotions.
2. Demonstrates increased periods of stability.
3. Takes on new roles and responsibilities.
4. Has energy to invest in new endeavors.
5. Remembers both positive and negative aspects of the deceased loved one.
6. Brief periods of intense emotions might occur at significant times, such as anniversaries and holidays.

Data from Gorman, L.M., Sultan D.F., & Raines, M.L. (1996). *Davis's manual of psychosocial nursing for general patient care*. Philadelphia: FA Davis.

---

●In addition to NANDA International

*Short-Term Goals*

- The bereaved will state the names of two support people he or she can share painful feelings and memories with
- If the bereaved demonstrates signs of dysfunctional grief reaction, he or she will agree to seek support and treatment
- The bereaved will express feelings about the loss within 2 days
- The bereaved will verbalize reality of the loss within 1 week
- The bereaved will express spiritual beliefs about death

*Interventions and Rationales*

| Intervention | Rationale |
|---|---|
| **Outside the Hospital**<br>1. Employ methods that can facilitate the grieving process (Robinson, 1997): | |
| a. Giving your full presence: use appropriate eye contact, attentive listening, and appropriate touch. | a. Talking is one of the most important ways of dealing with acute grief. *Listening patiently* helps the bereaved express all feelings, even ones he or she thinks are negative. *Appropriate eye contact* helps to let him or her know you are there and sharing his or her sadness. *Suitable human touch* can express warmth and nurture healing. Inappropriate touch can leave a person confused and uncomfortable. |
| b. Be patient with the bereaved in times of silence. Do not fill silence with empty chatter. | b. Sharing painful feelings during periods of silence is healing and conveys your concern. |

| Intervention | Rationale |
|---|---|
| 2. Avoid the use of euphemisms. We use euphemisms in the hope they will stave off or soften the intrusive vulgarity of the death (e.g., "passed away," "You lost your husband."). Instead say something like, "I am really sorry to hear that James died." | 2. Euphemisms can do harm:<br>a. Can cause the bereaved to think we have not caught the gravity of the situation.<br>b. Wanting at one level to deny what is happening, the bereaved might use euphemisms to help postpone facing the painful feelings they desperately need to work through. |
| 3. Avoid banal advice and philosophical statements such as, "He's no longer suffering"; "You can always have another child"; or "It's better this way." It is *more helpful* to put into words acknowledgment of the bereaved's painful feelings, such as:<br>a. "His death will be a terrible loss."<br>b. "No one can replace her."<br>c. "He will be missed for a long time." | 3. Gives the bereaved the impression that their experience is not understood, and that you are minimizing the experience and pain. The fact that the deceased is no longer suffering does not mean that the bereaved is not experiencing a devastating, painful loss. |
| 4. Encourage the support of family and friends. If no supports are available, refer the bereaved to a community bereavement group. (Bereavement groups are helpful even when a person has many friends and/or family support.) | 4. There are routine matters that friends can help with, for example:<br>a. Getting food to the house<br>b. Making phone calls<br>c. Driving to the mortuary<br>d. Taking care of kids or other family members |

| Intervention | Rationale |
|---|---|
| 5. Offer spiritual support and/or referrals when needed. | 5. Dealing with an illness or catastrophic loss can cause the most profound spiritual anguish (Zerbe, 1999). |
| 6. When intense emotions are in evidence, show understanding and support (see Box 18-2 for guidelines). | 6. Empathetic words that reflect acceptance of a bereaved individual's feelings are always healing (Robinson, 1997). |

## DYSFUNCTIONAL GRIEVING

Extended unsuccessful use of intellectual and emotional responses by which individuals, families, and communities attempt to work through the process of modifying self-concept based upon the perception of loss

---

### Box 18-2 Guidelines for What to Say

| When you sense an overwhelming *sorrow:* | "This must hurt terribly." |
|---|---|
| When you hear *anger* in the bereaved's voice: | "I hear anger in your voice. Most people go through periods of anger when their loved one dies. Are you feeling anger now?" |
| If you discern *guilt:* | "Are you feeling guilty? This is a common reaction many people have. What are some of your thoughts about this?" |
| If you sense a *fear* of the future: | "It must be scary to go through this." |
| When the bereaved seems *confused:* | "This can be a bewildering time." |
| In almost any *painful situation:* | "This must be very difficult for you." |

Adapted from Robinson, D. (1997). *Good intentions: The nine unconscious mistakes of nice people.* New York: Warner Books, p. 249; reprinted by permission. Copyright 1997 by Duke Robinson.

## Related To (Etiology)

- ▲ Loss of support systems
- ▲ Loss or perceived loss/change (specific)
- ● Presence of factors identified in history (e.g., substance abuse, multiple losses, poor physical health, other mental health risks)

## As Evidenced By
## (Assessment Findings/Diagnostic Cues)

- ▲ Verbal expression of distress or loss or denial of loss *and* one of the following:
  - • Arrested grieving process before resolution
  - • Prolonged grieving beyond expected time for cultural group
  - • Emotional response more exaggerated than expected for cultural group (severity of reaction)
- ▲ Expression of unresolved issues
- ▲ Interference with life functioning
- ● Suicidal ideation
- ● Prolonged panic attacks
- ● Prolonged depression
- ● Engagement in self-destructive activities
- ● Self-neglect
- ● Protracted social withdrawal

## Outcome Criteria

- • Express optimism about the future
- • Expressions of feeling socially engaged
- • Takes on new roles and responsibilities

## Long-Term Goals

Bereaved will:
- • Resolve blocks to the grieving process (maladaptive avoidance, extreme prolonged denial), and the stages of mourning will be reactivated during grief counseling
- • Demonstrate initial integration into their life within 6 months

---

▲ NANDA International accepted; ● In addition to NANDA International

- Demonstrate physical recuperation from the stress of loss and grieving within 6 months
- Demonstrate reestablished relationships and social supports within 4 weeks

## Short-Term Goals

Bereaved will:
- Be free of self-directed harm
- Demonstrate decreased suicidal, aggressive, depressive, or withdrawn behaviors within 2 weeks
- Express feelings, verbally and nonverbally
- Establish or maintain an adequate balance of rest, sleep, and activity with help from nurse and family
- Establish or maintain adequate nutrition, hydration, and elimination within 2 weeks

## Interventions and Rationales

| Intervention | Rationale |
|---|---|
| 1. Always assess for presence of suicidal thoughts or ideation. | 1. Severely depressed or suicidal individuals might require hospitalization and protection from self-harm and severe self-neglect. |
| 2. Talk with the bereaved in realistic terms. Discuss concrete changes that have occurred in the person's life after the death and how it might affect the person's future. | 2. Discussing the death and how it has and will continue to affect the person's life can help the death become more concrete and real. |
| 3. If the bereaved cannot talk about the death initially, encourage other means of expression (e.g., keeping a journal, drawing, reading about the experience of grief). | 3. Talking is usually the most important tool for resolving initial pain; however, any avenue for the expression of feelings can help the bereaved identify, accept, and work through their feelings. |

| Intervention | Rationale |
|---|---|
| 4. Stress that people often have strong feelings of anger (even hate) at the deceased, feel guilty, harbor strong feelings of resentment, and the like. | 4. Understanding that strong "negative" feelings are, in fact, normal and experienced by most people can make the bereaved aware of such feelings and then work through them. |
| 5. Encourage the person to recall memories (happy ones, sad ones, difficult ones); listen actively; and stay silent when appropriate. | 5. Reviewing past memories is an important stage in mourning. Being with the bereaved and sharing painful feelings can be healing. |
| 6. Encourage the person to talk to others individually, in small groups, or in community bereavement groups. | 6. Talking and listening are the most important activities that can help resolve grief and reactivate the mourning process. |
| 7. Carefully avoid false reassurances that everything will be okay as time passes. | 7. For some, separation through death is never okay; even when the grieving process is complete, the person might be sorely missed. |
| 8. Assess the need for psychotherapy "re-grief" work. | 8. Many people find brief counseling (6 to 10 sessions) useful during the work of mourning. |
| 9. Identify religious/spiritual background, and determine if the bereaved would be receptive to a spiritual advisor. | 9. For many people, spiritual needs and support are extremely comforting at this time, and sharing feelings with a trusted and empathetic religious figure might be comforting. |

| Intervention | Rationale |
|---|---|
| 10. Offer written guidelines for coping with overwhelming grief. | 10. When grieving, even simple tasks can become monumental, life becomes confusing, and normal routines are often interrupted. These guidelines offer simple reminders and help validate the bereaved's experience. |

## GUIDELINES FOR COPING WITH GRIEF

Box 18-3 suggests guidelines that can help the bereaved through this period.

---

**Box 18-3 Client Guidelines for Coping with Catastrophic Loss**

1. **Take the time you need to grieve.** The hard work of grief uses psychological energy. Resolution of the "numb state" that occurs after loss requires a few weeks at least. A minimum of 1 year, to cover all the birthdays, anniversaries, and other important dates without your loved one, is required before you can "learn to live" with your loss.

2. **Express your feelings.** Remember that anger, anxiety, loneliness, and even guilt are normal reactions and that everyone needs a safe place to express them. Tell your personal story of loss as many times as you need to—this repetition is a helpful and necessary part of the grieving process.

3. **Make a daily structure and stick to it.** Although it is hard to do, keeping to some semblance of structure makes the first few weeks after a loss easier. Getting through each day helps restore the confidence you need to accept the reality of loss.

4. **Don't feel that you have to answer all the questions asked of you.** Although most people try to be kind, they might be unaware of their insensitivity. At some point, you might want to read books about how others have dealt with similar circumstances. They often have helpful suggestions for a person in your situation.

---

### Box 18-3 **Client Guidelines for Coping with Catastrophic Loss—cont'd**

5. **As hard as it is, try to take good care of yourself.** Eat well, talk with friends, get plenty of rest. Be sure to let your primary care clinician know if you are having trouble eating or sleeping. Make use of exercise. It can help you let out pent-up frustrations. If you are losing weight, sleeping excessively or intermittently, or still experiencing deep depression after 3 months, be sure to seek professional assistance.

6. **Expect the unexpected.** You may begin to feel a bit better, only to have a brief "emotional collapse." These are expected reactions. Moreover, you might dream, visualize, think about, or search for your loved one. This, too, is a part of the grief process.

7. **Give yourself time.** Do not feel that you have to resume all of life's duties right away.

8. **Make use of rituals.** Those who take the time to "say good-bye" at a funeral or a viewing tend to find it helps the bereavement process.

9. **If you do not begin to feel better within a few weeks, at least for a few hours every day, be sure to tell your doctor.** If you have had an emotional problem in the past (e.g., depression, substance abuse), be sure to get the additional support you need. Losing a loved one puts you at higher risk for relapse of these disorders.

---

From Zerbe, K.J. (1999). *Women's mental health in primary care.* Philadelphia: WB Saunders, pp. 207–208; reprinted with permission.

## NURSE, CLIENT, AND FAMILY RESOURCES

## BOOKS

*For People with a Terminally Ill Family Member*
Callahan, M. & Kelley, P. (1997). *Final gifts: Understanding the special awareness, needs and communication of the dying.* New York: Poseidon.

*For Survivors of Suicide*
Chance, S. (1992). *Stronger Than Death.* New York: WW Norton.

*For Widows*
Brothers, J. (1990). *Widowhood*. New York: Ballantine.
Caine, L. (1988). *Being a widow*. New York: Penguin.

*For Bereaved Parents*
Rosof, B.D. (1994). *The worst loss: How families heal from the death of a child*. New York: Henry Holt.

*For Children*
Lionni, L. (1995). *Little blue and little yellow*. New York: Mulberry.

*About Death*
O'Gorman, S. (1998). Death and dying in contemporary society: An evaluation of current attitudes and rituals associated with death and dying and their relevance to recent understandings of health and healing. *Journal of Advanced Nursing, 27*, 1127-1135.

## EDUCATIONAL RESOURCES

*About Dying*
**National Hospice Foundation**
1700 Diagonal Road, Suite 625
Alexandria, VA 22314
(800) 646-6460
http://www.hospiceinfo.org

## INTERNET SITES

**American Academy of Hospice and Palliative Medicine**
http://www.aahpm.org

**Approaching Death: Improving Care at the End of Life**
http://nap.edu/book/html/approaching
Online publication
**Hospice Foundation of America**
http://www.hospicefoundation.org

**National Institute on Aging**
http://www.nia.nih.gov

# PART IV

# CHALLENGING
# BEHAVIORS

# CHAPTER 19

# Manipulative Behaviors

## OVERVIEW

Healthy manipulation is essentially purposeful behavior directed at getting needs met. It (1) is goal oriented and used only when appropriate, (2) considers others' needs, and (3) is only one of several coping mechanisms used.

Individuals manipulate events every day to manage their lives (e.g., carry out financial obligations, optimize social activities, ensure the welfare of their families) and to keep their lives and the lives of those they care about as secure and stable as possible. Most nurses are good at organizing their daily schedules to provide the optimum care to their clients. This includes consults with other health care professionals, changing time schedules, organizing care into priorities, and countless other ways to ensure quality care. These are all healthy uses of manipulation. Nurses manipulate situations and events not just to complete their assignment, but to best serve their clients.

**Manipulation** is **maladaptive** when (Chitty & Maynard, 1986):

- It is the primary method used for getting needs met.
- The needs, goals, and feelings of others are disregarded.
- Others are treated as objects to fulfill the needs of the manipulator.

Manipulation is, in effect, a matter of gaining a sense of control. When manipulation is used in a maladaptive manner, individuals say or do almost anything to get what they want, even if it is at the expense of others.

*Maladaptive manipulation* in the health care system presents a real challenge to staff. The staff is most effective when all are working together on intervention for manipulation. One situation in which staff members should be alert to possible manipulation is when each staff member views and experiences the client in extremely different ways. This inevitably results in staff confusion and disagreements. Infighting can result when discussing caring for the client. Variations in experiences can occur between nurses and physicians, between shifts, between individuals on the nursing staff, and/or between administrators and staff (Gorman et al., 1996).

Potential for staff manipulation is particularly high among individuals who:

- Have personality disorders (PDs) (especially borderline and antisocial PDs)
- Have a chemical dependence
- Are in the manic phase of bipolar disorder
- Have long histories of physical complaints without physical cause
- Are children or adolescents who have the diagnosis of conduct disorder

People who manipulate might be trying to gain a variety of different things, although a need for control is usually the underlying force. For example, people might manipulate to get nurturance, power over a situation or person, possessions, or some other material gratification.

Clients manipulate by the use of pitting one person or group against another person or group:

> "Nurse X really understands my situation, so she lets me take my own medications. Why can't you? Please don't tell anyone I told on Nurse X. I don't want her to get into trouble."

Or, when talking to a member of the day staff, a manipulative client might say something like:

> "The night staff is awful. They just sit around and drink coffee, yell at the patients when they ring their bells, and really say some nasty stuff about you day people."

Once staff is all stirred up and angry with each other, the client is better able to get what he or she wants without interference. Staff splitting is a real challenge in the health care setting. Clients also manipulate when they flatter and behave in such a way as to give the impression of sincerity, caring, and appreciation when their only goal is to get their needs met in any manner possible:

"You are the kindest nurse on the unit, and the only one here who cares enough to understand me. You know how much I need to go out on pass even if I did come in late yesterday. I know I'm not supposed to but please trust me just this once. I promise I will be on time."

Clients with *chemical dependence* problems are used to soothing anxiety and denying or postponing unattractive realities through use of their substance. Clients learn to manipulate others through anger, threatening, swindling, cajoling, instilling guilt, flattering, or any other method to get their drugs. For most people dependent on a drug, the drug is the only thing in the world they care about.

Another form of manipulation is seen in clients who are profane, fault finding, and adept at exploring others' vulnerabilities. They constantly push limits. Their manipulative behaviors often alienate family, friends, employers, health care providers, and others.

## ASSESSMENT

### Assessing History

A positive history might include some of the following:
- A history of a personality disorder PD (borderline, antisocial, passive-aggressive)
- A history of mania
- A history of substance use or dependence
- A history of unreliable or immature behaviors marked by instability, frequent changes in jobs, relationships, and physicians
- A long history of unsubstantiated physical complaints

### Presenting Signs and Symptoms

- Manipulation of staff, family, and others
- Playing one person against another (nurse against nurse, family member against staff, therapist against family member)
- Attempts to get special treatment or privileges
- Attention-seeking behaviors
- Use of somatic complaints to get out of doing things
- Lacks insight
- Denies problems

- Focuses on other people's problems (clients, staff, unit dynamics)
- Uses intimidation to control or feel superior
- Demanding (the more staff try to cater to client's demands, the more they escalate)
- Frustration causes more intense manipulative behavior
- Lies, cheats, steals
- Exploitive with little concern for others
- Quick to recognize vulnerability in others
- Devalues others to feel good about self
- Resists limits set on negative behaviors

## Assessment Guidelines
### Manipulation

1. Assess for history of physical or psychosocial problems.
2. Identify client's usual coping responses.
3. Assess medications client is taking.
4. Assess for a history of substance use or dependence, spouse abuse, legal difficulties, violent behavior.
5. Assess client's strengths as well as weaknesses.
6. Who does the client trust?
7. What does he do when he does not get his own way?
8. Is the client at risk for suicide? Homicide?
9. Is the client abusing others? Child? Spouse? Elder? Other?

# NURSING DIAGNOSES WITH INTERVENTIONS

## Discussion of Potential Nursing Diagnoses

Clients who employ manipulation as a primary means of getting their needs met often have no motivation to change, as long as they can get what they want when they want it, even if it is at the expense of others. **Impaired Social Interaction** is usually present because the individual's actions usually impact negatively on others. People who employ maladaptive manipulation in their relationships with others usually present with a history of interpersonal difficulties and unstable relationships. The manipulative individual feels no compunction about lying, stealing, cheating, threatening, tormenting, devaluing, demeaning, or swindling to get what he or she wants.

Staff working with manipulative clients are best pre-pared when they establish firm rules that are rigidly inter-preted and consistently enforced among all members of the health care team. Frequent discussions regarding the client's progress can help reduce staff frustration and isola-tion, and minimize the client's attempts at staff splitting. Smith (1994) identifies important guidelines when inter-vening with manipulative behaviors:

• Ignoring manipulative behaviors will not make them go away; they get worse when ignored.
• Interventions such as employing limit-setting techniques help reduce stress and hostility for both client and staff.
• To successfully limit problem behavior, limits must be consistent and reinforced by everyone, including all health care personnel as well as family.

Therefore, **confronting** unacceptable, inappropriate, or harmful behavior needs to be done immediately, and **setting limits** on client behaviors is the pivotal intervention when working with manipulative clients. Clear, enforce-able consequences of continuing unacceptable behaviors need to be clearly spelled out and consistently and matter-of-factly enforced by all staff involved in the client's care.

Schultz and Videbeck (2005) point out that it is not the nurse's purpose to be a friend to the client, nor the client a friend to the nurse. The most effective approach with the client is to maintain a professional therapeutic relationship with clear boundaries. A professional relationship is based on the client's therapeutic needs, not on being liked or the nurse's personal feelings. People who manipulate others need clear and firm boundaries with clear and firm conse-quences identified for overstepping those boundaries.

Manipulative clients often have great difficulty with impulse control, become inappropriately angry, might become a risk to others, and are aggressive with little or no provocation when they cannot get their own way. Therefore, anger management is often useful and important for nurses to learn and employ. Refer to Chapter 17.

## Overall Guidelines for Nursing Interventions

### Manipulation

1. Anger is a natural response to being manipulated. Deal with your own feelings of anger toward client. Peer supervision can be useful.

2. Assess your feelings toward clients who use manipulation, and work on being assertive in stating limits. Workshops in assertiveness can be very helpful for nurses.

3. State limits and the behavior you expect from the client in a matter-of-fact, nonthreatening tone.

4. Be sure the limits are:
   - Appropriate, not punitive
   - Enforceable
   - Stated in a nonpersonal way (e.g., "Alcohol is not allowed," *not* "I don't want you to drink alcohol on the unit.")

5. State the consequences if behaviors are not forthcoming. Written limits and consequences can be useful (one copy for client and one for staff).

6. Be sure all staff members understand the expectations, limits, and consequences discussed with the client to provide consistency. A written copy should be in Kardex or client folder.

7. Follow through with the consequences.

8. Enforce all unit, hospital, group, or community center policies. State reasons for not bending the rules.

9. Be direct and assertive, if necessary, in a neutral, factual manner, not in anger.

10. Do *not:*
    - Discuss yourself or other staff members with the client
    - Promise to keep a secret for the client
    - Accept gifts from the client
    - Attempt to be liked, "the favorite," or popular with the client

11. Withdraw your attention when client's behavior is inappropriate.

12. Give attention and support when the client's behavior is appropriate and positive.

13. Emphasize the client's feelings, not his or her rationalizations or intellectualizations.

14. Encourage the expression of feelings.

15. Set limits on frequency and time of interactions with the client, especially those that involve therapists who are significant to the client.

16. Encourage identification of feelings or situations that trigger manipulative behaviors.

17. Role-play situations so that the client can practice more direct and appropriate ways of relating.

18. Provide positive feedback when the client interacts without use of manipulation.
19. Where appropriate, see that clients and families have names and numbers of appropriate community resources (e.g., Alanon, Alcoholics Anonymous, Parents Anonymous, Tough Love).
20. Keep detailed records in client's chart as to client's responses to limit setting and any increase or decrease in undesirable, unacceptable, maladaptive manipulative behavior. Identify what seems to work and what does not seem to work. Share information with all staff members.

## Selected Nursing Diagnoses and Nursing Care Plans

### IMPAIRED SOCIAL INTERACTION

Insufficient or excessive quantity or ineffective quality of social exchange

### Related To (Etiology)

- Longstanding patterns of maladaptive behaviors
- Biochemical/neurologic imbalances
- Impulsive and chronic need for immediate gratification without regard to consequences to others
- Inability or unwillingness to respect the rights and wishes of others

### As Evidenced By (Assessment Findings/Diagnostic Cues)

- ▲ Observed use of unsuccessful social interactions
- ▲ Dysfunctional interaction with peers, family, and/or others
- Use of forms of coping that impede adaptive behavior
- Destructive behavior toward self or others
- Inability to meet role expectations
- Inability to take responsibility for own actions
- Lack of remorse when actions hurt or hinder others

---

▲ NANDA International accepted; ● In addition to NANDA International

## Outcome Criteria

- Increase in assertive ways to get needs met
- Decrease in manipulative behaviors to get needs met
- Demonstrate responsible behaviors when dealing with others

## Long-Term Goals

Client will:
- Respond in a positive manner to confrontation and limit setting
- Learn and master at least three skills that facilitate adaptive behaviors (particularly anger management)
- Demonstrate an increase in responsible behavior in dealing with others as witnessed by staff and stated by others (clients, family, acquaintances)
- Use acceptable methods of getting needs met
- Participate in ongoing management of anger, impulsivity, control issues, and the like
- Demonstrate a decrease in manipulative, attention-seeking, or passive-aggressive behaviors as reported by staff, family, and peers within 6 months

## Short-Term Goals

Clients will:
- Participate in treatment program, activities, responsibilities, and the like within 1 to 3 days
- State they understand the unit (community center/rehabilitation program, etc.) rules and the consequences of breaking them by first day
- Sign and discuss the content of a contract defining staff and client expectations by first day
- Participate in articulating a contract to modify specific inappropriate and unacceptable behaviors that spells out the consequences of continuing behaviors by first or second day (a copy goes to the client and the Kardex/community center/rehabilitation counselor, etc.)
- Target two inappropriate behaviors to work on learning alternative ways of behaving within 2 to 3 days
- Role play with nurse new skills in dealing with targeted behaviors (ongoing)

*Interventions and Rationales*

| Intervention | Rationale |
|---|---|
| 1. Assess your own reactions toward client. If you feel angry, discuss with peers ways to reframe your thinking to defray feelings of anger. | 1. Anger is a natural response to being manipulated. It is also a block to effective nurse-client interaction. |
| 2. Assess client's interactions for a short period before labeling them manipulative. | 2. A client might respond to one particular, high-stress situation with maladaptive behaviors, but use appropriate behaviors in other situations. |
| 3. Approach client in a calm, neutral manner when confronting client with unacceptable behavior. Focus on the behavior, not the client (e.g., "Drinking alcohol is not allowed here," *not* "I don't want you to drink alcohol on this unit."). | 3. Focusing on behavior (drinking) is less accusing than personalizing the behavior (your drinking). |
| 4. State clearly the limits and behavior the staff expects of client. | 4. Client needs to be aware of specific expectations and boundaries. |
| 5. Limits are:<br>a. Appropriate, not punitive.<br>b. Enforceable.<br>c. Stated in a nonpunitive manner.<br>d. Written with consequences of nonadherence clearly stated. Make one copy for client, and one copy for client's record (e.g., Kardex). | 5. Clear, enforceable limits give client specific boundaries of expected behaviors. |

| Intervention | Rationale |
|---|---|
| 6. Meet with client to formulate a written contract detailing specific, undesirable behaviors that are to be changed, alternatives to those behaviors, and specific consequences of nonadherence. | 6. Encouraging clients to participate in contract drafting might encourage compliance. |
| 7. Both nurse and client sign the contract; one copy goes to client and another copy goes to nurse (Kardex). | 7. Validates that the contract is a serious document and will be a guideline for all staff, and a reminder for the client. |
| 8. Communicate frequently to all staff about specific limits and consequences set for clients. Post copy on Kardex. | 8. Limits and consequences have to be adhered to by all of the staff to be effective means for modifying behavior. |
| 9. Follow through with consequences in a nonpunitive manner (e.g., "The unit rules we went over together when you arrived, Mr. Miller, clearly stated that clients were not to have alcohol on the unit or their weekend passes were to be cancelled. Because you brought alcohol to the unit, your weekend pass is canceled."). | 9. Clients begin to understand that they will be taking responsibility for their behavior. In this example, the client chose to drink on the unit, but by doing so, he has also chosen to forgo his weekend pass. |

| Intervention | Rationale |
|---|---|
| 10. Discuss with clients their thoughts and feelings immediately before the undesirable behavior. | 10. Identifies specific thoughts and feelings that can be discussed and dealt with in alternative ways. |
| 11. Discuss with clients alternative behaviors they could use to effectively deal with these kinds of thoughts, feelings, or situations in the future. | 11. Clients might not be aware of what they are feeling (anger, anxiety, and sadness) or the thinking that triggers specific maladaptive behaviors. |
| 12. Teach or refer client to an appropriate place to learn needed coping skill (e.g., anger management, assertiveness training). | 12. If clients are *not to do* a specific maladaptive behavior, they need to learn *what to do* to deal with intense thoughts/feelings and impulsive behaviors. |
| 13. Role play situations so that client can practice the use of new behaviors. | 13. Gives client chances to practice more direct and appropriate ways of relating and getting needs met. |
| 14. Be vigilant; avoid:<br>a. Discussing yourself or other staff members with client<br>b. Promising to keep a secret for the client<br>c. Accepting gifts from the client<br>d. Doing special favors for the client | 14. Client can use this kind of information to manipulate you and/or split staff. Decline all invitations in a firm, but matter-of-fact manner; for example:<br>a. "I cannot keep secrets from other staff. If you tell me something I may have to share it."<br>b. "If you want to know about Ms. Williams, you will have to ask her."<br>c. "I am here to focus on you." |

| Intervention | Rationale |
|---|---|
| | d. "You are to return to the unit by 4 PM on Sunday, period." |
| 15. Meet frequently with staff to discuss client's care plan and progress. Revise care plan as a team. | 15. Helps ensure consistency of enforcing limits, and minimizes staff splitting. |
| 16. Give client attention and support when behavior is appropriate and positive. | 16. Reinforces appropriate behaviors. |
| 17. Withdraw attention when client's behavior is inappropriate (unless there is a need to enforce consequences). | 17. Client learns that inappropriate behavior will not be rewarded with the attention he or she might be seeking. |
| 18. Maintain a neutral manner at all times. Avoid power struggles or trying to outmanipulate client. | 18. You cannot win a power struggle or outmanipulate a manipulative client. In any case, this is not a game. |
| 19. Provide positive feedback when client interacts without use of manipulation. | 19. Encourages and reinforces appropriate behaviors. |
| 20. Keep detailed and accurate notes on: a. Client's behaviors b. Frequency of behaviors c. Limits set d. Consequences enforced | 20. Helps staff identify what is working and not working. Can minimize manipulation of staff. |
| 21. Include family in client education. | 21. The same skills used when working with the client might be useful for the family. |

# NURSE, CLIENT, AND FAMILY RESOURCES

## JOURNAL ARTICLES

Bowers, L. (2003). Manipulation: Description, identification, and ambiguity. *Journal of Psychiatric Mental Health Nursing, 10,* 23-28.

## INTERNET ARTICLES

Trimble, T. Recognizing manipulative behaviors by patients.
*Emergency Nursing World.*
http://ENW.org/BSQ.htm

*Managing Challenging Behaviors*
http://www.rnceus.com/hiv/challenging.htm
This 4-page article, although targeted to a client with HIV, is relevant for working with a client with manipulative behaviors in the hospital and offers clear-cut useful strategies. It can be especially helpful for caregivers.

*Tools for Handling Control Issues: Eliminating Manipulation*
http://www.coping.org/control/manipul.htm
This 8-page article defines manipulation and its negative effects and offers ways to help eliminate manipulation in relationships and life. Included is a "Manipulative Behavior Inventory."

# CHAPTER 20

# Nonadherence to Medication or Treatment

## OVERVIEW

Nonadherence to prescribed health care is thought to be a frequent phenomenon. In fact, it is estimated that up to 50% of clients fail to adhere to their prescribed health care regimen (Postrado & Lehman, 1995).

When clients do not follow medication and treatment plans, they are often labeled as "noncompliant." The term *noncompliant* applied to clients often brings with it negative connotations. The term *compliance* refers to the extent to which a client obediently and faithfully follows health care providers' instructions. "That client is noncompliant" often translates into he or she is "bad" or "lazy." The "noncompliant" client is then open to blame and criticism. The situation often results in a power struggle between the health care worker and client that can leave both frustrated and angry. Clients who are labeled as noncompliant are often seen as "deviant," and the term is invariably judgmental.

By contrast, the term *adherence* implies a more active, voluntary, and collaborative involvement of the client in a mutually acceptable course of behavior (Meichenbaum & Turk, 1987). Lerner (1997) suggests that, rather than seeing the health care worker's role as trying to "get a noncompliant client to comply," we should emphasize the importance of negotiation and accommodation within the client–health care worker relationship. Therefore, the term *nonadherence* has less of a negative connotation, and frames the behavior more as a problem to be solved, and not so much willful, negative behavior. For that reason, the term *nonadherence* is used here.

The reasons clients do not adhere to their treatment of care, although they fully understand their health care regimen, are many and complex. Nonadherence to medications and treatment alone is not the problem. Nonadherence is usually a *symptom* of more complex, underlying problems. Although inadequate client education is a common reason for nonadherence to a medical regimen, it is certainly not the only reason.

Many complex issues can complicate a person's willingness to follow a path leading to increased health or health maintenance. These issues, once addressed, can increase a person's adherence toward their health care regimen. Table 20-1 presents some factors that will need to be uncovered and dealt with before medical compliance can be a reality.

## ASSESSMENT

### Assessing History

A positive history includes:
- A history of not keeping appointments
- A history of not taking medications
- Escalation of signs and symptoms despite the availability of appropriate medication
- A history of emergency visits that are effectively treated with prescribed medication or treatment
- Religious or cultural beliefs that contradict medical/psychologic health care regimen
- A poor outcome from past medical/psychologic treatments
- A history of poor relationships with past health care providers
- A history of leaving the hospital against medical advice (AMA)

### Presenting Signs and Symptoms

- Objective tests (e.g., blood and urine) inconsistent with reported medication intake (e.g., low lithium levels, low neuroleptic blood levels, high sugar levels)
- Family members or friends state that client is not adhering to prescribed regimen

Table 20-1 **Selected Factors That Contribute to Nonadherence**

| Factor | Suggested Interventions |
| --- | --- |
| Use of power struggles to gain a sense of control | Devise ways to give client more control over regimen by giving alternate, effective treatment options. |
| Reluctance to give up a behavior that is a usual coping mechanism (e.g., smoking, diet, drugs/alcohol) | Teach client alternative coping strategies (relaxation, exercise, creative pursuits) and role-play ceasing the one and employing another. |
| Secondary gains from the "sick" role | Teach family and staff to give positive reinforcement for healthy behavior and use of healthy coping skills, and draw away from giving attention to problem behavior. |
| Self-destructive behavior (e.g., suicide, anorexia, bulimia, drugs) | Perform good nursing assessment and work or refer client to competent specially trained clinician. |
| Negative family influence related to denial, lack of understanding, or need for client to maintain sick role | Family teaching and possibly family therapy to clarify issues, identify long-range consequences of nonadherence, and involve them in treatment plan. |
| Lack of economic resources (e.g., cannot afford medications or time off to keep appointments) | Refer to social services; identify community resources that might be helpful. |
| Lack of transportation | Refer to social services. |
| Unsatisfactory relationships with health care personnel | Work to establish a partnership with client showing concern and interest; avoid power struggles. |
| Cultural and/or religious beliefs | Identify specific concerns. Emphasize what can happen when regimen is not followed. Attempt to engage client, family/friends to problem-solve alternative solutions. |
| Language problems, inability to read or understand instructions | Obtain an interpreter, and involve other members of the family who have more facility with English. Have written instructions in client's primary language. |

Table 20-1 **Selected Factors That Contribute to Nonadherence—cont'd**

| Factor | Suggested Interventions |
| --- | --- |
| Uncomfortable side effects | Encourage client and family to share untoward reactions to drug so that adjustments can be made before client stops taking medication or treatment. |
| Lack of skills to adhere to treatment regimen | Assess and identify needed skills. Some of these skills include decision-making skills, relaxation skills, assertiveness training skills, relapse prevention techniques. |
| Conflict with self-image, especially children and adolescents (e.g., taking medication or imposing limits on activity) | Refer and encourage client to join a group with others grappling with similar issues. |
| Confusion about (1) taking the medication, (2) when to take it, or (3) if he or she has already taken medication | Set up a concrete system for taking medications (e.g., cross-off chart, pillbox with separate compartments). Try to enlist help from family or others if available. |

Data from Gorman, L.M., Sultan D.F., & Raines, M.L. (1996). *Davis's manual of psychosocial nursing for general patient care.* Philadelphia: FA Davis, pp. 243-245; and Schultz, J.M., & Videbeck, S.D. (2005). *Lippincott's manual of psychiatric nursing care plans.* 7th ed. Philadelphia: JB Lippincott.

- Progression of disease/behaviors despite appropriate medication/treatment ordered
- Fails to follow through with referrals
- Fails to keep appointments
- Denies the need for medication or treatment

## Assessment Guidelines

### Nonadherence

1. Identify any ethnic and/or cultural beliefs that might conflict with the client adhering to medical management.
2. Does the taking of medication pose a financial problem?
3. Evaluate age-related issues interfering with adherence to medication/treatment protocols (see Table 20-1).

4. Assess presence of side effects of medications/treatments and how they affect client's lifestyle. What would he/she like to change?
5. Does client believe that the medications/treatments are really necessary?
6. Are the directions for taking medications in client's own language?
7. What does client identify as being the most difficult aspect of following through with medication/treatment regimen?

# NURSING DIAGNOSES WITH INTERVENTIONS

## Discussion of Potential Nursing Diagnoses

Nonadherence to medications or treatment can be voluntary, or a result of a variety of factors that make adherence difficult. The nursing diagnosis of **Noncompliance** coincides with the *active decision of an individual or family to fully or partially nonadhere to an agreed-on medication/treatment regimen*. In contrast, **Ineffective Therapeutic Regimen Management** refers to the *difficulty or inability to regulate or integrate a medication/treatment plan into daily life*. A distinction between the two is important in obtaining desired results.

The position taken in this chapter is that **Noncompliance** is used to identify *voluntary nonadherence* to a medical/psychiatric treatment regimen, and **Ineffective Therapeutic Regimen Management** refers to those situations in which the client *might be willing to comply, but is having difficulty* integrating the therapeutic regimen into his or her life or lifestyle.

## Overall Guidelines for Nursing Interventions

### Enhancing Adherence

1. Establish an open and honest relationship with the client. A *partnering* relationship rather than an *authoritative* one can significantly enhance accurate reporting of adherence difficulties.
2. Educate the client. Provide information on the disorder, the treatment options, medication side effects, and toxic effects, using booklets, handouts, phone numbers, and websites for further information.

3. After teaching, evaluate client understanding to clarify misunderstandings and reinforce requests.
4. Keep active follow-up appointments; call if appointment is missed. Definite follow-up appointments enhance adherences.
5. Identify issues that might impede compliance with medications, and work out a needed intervention. For example, weight gain is often associated with many psychotropic agents. Dietary teaching is essential because many medications alter metabolism and predispose the client to obesity, diabetes, and/or heart disease.
6. Provide feedback on progress and acknowledge and reinforce efforts to adhere.
7. Refer client and family to a variety of outside resources for education, support, and assistance (e.g., pharmacists, health educators, medication groups, and selfhelp groups) (Kobayashi, Smith, & Norcross, 1998).

## Selected Nursing Diagnoses and Nursing Care Plans

### NONCOMPLIANCE

Behavior of person and/or caregiver that fails to coincide with a health-promoting or therapeutic plan agreed on by the person (and/or family and/or community) and health care professional. In the presence of an agreed-on, health-promoting, or therapeutic plan, person's or caregiver's behavior is fully or partially nonadherent and may lead to clinically ineffective or partially ineffective outcomes

### *Related To (Etiology)*

▲ Health care plan
  • Duration
  • Significant others
  • Cost
  • Intensity
  • Complexity

▲ NANDA International accepted

▲ Individual factors
  • Personal and developmental abilities
  • Health beliefs and cultural influences
  • Spiritual values
  • Individual value system
  • Knowledge and skill relevant to the regimen behavior
  • Motivational forces
▲ Health system
  • Satisfaction with care
  • Credibility of provider
  • Access and convenience of care
  • Financial flexibility of plan
  • Client-provider relationships
  • Provider reimbursement of teaching and follow-up
  • Provider continuity and regular follow-up
  • Individual health coverage
  • Communication and teaching skills of the provider
▲ Network
  • Involvement of members in health plan
  • Social value regarding plan
  • Perceived beliefs of significant others

*As Evidenced By*
*(Assessment Findings/Diagnostic Cues)*

▲ Behavior indicative of failure to adhere (by direct observation or by statements of patient or significant others)
▲ Evidence of development of complications
▲ Evidence of exacerbation of symptoms
▲ Failure to keep appointments
▲ Failure to progress
▲ Objective tests (blood, urine, physiologic markers)

*Outcome Criteria*

• Uses health services congruent with needs
• Reports following prescribed regimen
• Seeks external reinforcement for performance of health behaviors

---

▲ NANDA International accepted

## Long-Term Goals

Client will:
- State correct information about his/her condition, benefits of treatment, risks of treatment, and treatment options each time changes are made to their treatment plan by (date)
- Participate in decision making concerning treatment plan on an ongoing basis
- Demonstrate adherence to the treatment plan by (date)
- Follow behavioral contract in assuming his/her responsibility for self-care on an ongoing basis

## Short-Term Goals

Client will:
- Discuss the impact of illness on lifestyle (ongoing)
- Discuss fears, concerns, and beliefs that influence non-compliance (ongoing)
- Identify one barrier to compliance (by end of session)
- With family, problem-solve ways to minimize or erase barrier (within 1 week)
- With family, discuss with nurse the potential undesirable consequences of nonadherence to therapeutic regimen (within 1 week)
- Negotiate acceptable changes in the treatment plan that he/she is willing to follow (ongoing)
- Participate in one decision regarding his/her treatment plan (by end of first session)
- Sign a behavioral contract defining his/her mutual participation and responsibility for care (at end of session and review/update frequently)

## Interventions and Rationales

| Intervention | Rationale |
|---|---|
| 1. Explore with clients their feelings about the illness/disorder and the need for ongoing treatments (medications). | 1. Setting up a rapport with clients who believe you are interested in them encourages understanding of client's perspective. |

| Intervention | Rationale |
|---|---|
| 2. Use therapeutic nursing techniques to encourage client to share feelings in an atmosphere of acceptance. | 2. When clients feel understood, they are less likely to feel defensive and more likely to be open to suggestions and information regarding optimizing their health. |
| 3. Identify communication barriers that might impede client's (family's) comprehension. Identify need for:<br>a. Interpreters<br>b. Use of nontechnical language<br>c. Need for written material<br>d. Understanding religious barriers<br>e. Ascertaining attitudes toward the health care system | 3. When we make assumptions according to what we teach clients, and not what they might or might not understand, the potential for miscommunication is enhanced. |
| 4. Assess client's (family's) understanding about the illness/disorder, treatment options, how medications work, and side and toxic effects. | 4. Client (family) misperceptions about disease/disorder or treatments result in faulty decision making. |
| 5. Assess how the client's disease/disorder and subsequent treatments/medications impact upon client's (and family's) lifestyle. | 5. Age, religion, cultural beliefs, and expectations of others all impact on our value system and factor into how we make decisions. |
| 6. Ask client to share his/her rationale for nonadherence to medical/psychosocial regimen. | 6. Identifies areas of misunderstanding. |

| Intervention | Rationale |
|---|---|
| 7. Do not argue with clients about the value of their beliefs; rather, point out the negative outcomes these beliefs might cause. | 7. Arguing or getting into power struggles with clients makes them defensive and not open to alternative actions. |
| 8. Engage family, friends, caregivers to explain negative actions of nonadherence to treatment regimen. | 8. Those whom client trusts, and who are from similar background, culture, and the like, might inspire trust and open the way for negotiation. |
| 9. Encourage clients to participate in the decision-making process regarding their plan of care. | 9. Can give clients a sense of control, and give them the opportunity to choose those interventions they might decide to try. |
| 10. Give the client a range of assignments from which to choose. | 10. Giving client choices in making a decision increases client involvement in treatment planning. |
| 11. Negotiate with clients one or two areas they will comply with, if client refuses the whole treatment plan outright. | 11. Clients may "try" one or two items from the treatment regimen to comply with at first. Hopefully this can form a base for further adherence. |
| 12. Negotiate a behavioral contract with client, and review it periodically. Give a written copy to client and file one in client's chart. | 12. Contracts have been found to enhance adherence in both adults and children (Kobayashi, Smith, & Norcross, 1998). |
| 13. Reduce the complexity of the treatment plan (prioritize, facilitate schedules, fit to client lifestyle). | 13. The more complicated a treatment plan, the more likely is nonadherence. |

| Intervention | Rationale |
|---|---|
| 14. When appropriate, encourage support groups. | 14. While giving support, groups also share information, and encourage healthy choices. |
| 15. Determine if a different medication or a different type of therapy might be acceptable to the client. | 15. Client might engage in treatment if alternative but equally effective treatment options are available. |
| 16. Recognize that it might not be possible to alter strong cultural or religious beliefs. | 16. Ultimately, the final choice is with the client. Our job is to provide information and effective treatment options that best suit the client's lifestyle. |

### Medication Nonadherence

| | |
|---|---|
| 1. Assess if client believes he/she needs the medication. Identify need for teaching. | 1. If client denies need for medication, motivation for adherence is lacking. |
| 2. Use a variety of teaching strategies for client and family members (e.g., pamphlets, videotapes, role playing, group teaching with others in similar circumstances, support groups). | 2. Knowledge and understanding can increase adherence to treatment regimen. |
| 3. If client stops taking medication when he/she feels "better," more client teaching is needed. | 3. People need to know that, in most instances, medications cannot cure them, but they can help stabilize their symptoms with time. |

| Intervention | Rationale |
|---|---|
| 4. Encourage reporting side effects (e.g., "Do these medications affect your ability to function sexually? They affect many people that way."). | 4. Physician can lower dose, or give client an alternative medication, when side effects are affecting adherence. |
| 5. Encourage client to report any disturbing side effects right away, rather than stopping medication. | 5. Some side effects can be minimized through simple actions. |

## INEFFECTIVE THERAPEUTIC REGIMEN MANAGEMENT

Pattern of regulating and integrating into daily living a program for treatment of illness and the sequelae of illness that is unsatisfactory for meeting specific health goals

### *Related To (Etiology)*

▲ Perceived barriers
▲ Social support deficits
▲ Mistrust of regimen and/or health care personnel
▲ Knowledge deficits
▲ Family patterns of health care
▲ Economic difficulties
▲ Complexity of therapeutic regimen
▲ Inadequate number and types of cues to action

### *As Evidenced By*
### *(Assessment Findings/Diagnostic Cues)*

▲ Choices of daily living ineffective for meeting the goals of a treatment or prevention program
▲ Verbalized that they did not take action to reduce risk factors for progression of illness and sequelae

---

▲ NANDA International accepted

▲ Verbalized difficulty with regulation/integration of one or more prescribed regimens for treatment
▲ Acceleration of illness symptoms
▲ Verbalized that they did not take action to include treatment regimens in daily routines

## *Outcome Criteria*

- Describes diminished barriers to following through with health care regimen (e.g., financial, transportation, family/friends, knowledge and understanding)
- Perceived support of health care workers
- Demonstrates adherence to treatment regimen

## *Long-Term Goals*

Client will:
- Verbalize acceptance and adherence to the treatment plan by (date)
- Keep follow-up appointments by (date)
- Demonstrate skills or knowledge needed for adherence by (date)
- Establish a network of referrals to call upon if and when difficulties with carrying out treatment regimen arise
- Participate in adjunctive services when appropriate

## *Short-Term Goals*

Client will:
- Establish a supportive, therapeutic partnership with health care workers
- Identify obstacles that interfere with carrying out treatment plan
- Identify resources needed to ensure compliance
- Negotiate acceptable changes in the treatment plan that he or she is willing to follow

---

▲ NANDA International accepted

*Interventions and Rationales*

| Intervention | Rationale |
|---|---|
| 1. Establish an open and supportive partnership with client. | 1. Adherence is positively correlated with client's perception of health care personnel's caring and interest (DiMatteo & DiNicola, 1982) |
| 2. Identify areas in the treatment regimen that interfere with adherence:<br>a. Economic<br>b. Transportation<br>c. Knowledge barrier<br>d. Language barrier<br>e. Lack of or negative family involvement<br>f. Lack of appropriate skills | 2. Targets areas for interventions. |
| 3. Involve adjunctive services when appropriate, for example:<br>a. Social services for financial or transportation problems<br>b. Interpreters if language difficulties<br>c. Family teaching and/or alternative teaching strategies if knowledge deficit<br>d. Skills training | 3. Nonadherence is often a symptom of an underlying problem. That problem must be identified. |
| 4. Teach needed skills (e.g., problem-solving skills, assertiveness skills, relaxation skills, decision-making skills). | 4. Skills training can help foster adherence to health care regimen. |
| 5. Keep the treatment plan as clear and simple as possible. | 5. The easier the regimen is to follow, the greater the likelihood of compliance. |

| Intervention | Rationale |
|---|---|
| 6. Evaluate client comprehension by having client repeat or demonstrate what is to be done. | 6. Clarifies misunderstandings and reinforces learning. |
| 7. Use behavioral reminders for follow-up:<br>a. Calendars<br>b. Linking appointments<br>c. Written reminders on refrigerators<br>d. Sending reminder postcards | 7. Behavioral reminders have proved successful for long-term adherence (Kobayashi, Smith, & Norcross, 1998). |
| 8. Facilitate short-term goal-setting with client (explicitly defined, achievable goals). | 8. Clients who use short-term goals rather than long-term goals are most successful at maintenance (Meichenbaum & Turk, 1987). |
| 9. Provide feedback on client's progress and develop positive reinforcers for self-regulation. | 9. Encouragement and recognition by clinician as to progress of goals can act as a motivator for positive change. |
| 10. Tailor treatment plan to be congruent with client's social, cultural, and environmental milieus. | 10. Optimizes client feeling comfortable with adhering to medications/treatments. |
| 11. Teach relapse prevention skills. | 11. Helps clients learn behavioral cues to potential relapse and how to cope with relapse. |
| 12. Repeat everything. | 12. Information that is repeated is more likely to be retained than information that is not repeated. |

# 🖼 NURSE, CLIENT, AND FAMILY RESOURCES

## JOURNAL ARTICLES

Kemppainen, J.K., et al. (2003). Psychiatric nursing and medication adherence. *Journal of Psychosocial Nursing and Mental Health Services, 2,* 38-49.

# PART V

# PSYCHOPHARMACOLOGY

# CHAPTER 21

# Major Psychotropic Interventions and Client and Family Teaching

## OVERVIEW

Although the origins of a psychiatric illness are influenced by a number of factors (genetic, neurodevelopment, psychosocial experience, infections, drugs), there will eventually be an alteration in cerebral function that accounts for disturbances in the client's behavior and mental experience (Raynor, 2005). These physiologic alterations are the targets of the psychotropic drugs, and reversal of these alterations are goal of treatment (Raynor, 2005).

All activities of the brain involve the actions of neurons, neurotransmitters, and receptors. It makes sense, therefore, that it is the neurotransmitters and receptor sites in the brain that are the targets of pharmacologic intervention. Therefore, most psychotropic drugs act by either increasing or decreasing the activity of certain transmitter-receptor systems. Furthermore, different transmitter-receptor systems are dysfunctional in different psychiatric conditions. For example, it was found that most agents that were effective in reducing the hallucinations and delusions in clients with schizophrenia also blocked the dopamine ($D_2$) receptors in the brain (Raynor, 2005). Therefore, it was concluded from this information that an overactivity of dopamine at the dopamine receptor sites resulted in hallucinations and delusions.

Ideally clinicians want a drug that will relieve the mental disturbance of clients, without resulting in either mental or physical adverse effects. Unfortunately, as with all medications, the effectiveness of a specific psychotropic drug might be accompanied by certain adverse or toxic effects. Therefore, it is important for nurses to understand which drugs help target specific mental symptoms, the potential adverse and toxic effects, and, of course, how to counsel clients and their families as to:

- What potential adverse reactions might occur
- Recognizing potential toxic effects and when to notify the health care provider
- Situations in which these drugs are contraindicated or should be used with great caution
- Any dietary or medication restrictions associated with a specific drug
- How and when to take the medication to optimize the action of the drug and minimize the side/toxic effects

Some important guidelines listed in Box 21-1 might enhance clients' medication compliance.

Two adverse effects of psychotropic agents that negatively impact medication compliance are weight gain and sexual dysfunction. Nurses have a role in monitoring, recording, reporting, and managing *weight gain* associated with psychotropics (e.g., clozapine, olanzapine). Dietary teaching is essential when medication alters metabolism and predisposes the client to obesity, diabetes, and/or heart disease (personal communication from Dorothy A. Varchol, June 2003).

Assessing *sexual dysfunction* secondary to a psychotropic agent and substituting an alterative agent can increase potential for compliance and increase the person's quality of life.

In this chapter, the major classes of psychotropic drugs are reviewed. Within each class of drugs, the neurotransmitters targeted are identified. The neurotransmitter's (increase or decrease) is responsible for the alleviation of symptoms; however, that same alteration of a specific neurotransmitter can also affect other systems and result in adverse effects. These adverse effects will be identified as well. To encourage client compliance to medication treatment and protect the client's safety, client and family teaching is vital. To aid in client and family teaching, specific guidelines are provided for each of the major classes of psychotropic medications.

---

Box 21-1 **Nursing Guidelines for Medication Management**

1. **Clients should be active partners** in managing their symptoms with psychopharmacologic agents. Nurses who listen carefully in taking a medication history and educating individuals in how to be proactive in this process might be more successful with client compliance.
2. **Side effects can cause noncompliance.** Identify with your clients what problems they are having with the medication, and make adjustments. Without examining these issues, the assumption might be made that the drug is not working, not that the client is not taking the drug because of troublesome side effects.
3. **Psychosocial rehabilitation** can optimize the outcomes of psychopharmacology.
4. **Sleep hygiene** can enhance psychopharmacologic treatment (e.g., avoid napping; avoid stimulants such as exercise, television, computer, and alcohol at bedtime).
5. **Evidence-based guidelines** should be used when available.
6. **Individual responses** to medications should be monitored closely in those not responding well to treatment.
7. **Liability** might be an issue for the advanced practice nurse if the diagnosis is incorrect and if the client is treated from the incorrect medication group.
8. **Full remission** might be expected with medications for anxiety or mood, but outcomes are not as good for psychotic disorders or dementia.

---

Personal communication from Dorothy A. Varchol, June 2003.

Refer to Figures 21-1 and 21-2 later in this chapter to understand how specific psychotropics (antidepressants, antipsychotics) can affect various neurotransmitters and how these effects (increase or decrease) are responsible for a wide range of undesirable and sometimes dangerous effects.

# ANTIANXIETY/ANXIOLYTIC MEDICATIONS

This section introduces:
- Benzodiazepines
- Non-benzodiazepines—azapirones (buspirone)

## Benzodiazepines

*Therapeutic Uses* The benzodiazepines (BZs) have three main indications for use: (1) anxiety, (2) insomnia, and (3) seizure disorders. BZs are also used for alcohol withdrawal.

All BZs share the same pharmacologic properties and produce a similar spectrum of responses. However, they differ significantly from one another with respect to time course or action. They also differ in onset and duration of action, and tend to accumulate with repeated dosing. Therefore, because of these differences, individual BZs differ in clinical applications (Lehne, 2001). The downside of the BZs is that they are associated with impaired psychomotor function and the development of tolerance and dependence. For these reasons, they should only be used on a **short-term** basis.

- **Anxiety disorders:**
  - **Panic disorder:** Alprazolam (Xanax) and clonazepam (Klonopin) have the most specific antipanic effect.
  - Generalized anxiety disorder (GAD): The BZs are still the most widely used drugs in the treatment of GAD. Most are effective, although different dosages are needed for different clients. Buspirone is often attempted initially before BZ treatment begins.
  - **Acute anxiety:** For short-term, limited use when reassurance is not effective.

In the treatment of anxiety disorders, Papp (1999) states that **high-potency benzodiazepines should be considered only if the adverse effects of all other alternatives are unacceptable to the client, or if the client is unwilling or unable to wait out the 4- to 6-week delay in response associated with most antidepressants (selective serotonin reuptake inhibitors [SSRIs] or buspirone**. Refer to Chapter 5 for a list of antianxiety/anxiolytic medications and the specific medications and treatments that have been found most effective with specific anxiety disorders.

- Used in the treatment of **acute mania**: Clonazepam (Klonopin) and lorazepam (Ativan)
- **Short-term hypnotic:** Useful when used short-term to help induce sleep (e.g., temazepam (Restoril), estazolam (ProSom), quazepam (Dural), Zolpidem (Ambien), and Zaleplon (Sonata)
- **Muscle spasms:** Relaxes muscles (Valium)
- **Seizure disorders:** Anticonvulsant properties help suppress seizure activity (intravenous Valium, Ativan, and Klonopin)

- Treatment of **sedative withdrawal syndromes:** Use long-acting BZs such as diazepam (Valium) or chlordiazepoxide (Librium)
- **Preoperative anesthesia** (midazolam)
- For those needing to drive or operate machinery in their work: The oxazobenzodiazepine mexazolam (Sedaxil, Melex) can be used in clinical trials

## Mechanism of Action

Benzodiazepines potentiate and intensify the actions of gamma-aminobutyric acid (GABA). GABA is an inhibitory neurotransmitter found throughout the central nervous system (CNS). GABA plays a role in inhibition by reducing aggression, excitation, and anxiety. GABA has anticonvulsant and muscle-relaxing properties and might play a role in pain perception. The BZ work by binding to specific receptors in a supramolecular structure known as the *GABA receptor-chloride channel complex*, thereby intensifying the effects of GABA in the CNS (Lehne, 2001).

## Clinical Dosage

For the usual daily doses for selected BZs, and usual daily doses for other anxiolytic agents, see Table 5-2.

## Metabolism

Benzodiazepines are metabolized by the liver. Oxidation can be impaired through hepatic cirrhosis, old age, or other drugs (cimetidine, estrogens, or isoniazid).

Benzodiazepines can be classified as long-acting or short-acting. The faster-acting BZs are more likely to be abused. The **long-acting BZs** (e.g., Librium, clorazepate [Tranxene], Valium, prazepam [Centrex]) have active metabolites with elimination half-lives of approximately 4 days. Therefore, the long-acting BZs can be discontinued suddenly without serious withdrawal symptoms. The **short-acting BZs** (Xanax, Ativan, oxazepam [Serax]), which are quickly eliminated, have the potential for serious withdrawal reactions.

## Adverse Effects

**Central Nervous System** Benzodiazepines *depress neuronal function* at multiple sites in the CNS and reduce anxiety through the effects on the limbic system. They promote sleep through *effects on cortical areas*, and on the sleep–wakefulness clock. Muscle relaxation is induced through effects on *supraspinal motor areas*, including the cerebellum. Two important side effects, confusion and anterograde amnesia, result from *effects on the hippocampus and cerebral cortex* (Lehne, 2001).

**Central nervous system side effects produce:**
- Psychomotor impairment and drowsiness.
  - Muscle weakness, ataxia, vertigo, confusion, sleepiness
  - Older clients are especially susceptible to psychomotor impairment and falls.
- Cognitive impairment. BZs impair memory.
  - Acute anterograde amnesia
  - Impaired long-term memory from interference with memory consolidation, especially with the elderly
- Sedative effects. When taken alone within the proper dose range, the BZs are relatively safe. However, the BZs augment the sedative side effects of other sedatives, such as narcotics, barbiturates, and alcohol. When BZs are taken in combination with other CNS depressants, the combination can lead to respiratory depression, coma, and death.

**Respiratory System** The BZs are weak respiratory muscle depressants and are usually safe when taken orally, and without other CNS depression. Respiratory depression is most marked in people with $CO_2$ retention; therefore, people with pulmonary disease should have blood gases taken to test their $PCO_2$ before a BZ is ordered. Respiratory depression is more apt to occur with IV administration of a BZ and, as mentioned earlier, in conjunction with other CNS depressants.

**Cardiovascular Effects** When taken orally, there is no effect on the heart or blood vessels. However, when taken intravenously, the BZs might produce profound hypotension and cardiac arrest (Lehne, 2001).

**Potential for Abuse** Although it is rare that the average person with brief exposure to the drug becomes an abuser, the BZs are potentially drugs of abuse. Addicted-prone individuals are more likely to become physically dependent. Benzodiazepines should be prescribed for short-term use and be prescribed with caution.

**Overdose** Death from BZs alone is rare; however, as previously emphasized, in combination with other CNS depressants, death from overdose can occur. **Flumazenil (Mazicon), a benzodiazepine receptor antagonist,** can reverse excessive sedation and psychomotor impairment.

**Discontinuing Benzodiazepines** The long-acting BZs will often self-taper, however, the short-acting BZs (e.g., Xanax) should be tapered over several weeks or months. Slowly tapering the BZ helps to prevent withdrawal symptoms (e.g., anxiety, insomnia, headache, muscle irritability, blurred vision, dizziness, delirium, paranoia, psychosis). This is especially true if the client has been taking high doses over a long period of time.

**Pregnancy** The use of BZs is thought to cause a risk of congenital malformations in the fetus. Such risks include cleft lip, inguinal hernia, cardiac anomalies, and CNS depression. Benzodiazepines enter breast milk, and, therefore, these drugs should be avoided by nursing mothers.

## Drug Interactions

**Drugs That Increase Benzodiazepine Levels**
- Fluoxetine (Prozac)
- Cimetidine (Tagamet)
- Low-dose estrogens
- Disulfiram (Antabuse)
- Isoniazid (INH)

**Drugs Whose Levels Might Be Increased by Benzodiazepines**
- Phenytoin (Dilantin)
- Warfarin (Coumadin)
- Digoxin (Lanoxin)

**Drugs That Might Impair Benzodiazepine Absorption**
- Antacids
- Anticholinergics

**Drugs That Potentiate Central Nervous System Depressant Properties**
- Alcohol and other CNS depressants
- Kava Kava

## Use with Caution

- Elderly should be started with lower doses, **"start low, go slow"**; assess potential for falls and confusion/memory loss
- Clients with pulmonary disease should be medically evaluated (e.g., $PCO_2$ level)
- Used with caution in clients with hepatic or renal disease
- Assess client safety in depressed or suicidal clients
- Evaluate for drug interactions

## Contraindications

- Driving or around machinery
- Pregnant and nursing women
- History of substance abuse
- Women of childbearing age if they become pregnant
- Narrow-angle glaucoma
- Concurrent alcohol or other CNS depressants

## Client and Family Teaching

See Box 21-2 for medication teaching guidelines for clients with anxiety disorders.

## Non-Benzodiazepine Antianxiety: Azapirones (Buspirone [BuSpar])

### Therapeutic Uses

The azapirone group is represented by buspirone (BuSpar). Buspirone differs from other anxiolytics in that it does not cause sedation, has no abuse potential, does not enhance CNS depression, and does not significantly interact with other drugs (except monoamine oxidase inhibitors [MAOIs] and haloperidol). For these reasons, buspirone is particularly useful in treating anxiety or mixed anxiety/depression (Keltner and Folks, 2001). Its major disadvantage is that its anxiolytic effects can take several weeks to become effective. Therefore, it cannot be used as an as needed (prn) medication.

- **Anxiety**
  - General anxiety disorder (GAD)
  - General anxiety with accompanying depressive symptoms.

> ### Box 21-2 **Client and Family Teaching: Anxiety Disorders**
>
> 1. Caution the client:
>    - Not to increase the dose or frequency of administration without previous approval of therapist.
>    - That these medications reduce ability to handle mechanical equipment (e.g., cars, saws, and machinery).
>    - To refrain from drinking alcoholic beverages or taking other antianxiety drugs because depressant effects of both would be potentiated.
>    - To avoid drinking beverages containing caffeine because they decrease the desired effects of the drug.
> 2. Recommend that the client avoid becoming pregnant because taking benzodiazepines increases the risk of congenital anomalies.
> 3. Advise the client not to breastfeed because the drug is excreted in the milk and will have adverse effects on the infant.
> 4. Teach the client that:
>    - Stoppage of the benzodiazepines after 3 to 4 months of daily use can cause withdrawal symptoms (e.g., insomnia, irritability, nervousness, tremors, convulsions, confusion).
>    - Medications should be taken with, or shortly after, meals or snacks to reduce gastrointestinal discomfort.
>    - Drug interaction can occur: Antacids delay absorption; cimetidine interferes with metabolism of benzodiazepines, causing increased sedation; central nervous system depressants (e.g., alcohol, barbiturates) cause increased sedation; serum phenytoin concentration can build up because of decreased metabolism.
> 5. Lower doses should be considered for elderly clients.

Adapted from Varcarolis, E. (2002). *Foundations of psychiatric mental health nursing* (4th ed.). Philadelphia: WB Saunders, p. 330.

- **Other uses** (Goldberg, 1998)
  - Augments response to antidepressants
  - Augments response to drugs that treat obsessive compulsive disorder (OCD)
  - Might reduce the frequency and severity of episodic aggression in some populations with brain damage (developmentally disabled and demented)

## Mechanism of Action

The mechanism for action has not yet been determined. Buspirone does *not* seem to bind to receptors for GABA as do the benzodiazepines, but seems to show a high affinity for serotonin receptors (5-HT) in the CNS and a low affinity for dopamine ($D_2$ receptors).

## Clinical Dosage

The dosage range for anxiety is between 20 and 40 mg/day, starting at 5 to 10 mg three times/day (tid). Antidepressant effects are usually seen at 40 to 80 mg/day, starting at 10 mg tid.

## Metabolism

Buspirone undergoes extensive hepatic metabolism. Its metabolites are excreted primarily in the urine, and, to a lesser extent, in the feces. The elimination of a half-life of buspirone might be prolonged in people with renal impairment and those with cirrhosis. These clients might require lower doses.

## Adverse Effects

Buspirone is well tolerated. The most common reactions (5% to 10% incidence) are as follows:

**Central Nervous System** Reactions include dizziness, drowsiness, headache, lightheadedness, and excitability.

**Gastrointestinal** Reactions include nausea and, to a lesser extent, dry mouth, diarrhea, constipation, and vomiting.

**Other Systems** Buspirone has little, if any, effect on respiratory system, platelet, smooth muscle, or autonomic nervous system functions.

NOTE: As previously stated, buspirone does *not* seem to instigate a physical or psychological dependency. No withdrawal symptoms seem to occur when the drug is discontinued nor is there a cross-tolerance or cross-dependency with other sedative-hypnotics.

## Drug Interactions

- Do not take with MAOIs
- Might increase haloperidol levels

### Use with Caution
- Clients who are pregnant or breastfeeding
- Clients who are elderly or debilitated
- Clients who have hepatic or renal dysfunction

### Contraindications
- Main contraindication: clients with a history of hypersensitivity to buspirone
- Clients taking MAOIs or haloperidol

### Client and Family Teaching
Because of the lag time of several weeks, clients need to be supported through the first few weeks. They need to be told to continue taking the drug, although they are not experiencing any changes as yet.

# ANTIDEPRESSANT MEDICATIONS
Currently there is no conclusive evidence to demonstrate the clinical superiority of one group of antidepressants (Mendelowitz, 2000). The choice of medication is usually based on the side effect profile and ease of administration. For example, if a client is suffering from insomnia, a more sedative antidepressant might be ordered. Conversely, if the client is sleeping and lethargic, a more energizing antidepressant would be suitable. It might, however, take trial and error to find a drug that will suit a particular client. There are other considerations as well.
- The (SSRIs) and other newer generation antidepressants are usually better tolerated than the tricyclic antidepressants (TCAs) and are safer in overdose.
- **Safety for the use in depressed individuals under 18 is presently heatedly debated.** The FDA has issued a supplementary warning to follow all individuals closely who are on antidepressants.
- When cost is a consideration, the generic products are less expensive.
- Past experience with a drug or the response of a first-degree relative can be a predictor of an effective medication regimen.

- Most antidepressants are effective in the depressive phase of bipolar disorder; however, use caution, because they all carry a risk for inducing mania.
- If a single antidepressant action on serotonin **(5-HT)** or norepinephrine **(NE)** receptor is ineffective, a synergistic effect can occur when two independent antidepressant drugs are combined. Therefore, two antidepressants may be prescribed to target specific symptoms.
- Antidepressant medications can take from 1 to 3 weeks or longer before symptoms are relieved.
- Suicide is always a consideration when treating depression. Some clients might be given a limited supply initially to minimize taking an overdose. A precaution in hospitals is to make sure that the medication is taken and not "cheeked."

An overall guide to an effective choice of antidepressants in clients with special needs is presented in Table 21-1.

Table 21-1 **Special Problems and Medications of Choice**

| Problem | Drugs of Choice |
| --- | --- |
| 1. High suicide risk | 1. Trazodone, SSRIs, bupropion, venlafaxine |
| 2. Concurrent depression and panic attacks | 2. Phenelzine (MAOI), imipramine (TCA), SSRIs |
| 3. Chronic pain with or without depressio | 3. Amitriptyline, doxepin, venlafaxine |
| 4. Weight gain on other antidepressants | 4. Bupropion, SSRIs |
| 5. Sensitivity to anticholinergic side effects | 5. Trazodone, phenelzine, tranylcypromine, bupropion, SSRIs (except paroxetine) |
| 6. Orthostatic hypotension | 6. Nortriptyline, bupropion, sertraline |
| 7. Sexual dysfunction | 7. Bupropion, nefazodone, citalopram |

From Preston, J., & Johnson, J. (2004). *Clinical psychopharmacology made ridiculously simple* (5th ed.). Miami, Fla: MedMaster, Inc.

*MAOI,* Monoamine oxidase inhibitor; *SSRI,* selective serotonin reuptake inhibitor; *TCA,* tricyclic antidepressant.

**NOTE:** Most antidepressants are quite toxic when taken in an overdose. Extreme caution should be taken in prescribing to high-risk suicidal patients. Of the existing antidepressants, trazodone appears to have the lowest degree of cardiotoxicity.

- **First-Line Agents**
  - SSRIs
  - Novel (atypical) new antidepressants
  - TCAs
- **Second-Line Agents**
  - MAOIs

Each group of antidepressant medications targets different receptors. Figure 21-1 illustrates some of the effects of receptor binding among the various antidepressant agents.

# FIRST-LINE AGENTS

## Selective Serotonin Reuptake Inhibitors

Selective serotonin reuptake inhibitors are as effective as the TCAs, but do not have the troubling side effects of the TCAs; for example, hypotension, sedation, or anticholinergic effects. Overdose does not cause cardiotoxicity (Lehne, 2001). The SSRIs are specific for **serotonin (5-HT)** reuptake blockage. The SSRIs currently carry an FDA supplemental warning for individuals under 18 years of age.

### *Therapeutic Uses*

- Major depression: All, except for fluvoxamine (Luvox)
- Obsessive compulsive disorder (OCD): Fluoxetine (Prozac), sertraline (Zoloft), fluvoxamine (Luvox), paroxetine (Paxil)
- Bulimia nervosa: Fluoxetine (Prozac)
- Panic disorder: Sertraline (Zoloft), paroxetine (Paxil), fluoxetine (Prozac), citalopram (Celexa)
- Social anxiety disorder: Paroxetine (Paxil)

### Unlabeled Uses
- Premenstrual syndrome: Fluoxetine (Prozac)

### Investigational Uses
- Fluoxetine (Prozac): Alcoholism, attention-deficit/hyperactivity disorder, bipolar disorder, migraine, Tourette's syndrome, and obesity.

### *Mechanism of Action*

As mentioned, the SSRIs specifically block the reuptake of 5-HT into the presynaptic cell from which it was originally

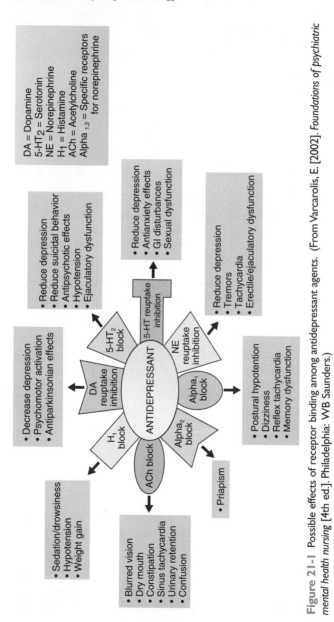

**Figure 21-1** Possible effects of receptor binding among antidepressant agents. (From Varcarolis, E. [2002]. *Foundations of psychiatric mental health nursing* [4th ed.]. Philadelphia: WB Saunders.)

released. Because these drugs are specific to serotonin and have little or no ability to block muscarinic and other receptors, they tend to have fewer untoward autonomic effects than the TCAs. They also do not cause as much sedation or have cardiac toxicity.

## Metabolism

The primary pathway is hepatic metabolism. Impaired hepatic function is associated with impaired metabolism of the SSRIs. There is also metabolic impairment with renal dysfunction. For this reason, a dosage adjustment is made for the elderly and those with hepatic impairment.

## Adverse Effects

**Central Nervous System** Common potential side effects include agitation, anxiety, sleep disturbance, tremor, sexual dysfunction (anorgasmia), and headache.

**Autonomic Nervous System Reactions** Common potential side effects are dry mouth, sweating, weight change, mild nausea, and loose bowel movement.

**Withdrawal Syndrome** Abrupt discontinuation of the SSRIs can cause a withdrawal syndrome. Symptoms begin within days to weeks of discontinuing the medication. Therefore, tapering off of the SSRI is necessary. Withdrawal symptoms include dizziness, headache, nausea, sensory disturbances, tremors, anxiety, and dysphoria.

**Central Serotonin Syndrome** Central serotonin syndrome is a rare and life-threatening event related to overactivation of the central serotonin receptors. This can occur when MAOIs or other drugs that increase the levels of serotonin in the brain are taken concurrently or within 2 weeks of each other. Symptoms include abdominal pain, diarrhea, fever, tachycardia, elevated blood pressure, delirium, myoclonus, increased motor activity, irritability, hostility, and mood change. Severe manifestations can induce hyperpyrexia, cardiovascular shock, and death. For an overview of the adverse and toxic effects, see Table 21-2.

Table 21-2 **Adverse and Toxic Effects of Selective Serotonin Reuptake Inhibitors**

| Adverse Effects | Comments |
|---|---|
| 1. Rash or allergic reaction | 1. Discontinue drug; ask your health care provider about treatment with antihistamines or steroids. |
| 2. Anxiety, nervousness, insomnia | 2. Discontinue the drug. Giving the drug in AM might help decrease insomnia. |
| 3. Anorexia, weight loss, nausea | 3. Particularly common in underweight, depressed clients. If significant weight loss occurs, ask your health care provider about changing to a different drug. |
| 4. Tremors, sweating, dizziness, lightheaded-ness | 4. Most of the effects listed in 4, 5, and 6 are transient and disappear when drug is discontinued. |
| 5. Drowsiness and fatigue | 5. SSRIs can affect cognitive and motor ability. |
| 6. Decreased or altered libido/erectile dysfunction | 6. If change in libido or ability to perform becomes a problem, ask your health care provider about changing the drug. |
| 7. Weight gain | 7. Weight gain is a reason for nonadherence to medication in most women and some men. **Dietary teaching is essential when medications alter metabolism and predispose to obesity, diabetes, and/or heart disease** (personal communication from Dorothy A. Varchol, June 2003). |
| 8. Nonadherence to drug | 8. Approximately 33% of clients experience sexual dysfunction. |

Serotonergic Syndrome: Toxic Effects
1. Hyperactivity/restlessness
2. Tachycardia→cardiovascular shock
3. Fever→hyperpyrexia
4. Elevated blood pressure
5. Confusion→delirium

Table 21-2 **Adverse and Toxic Effects of Selective Serotonin Reuptake Inhibitors—cont'd**

| Adverse Effects | Comments |
| --- | --- |
| Serotonergic Syndrome: Toxic Effects—cont'd | |
| 6. Irrationality, mood swings, hostility | |
| 7. Generalized seizures | |
| 8. Myoclonus, incoordination, tonic rigidity | |
| 9. Abdominal pain, diarrhea, bloating | |
| 10. Apnea→death | |

**NOTE:** Do not administer SSRIs to patients who are taking MAOIs. The drug interaction can result in serious or fatal reactions.

## Drug Interactions

- MAOIs: SSRIs should **not** be combined with the MAOIs; can produce serotonin syndrome
- Alcohol: CNS depressants antagonize CNS depressant effect
- Oral anticoagulants: Can displace highly protein-bound medications from protein-binding sites (e.g., warfarin [Coumadin])
- St. John's Wort, which may have harmful additive effects
- TCAs
- Lithium

## Use with Caution

- Clients with impaired renal or hepatic function
- Pregnant women: Safety in pregnancy has not been established; unknown if SSRIs cross the placenta or are distributed in breast milk
- Elderly: Often best to start at a lower dose in clients who are elderly
- Clients who are underweight or anorectic
- Clients who have abused drugs or are dependent on drugs
- Clients who are suicidal

## Contraindications

- Do not use within 14 days of MAOI ingestion.
- Do not use in clients who are hypersensitive to the SSRIs.
- Do not use with **St. John's Wort** (may be dangerous).

## Client and Family Teaching

For useful guidelines for family and client teaching, refer to Box 21-3.

## Box 21-3 Client and Family Teaching: Selective Serotonin Reuptake Inhibitors

SSRIs can cause sexual dysfunction or lack of sex drive. Inform your health care provider.

SSRIs can cause insomnia, anxiety, and nervousness. Inform your health care provider.

SSRIs can interact with other medications. Be sure physician knows other medications client is taking (digoxin, warfarin). SSRIs should not be taken within 14 days of the last dose of an MAOI.

Do not take any over-the-counter drugs without first notifying the physician.

Common side effects include fatigue, nausea, diarrhea, dry mouth, dizziness, tremor, fatigue, and sexual dysfunction or lack of sex drive.

Because of the potential for drowsiness and dizziness, client should not drive or operate machinery until these side effects are ruled out.

Avoid alcohol.

Client should have liver and renal function tests performed and blood counts checked periodically.

Do not discontinue medication abruptly. If side effects become bothersome, ask your health care provider about changing to a different drug, but be aware that the medication will have to be phased out over a period of time.

Report any of the following symptoms to your health care provider *immediately:*
- Rash or hives
- Rapid heart beat
- Sore throat
- Difficulty urinating
- Fever, malaise
- Anorexia/weight loss
- Unusual bleeding
- Initiation of hyperactive behavior
- Severe headache

## Novel (Atypical) New Generation Antidepressants

There are many drugs that have proved to have antidepressant qualities. The drugs and a brief side-effects profile are found in Table 21-3. Also see the drug monographs in Appendix G.

Table 21-3 **Novel/Atypical Antidepressants**

| Generic Name | Trade Name | Initial Dose (mg/day) | Dose after 4-8 Weeks (mg/day) | Side Effects Profile |
|---|---|---|---|---|
| Bupropion | Wellbutrin Wellbutrin SR Zyban | 100-150 | 200-450 | **Initial:** Nausea, headache, insomnia, anxiety/agitation; seizure risk<br>**Low:** Weight gain, sedation, sexual dysfunction |
| Trazodone | Desyrel | 50 | 150-400 | **Not recommended as a first-line treatment**<br>**Initial:** Sedation, **priapism**, dizziness, orthostasis<br>**High:** Sedation<br>**Low:** Weight gain, sexual dysfunction |
| **Dual-Action Reuptake Inhibitors (Serotonin and Norepinephrine) (SNRIs)** | | | | |
| Venlafaxine | Effexor Effexor XR | 50-75 | 75-375 | **Dual-action reuptake inhibitor: Can enhance chance of remission if both serotonin and norepinephrine reuptake are inhibited. (SNRIs)**<br>Dose-dependent hypertension<br>**High:** Sexual dysfunction<br>**Minimal:** Sedation<br>**Low:** Weight gain |

Not complete lists.

Adapted from Varcarolis, E. (2005). *Foundations of psychiatric mental health nursing* (5th ed.). Philadelphia: WB Saunders.

* Anticholinergic side effects include dry mouth, blurred vision, constipation, urinary retention, tachycardia, and possible confusion. Preston and associates, 2005.

** Not yet FDA approved, but use outside North America has been found effective against depression and panic disorders.

*Continued*

Table 21-3 **Novel/Atypical Antidepressants—cont'd**

| Generic Name | Trade Name | Initial Dose (mg/day) | Dose after 4-8 Weeks (mg/day) | Side Effects Profile |
|---|---|---|---|---|
| Duloxetine | Cymbalta | 40 | 60 | **Newest dual-action inhibitor**<br>Promise for severe depression<br>**High:** Anorexia, fatigue, insomnia, dizziness<br>**Less:** Acne, alopecia, anxiety, orgasmic disorder, ejaculation difficulty<br>**Low:** Abdominal/back pain; abnormal hepatic function tests, colitis, IBS, suicidal ideation, thrombocytopenia |
| Mirtazapine | Remeron | 7.5-15 | 15-45 | Anticholinergic*; might increase serum lipids; rare: peripheral edema, agranulocytosis; **high dose** can produce cardiovascular effects (severe postural hypotension, dizziness, tachycardia, palpitations, arrhythmias) |

**High:** Sedation even with low dose, weight gain
**Low:** Sexual dysfunction

**Energizing:** May improve concentration
**Moderate:** May cause sedation or anxiety
**Low:** Less sexual dysfunction, less weight gain

**Selective Noradrenaline Reuptake Inhibitor (SNRI)**

Reboxetine**    Edronax

Vestra

Adapted from Varcarolis, E. (2005). *Foundations of psychiatric mental health nursing* (5th ed.). Philadelphia: WB Saunders.

* Anticholinergic side effects include dry mouth, blurred vision, constipation, urinary retention, tachycardia, and possible confusion. Preston and associates, 2005.

** Not yet FDA approved, but used outside North America has been found effective against depression and panic disorders.

## Tricyclic Antidepressants

Tricyclic antidepressants have a long history of effectiveness in major depression. However, their main drawback is their side-effects profile, which can affect client adherence. These drugs can be sedating, cause orthostatic hypertension, and have anticholinergic effects (e.g., dry mouth, blurred vision, photophobia, constipation, urinary hesitancy, and tachycardia). The most hazardous effect is cardiac toxicity. Therefore, the TCAs might be poorly tolerated by some because of their side effects.

Because the TCAs have a narrow therapeutic index, there is significant risk for toxicity. A 1-week supply can be fatal in an overdose. A blood concentration higher than 1000 mg/dl is correlated with severe cardiac symptoms (prolonged QRS complex and arrhythmias) (Mendelowitz, 2000). The TCAs are commonly the drugs of choice in suicides (Mendelowitz, 2000).

### Therapeutic Uses

- Depression: Acute depression, prevention of relapse, and other depressive syndromes. The TCAs were the first group of drugs effective in the treatment of depression.
- Panic attacks: Imipramine (Tofranil), clomipramine (Anafranil), desipramine (Norpramin)
- Childhood enuresis: Imipramine (Tofranil)
- Bulimia nervosa: Imipramine (Tofranil), desipramine (Norpramin)
- Obsessive-compulsive disorder: Clomipramine (Anafranil) is the only TCA effective for OCD.

*Moderate evidence for:*
- Chronic pain: Several TCAs are useful in treating chronic pain—e.g., amitriptyline (Elavil), doxepin (Sinequan).
- Chronic insomnia: Amitriptyline (Elavil)
- Attention-deficit/hyperactivity disorder: Desipramine (Norpramin), imipramine (Tofranil) **(used with caution).**
- Migraine: Amitriptyline (Elavil)

### Mechanism of Action

The TCAs block NE and serotonin reuptake. Although the blockage is immediate, it takes several weeks for relief of symptoms to occur, as it does with all antidepressants. There is speculation that intermediary neurochemical effects are taking place during the lag time (Lehne, 2001). Along with the desired blockage of serotonin, the TCAs also cause blockage of the receptor sites for histamine ($H_1$), acetylcholine (ACh), and NE, which results in some of the negative side effects of these drugs. Refer to Figure 21-1.

## Metabolism

Clearance of tricyclic compounds is principally the result of hepatic metabolism. Renal clearance accounts for only a small portion of drug elimination. Elimination half-lives for most of the TCAs are approximately 24 hours. This allows for once-daily dosing.

## Adverse Effects

**Cardiovascular Effects** Orthostatic hypotension is one of the most common reasons for discontinuation of TCA treatment. Orthostatic hypotension can lead to dizziness, and increase risk of falls.

Most serious cardiovascular effects, especially in high doses, are **arrhythmias, tachycardia, myocardial infarction,** and **heart block.** Clients without conduction delay tolerate the tricyclics well. These drugs are used with caution and need to be evaluated in the elderly and in people with cardiac problems.

**Autonomic Nervous System Anticholinergic Effects** include dry mouth, blurred vision, tachycardia, constipation, urinary retention, and esophageal reflux. Urinary retention and severe constipation warrant immediate medical attention. The TCAs can cause ocular crisis in people with narrow-angle glaucoma.

**Central Nervous System** Tricyclics can produce confusion or delirium. These effects are dose related. Seizures also are possible side effects with all tricyclics and tetracyclic agents. A fine, rapid hand tremor can be a clinical indication of an elevated blood concentration.

**Hepatic Effects** Tricyclics can cause mild increases of liver enzymes and can be monitored safely. However, drug-induced acute hepatitis develops quickly and is associated with very high enzyme levels. This is a dangerous and potentially fatal condition.

**Sexual Dysfunction** A potential problem with many classes of antidepressants.

**Allergic Reactions** Tricyclics are sometimes associated with photosensitivity reactions. Rare reports of various blood dyscrasias have also been reported.

**Psychiatric** Confusion states (especially in the elderly), with hallucinations, disorientation, delusions, anxiety, restlessness, agitation, insomnia, and nightmares; hypomania; and exacerbation of psychosis may occur.

**Toxicity** Overdose with TCAs can be life-threatening. To avoid death by suicide, a client thought to be a risk for suicide should be given no more than a 1-week supply of TCAs.

## Drug Interactions

- Monoamine oxidase inhibitors, in combination with TCAs, lead to severe hypertension, hypertensive crisis, and potential death.
- Sympathomimetic drugs (e.g., epinephrine and norepinephrine) can lead to increased blood pressure and cardiac effects.
- Anticholinergic agents intensify anticholinergic effects of TCAs; for example:
  - Trihexyphenidyl (Artane)
  - Benztropine (Cogentin)
  - Diphenylamine (Benadryl)
  - Oxybutynin (Ditropan)
  - Propantheline (Pro-Banthine)
  - Meperidine (Demerol)
- CNS depressants (e.g., alcohol, antihistamines, opioids, and barbiturates). These can intensify the CNS depressant effects of the TCAs, increase respiratory depression, as well as decrease TCA effect.
- Phenothiazines might increase sedative and anticholinergic effects.
- St. John's Wort might have additive effects.

## *Use with Caution*

- Clients with:
  - History of urinary retention or obstruction
  - Glaucoma
  - Diabetes mellitus
  - History of seizures
  - Hyperthyroidism
  - Cardiac/hepatic/renal disease
  - Schizophrenia
  - Increased intraocular pressure
  - Hiatal hernia
- Clients who are elderly or debilitated
- Pregnant or lactating women (safety has not been established)

## *Contraindications*

- TCAs should not be taken during the acute recovery period following a myocardial infarction.
- TCAs should not be taken within 14 days of MAOI ingestion.

## *Client and Family Teaching*

See Box 21-4 for a useful tool in medication teaching.

# Second-Line Agents

## Monoamine Oxidase Inhibitors

Monoamine oxidase inhibitors are seldom first choice, but they are appropriate for those who do not respond to the SSRIs, atypical antidepressants, or the TCAs. The MAOIs can cause dangerous side effects. However, many believe they are the drug of choice for atypical depression and depression associated with anxiety, panic, and phobias (Lehne, 2001; Keltner & Folks, 2001).

## *Therapeutic Uses*

- Treatment-resistant major depression
- "Atypical" depression (characterized by anxiety, somatization, feeling better in the morning and worse as the

---

### Box 21-4 Client and Family Teaching: Tricyclic Antidepressants

1. Tell the client and the client's family that mood elevation can take from 7 to 28 days. It might take up to 6 to 8 weeks for the full effect to take place and for major depression symptoms to subside.
2. Have the family reinforce this frequently to the depressed family member because depressed people have trouble remembering, and they respond to ongoing reassurance.
3. Reassure the client that drowsiness, dizziness, and hypotension usually subside after the first few weeks.
4. When the client starts taking tricyclic antidepressants (TCAs), caution the client to be careful working around machines, driving cars, and crossing streets because of possible altered reflexes, drowsiness, and/or dizziness.
5. Alcohol can block the effects of antidepressants. Tell the client to refrain from drinking.
6. If possible, the client should take the full dose at bedtime to reduce the experience of side effects during the day.
7. If the client forgets the bedtime dose (or the once-a-day dose), the client should take the dose within 3 hours; otherwise, the client should wait for the next day. The client should *not* double the dose.
8. Suddenly stopping TCAs can cause nausea, altered heartbeat, nightmares, and cold sweats in 2 to 4 days. Clients should call their health care clinician or take one dose of TCA until the clinician can be contacted.
9. Client should have written information as to
   a. Side effects
   b. Possible toxic effects
   c. The telephone numbers of healthcare clinician and staff
10. Make a thorough assesment of how the client has been doing since the last visit.

---

Adapted from Varcarolis, E. (2005). *Foundations of psychiatric mental health nursing* (5th ed.). Philadelphia: WB Saunders; reprinted with permission.

day progresses, hyperphagia, weight gain, sensitivity to rejection, trouble falling or staying asleep)
- Treatment-resistant panic disorder
- Treatment-resistant mixed anxiety-depression

- Treatment-resistant depression in people with bipolar disorder
- Dysthymia not responsive to other antidepressants

## Mechanism of Action

The MAOIs inhibit the action of the monoamine oxidase (MAO) enzyme system at the CNS storage sites. There are two types of MAO in the body: MAO-A and MAO-B. In the brain, MAO-A inactivates NE and serotonin, whereas MAO-B inactivates dopamine.

The reduced MAO activity causes an increased concentration in epinephrine, NE, serotonin, and dopamine at neuron receptor sites producing antidepressant effects. These are all welcome effects.

The inhibition of MAO, therefore, can help relieve depression. But the MAOIs also inhibit the breakdown of the amine tyramine. When the amine tyramine increases and is not broken, these increased levels of tyramine can cause high blood pressure, hypertensive crisis, and, eventually, cerebrovascular accident. Tyramine is found in many foods. Therefore, when a person is on an MAOI, vigilance is required to avoid the long list of prohibited foods that are rich in tyramine. This avoidance extends to drugs as well.

## Metabolism

The MAOIs are absorbed from the gastrointestinal tract and metabolized in the liver. The metabolites are then excreted in the urine.

## Adverse Effects

**Hypertensive Crisis from Dietary Tyramine** This is by far the most dreaded side effect of the MAOIs that can occur if a client eats food that is rich in tyramine (see Table 21-4). MAOIs can also interact with many drugs (see Box 21-6). The increase in blood pressure can develop into intracranial hemorrhage, hyperpyrexia, convulsions, coma, and death.

Early symptoms include headache, stiff neck, palpitations, increase or decrease in heart rate (often associated with chest pain), nausea, vomiting, and increase in temperature. Immediate medical attention is crucial.

**Other Side Effects**
- Hypotension. This is the most critical of the side effects because it can lead to falls, especially in the elderly.
- Sedation, weakness, fatigue
- Insomnia
- Changes in cardiac rhythm
- Muscle cramps
- Anorgasmia or sexual impotence
- Urinary hesitancy or constipation
- Weight gain

*Use with Caution*
- Clients with:
  - Impaired renal function
  - History of seizures
  - Parkinson syndrome
  - Diabetes
  - Hyperthyroidism

*Contraindications*
- Clients older than 60 years
- Debilitated/hypertensive clients
- Clients with cerebrovascular/cardiovascular disease
- Foods containing tryptophan, tyramine, and dopamine (see Table 21-4)
- Certain medications (see Box 21-6)
- Pheochromocytoma
- Congestive heart failure (CHF)
- History of liver disease
- Abnormal liver function tests
- Severe renal impairment
- History of severe/recurrent headaches
- Children younger than 16 years of age

*Client and Family Teaching*
Box 21-5 can be used as a guideline for client and family teaching for a client on an MAOI. Table 21-4 is a list of forbidden foods, and Box 21-6 is a list of drugs that a person on MAOIs must be aware of and avoid.

---

### Box 21-5 Client and Family Teaching: Monoamine Oxidase Inhibitors

- Tell the client and the client's family to avoid certain foods and all medications (especially cold remedies) unless prescribed by and discussed with the client's health care provider/prescriber. Give client and family a written list of "forbidden" foods and drugs. (See Table 21-4 and Box 21-6.)
- Give the client a wallet card describing the monoamine oxidase inhibitor (MAOI) regimen.
- Instruct the client to avoid Chinese restaurants (sherry, brewer's yeast, and other products might be used).
- Tell the client to go to the emergency room right away if he or she develops a severe headache.
- Ideally, blood pressure should be monitored during the first 6 weeks of treatment (for both hypotensive and hypertensive effects).
- After stopping the MAOI, the client should maintain dietary and drug restrictions for 14 days.
- Document in detail how the client has been doing since the last visit (e.g., symptom changes, adverse reactions, drug having desired effect, change in quality of life).

Adapted from Varcarolis, E. (2005). *Foundations of psychiatric mental health nursing* (5th ed.). Philadelphia: WB Saunders, Reprinted with permission.

---

### Box 21-6 Drugs That Can Interact with Monoamine Oxidase Inhibitors

Drug restrictions that apply to clients taking a monoamine oxidase inhibitor include the following:
- Over-the-counter medications for colds, allergies, or congestion (any product containing ephedrine, phenylephrine, hydrochloride, or phenylpropanolamine)
- Tricyclic antidepressants (imipramine, amitriptyline)
- Narcotics
- Antihypertensives (methyldopa, guanethidine, reserpine)
- Amine precursors (levodopa, L-tryptophan)
- Sedatives (alcohol, barbiturates, benzodiazepines)
- General anesthetics
- Stimulants (amphetamines, cocaine)

From Varcarolis, E. (2005). *Foundations of psychiatric mental health nursing* (5th ed.). Philadelphia: WB Saunders, Reprinted with permission.

Table 21-4 **Foods That Can Interact with Monoamine Oxidase Inhibitors**

*Foods That Contain Tyramine*

| Category | Unsafe Foods (High Tyramine Content) | Safe Foods (Little or No Tyramine) |
|---|---|---|
| Vegetables | Avocados, especially if overripe; fermented bean curd; fermented soybean; soybean paste; sauerkraut | Most vegetables |
| Fruits | Figs, especially if overripe; bananas, in large amounts | Most fruits |
| Meats | Meats that are fermented, smoked, or otherwise aged; spoiled meats; liver, unless very fresh; beef and chicken liver | Meats that are known to be fresh (exercise caution in restaurants; meats might not be fresh) |
| Sausages | Fermented varieties; bologna, pepperoni, salami, others | Nonfermented varieties |
| Fish | Dried, pickled or cured fish; fish that is fermented, smoked, or otherwise aged; spoiled fish | Fish that is known to be fresh; vacuum-packed fish, if eaten promptly or refrigerated only briefly after opening |
| Milk, milk products | Practically all cheeses | Milk, yogurt, cottage cheese, cream cheese |

| | | |
|---|---|---|
| Foods with yeast | Yeast extract (e.g., Marmite, Bovril) | Baked goods that contain yeast |
| Beer, wine | Some imported beers, Chianti | Major domestic brands of beer, most wines |
| Other foods | Protein dietary supplements; soups (might contain protein extract); shrimp paste; soy sauce | |

*Foods That Contain Other Vasopressors*

| Food | Comments |
|---|---|
| Chocolate | Contains phenylethylamine, a pressor agent; large amounts can cause a reaction |
| Fava beans | Contain dopamine, a pressor agent; reactions are most likely with overripe beans |
| Ginseng | Headache, tremulousness, and manic-like reactions have occurred |
| Caffeinated beverages | Caffeine is a weak pressor agent; large amounts might cause a reaction |

From Lehne, R.A. (2001). *Pharmacology for nursing* (4th ed.). Philadelphia: WB Saunders.

# ANTIPSYCHOTIC/NEUROLEPTIC MEDICATIONS

This section presents:

1. **The Conventional/Standard Antipsychotic Agents.** Phenothiazines are used as the prototype for these drugs. They are usually less expensive; however, they have more troubling side effects than the newer generations of antipsychotics. They target predominantly the *positive symptoms* of schizophrenia (e.g., hallucinations, delusions, paranoia, abnormal thought formations).

2. **The Atypical (Novel) Antipsychotic Agents.** These newer agents have a better side effect profile than the conventional agents. Less troubling side effects can help to increase medication compliance. However, these new generation agents are much more expensive than the traditional agents. These newer agents target both the positive and *negative symptoms* (e.g., apathy, lack of motivation, social withdrawal, communication difficulties, and asocial behavior). By reducing the negative symptoms, many people are able to hold jobs, attend school, and interact with others in a positive and rewarding manner.

## Conventional/Standard Antipsychotic Agents

Refer to Table 8-3 in the chapter on schizophrenia for a list of the traditional antipsychotic medications and their dosages. The conventional/standard antipsychotic agents were the first effective drugs to treat schizophrenia. These neuroleptic agents are characterized by a relatively high tendency to produce extrapyramidal side effects (EPS) and anticholinergic side effects. Unfortunately, as mentioned, they have a poor effect on the negative symptoms of schizophrenia (refer to Chapter 8).

### *Therapeutic Uses*

- **Schizophrenia:**
  - Suppression of symptoms during the acute phase of illness (might take up to 4 weeks for full effects)
  - Taken long-term can decrease the risk of relapse

- Effective in targeting the positive symptoms of schizophrenia (e.g., hallucinations, delusions, disordered thinking, paranoia)
- Essentially does **not** target the troubling negative symptoms (e.g., social and emotional withdrawal, avolition [lack of motivation], anergia [lack of energy], blunted affect, poverty of speech)
- **Bipolar disorder:** During the acutely manic phase
- **Depression with psychotic symptoms**
- **Tourette's syndrome:** Helps suppress severe symptoms such as severe motor tics, barking cries, grunts, and outbursts of obscene language that are beyond the control of the individual (haloperidol [Haldol], pimozide)
- **Prevention of emesis:** Chlorpromazine (Thorazine)

**Investigational Uses**
- **Treatment of choreiform movements of Huntington's disease:** Haloperidol (Haldol)
- **Refractory hiccup:** Chlorpromazine (Thorazine)
- **Relief of acute intermittent porphyrin:** Chlorpromazine (Thorazine)
- **Nausea/vomiting associated with chemotherapy:** Haloperidol (Haldol)
- Psychosis associated with Parkinson's disease (Hodgson & Kizior, 2003; Keltner & Folks, 2001)

### Mechanism of Action

The conventional antipsychotic agents block a variety of receptors within and outside the CNS. The beneficial effects seem to be derived from the blockage of dopamine 2 ($D_2$) receptors in the mesolimbic and mesocortical areas of the brain. However, these drugs also block receptors for acetylcholine (ACh), histamine ($H_1$), and norepinephrine (NE). The wide variety of side effects associated with these drugs can be understood as a logical extension of their receptor-blocking activity (Figure 21-2).

### Clinical Dosage

Table 8-3 identifies the various standard/typical medications and the drug dosage. The drugs are listed from high potency to low potency. This is pertinent information because of what it tells us about the degrees of specific side effects; for example:

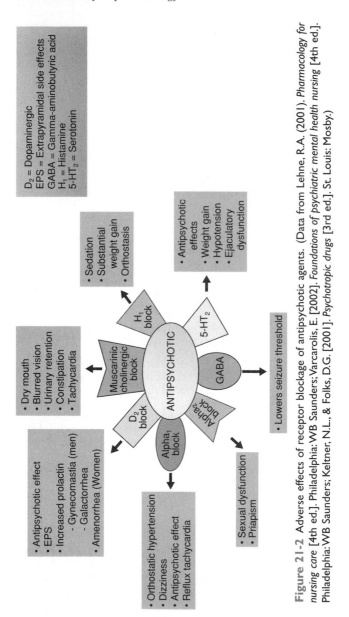

**Figure 21-2** Adverse effects of receptor blockage of antipsychotic agents. (Data from from Lehne, R.A. (2001). *Pharmacology for nursing care* [4th ed.]. Philadelphia: WB Saunders; Varcarolis, E. [2002]. *Foundations of psychiatric mental health nursing* [4th ed.]. Philadelphia: WB Saunders; Keltner, N.L., & Folks, D.G. [2001]. *Psychotropic drugs* [3rd ed.]. St. Louis: Mosby.)

- **Low Potency** = High Sedation + High ACh and Low EPS
- **High Potency** = Low Sedation + Low ACh and High EPS (e.g., akathisia)

## Metabolism

Neuroleptics undergo hepatic metabolism. All elderly clients should be given lower doses because of increased sensitivity to the side effects. Cigarette smoking significantly increases the metabolism of the conventional antipsychotic medications (e.g., thiothixene [Navane], fluphenazine [Prolixin].

## Adverse Effects

As previously mentioned, two side effects that contribute to nonadherence to medication regimen are weight gain (especially women) and sexual dysfunction (especially men). Agranulocytosis and neuroleptic malignant syndrome (NMS), both relatively rare, are serious, and can be fatal if the client is not monitored while taking the medication regimen. Refer to Table 21-5 for more information on the adverse and toxic reactions and the medical/nursing interventions.

### Central Nervous System
- Extrapyramidal side effects. The major neurologic side effects involve the extrapyramidal system. They occur in 50% to 75% of people taking the standard neuroleptics. EPS symptoms include: **acute dystonia, dyskinesia (pseudoparkinsonism), and akathisia.**
- Tardive dyskinesia (TD), also an EPS, is a movement disorder that can occur following long-term therapy and is often not reversible. See Table 21-5 for the EPS symptoms and medical/nursing interventions, as well as other untoward effects and nursing interventions for these.
- Lowers the seizure threshold.
- Sedation.

### Cardiovascular Symptoms
- Hypotension and postural hypotension and tachycardia might occur. Refer to Table 21-5.
- Prolongation of QTc interval is also possible, and pretreatment electrocardiograms should be checked in people older than 40 and those with a history of cardiac disease.

*Text continued on p. 611*

Table 21-5 **Nursing Measures for Side Effects of Standard/Conventional Antipsychotics**

| Side Effects | Onset | Nursing Measures |
|---|---|---|
| Anticholinergic Symptoms | | |
| 1. Dry mouth | | 1. Frequent sips of water and sugarless candy or gum. If severe, provide Xero-Lube, a saliva substitute. |
| 2. Urinary retention and hesitancy | | 2. Check voiding; try warm towel on abdomen; consider catheterization if this does not work. |
| 3. Constipation | | 3. Usually short-term. Stool softeners might be helpful. Assess for adequate water intake. |
| 4. Blurred vision | | 4. Usually abates in 1 to 2 weeks. If client has been prescribed thioridazine, do not give it, and check with health care provider. |
| 5. Photosensitivity | | 5. Encourage client to wear sunglasses. |
| 6. Dry eyes | | 6. Use artificial tears. |
| 7. Inhibition of ejaculation or impotence in men | | 7. Alert health care provider that client might need alternative medication. |

**Extrapyramidal Side Effects**

| | | |
|---|---|---|
| 1. **Pseudoparkinsonism:** Masklike faces, stiff and stooped posture, shuffling gait, drooling, tremor, "pill-rolling" phenomenon | >5-30 days | 1. Alert medical staff. An anticholinergic agent (e.g., trihexyphenidyl [Artane] or benztropine [Cogentin]) might be prescribed. |
| 2. **Acute dystonic reactions:** Acute contractions of tongue, face, neck, and back (tongue and jaw first) <br>• **Opisthotonos:** Titanic heightening of entire body, head and belly up <br>• **Oculogyric crisis:** Eyes locked upward | 1-5 days | 2. **First choice:** Diphenhydramine hydrochloride (Benadryl) 25-50 mg IM/IV. Relief occurs in minutes. <br>**Second choice:** Benztropine, 1-2 mg IM/IV. <br>**Prevent further dystonias** with ACh agent. Experience is very frightening. Take person to quiet area and stay with him or her until medicated. |
| 3. **Akathisia:** Motor inner-driven restlessness (e.g., tapping foot incessantly, rocking forward and backward in chair, shifting weight from side to side) | 5-60 days | 3. Health care provider may change antipsychotic agent or give antiparkinsonian agent. Tolerance does not develop to akathisia, but akathisia disappears when neuroleptic is discontinued. Propranolol (Inderal), lorazepam (Ativan), or diazepam (Valium) may be used. |

Adapted from Varcarolis, E. (2002). *Foundations of psychiatric mental health nursing* (4th ed.). Philadelphia: WB Saunders, pp. 550-551; reprinted with permission.

*IM,* Intramuscular; *IV,* intravenous.

*Continued*

## Table 21-5 Nursing Measures for Side Effects of Standard/Conventional Antipsychotics—cont'd

| Side Effects | Onset | Nursing Measures |
| --- | --- | --- |
| 4. **Tardive dyskinesia:**<br>• **Facial:** Protruding and rolling tongue, blowing, smacking, licking, spastic facial distortion, smacking movement<br>• **Limbs:**<br>**Choreic:** Rapid, purposeless and irregular movements<br>**Athetoid:** Slow, complex and serpentine movements<br>• **Trunk:** Neck, shoulder, dramatic hip jerks and rocking, twisting pelvic trusts | 6–24 mo to years | 4. **No known treatment.** Discontinuing the drug does not always relieve symptoms. Possibly 20% of patients taking the drug for >2 years develop tardive dyskinesia. **The health care provider should screen for tardive dyskinesia at least every 3 months.** (Refer to the AIMS Scale in Appendix D-14.) |
| **Cardiovascular Effects**<br>1. **Hypotension and postural hypotension** | | 1. Check blood pressure before giving; advise client to dangle feet before getting out of bed to prevent dizziness and subsequent falls. A systolic pressure of 80 mmHg when standing is an indication that the current dose should not be given. This effect usually subsides when drug is stabilized in 1 to 2 weeks. Elastic bandages might prevent pooling. If condition is serious, the health care provider can order volume expanders or pressure agents. |

2. Tachycardia

2. Clients with existing cardiac problems should *always* be evaluated before the antipsychotic drugs are administered. Haloperidol (Haldol) is usually the preferred drug because of its low ACh effects.

**Rare and Toxic Effects**

1. **Agranulocytosis:** Symptoms include sore throat, fever, malaise, and mouth sore. It is a rare occurrence, but one the nurse should be aware of; any flulike symptoms should be carefully evaluated.

Usually occurs suddenly and becomes evident in the first 12 weeks

1. Blood work is usually done every week, then every 2 months. Blood work is ordered to determine presence of leukopenia or agranulocytosis. If test results are positive, the drug is discontinued, and reverse isolation might be initiated. Mortality is high if the drug is not discontinued and if treatment is not initiated.

2. **Cholestatic jaundice:** Rare, reversible, and usually benign if caught in time; prodromal symptoms are fever, malaise, nausea, and abdominal pain; jaundice appears 1 week later.

2. Drug is discontinued; bed rest and high-protein, high-carbohydrate diet is given. Liver function tests should be performed every 6 months.

*Continued*

Table 21-5 Nursing Measures for Side Effects of Standard/Conventional Antipsychotics—cont'd

| Side Effects | Onset | Nursing Measures |
|---|---|---|
| 3. **Neuroleptic malignant syndrome:** Somewhat rare, potentially fatal<br>• **Severe extrapyramidal:** Severe muscle rigidity, oculogyric crisis, dysphasia, flexor extensor posturing, cog wheeling<br>• **Hyperpyrexia:** Elevated temperature (>103° F)<br>• **Autonomic dysfunction:** Hypertension, tachycardia, diaphoresis, incontinence | Can occur in the first week of drug therapy but often occurs later; rapidly progresses over 2 to 3 days after initial manifestation<br>RISK FACTORS:<br>• Using concomitant psychotropics<br>• Being older<br>• Being female (3:2)<br>• Having a mood disorder (40%)<br>• Undergoing rapid dose titration (Lieberman & Tasman, 2000) | 3<br>• Stop neuroleptic.<br>• Transfer to medical unit immediately.<br>• **Bromocriptine** can relieve muscle rigidity and reduce fever.<br>• **Dantrolene** might reduce muscle spasms.<br>• Cool body to reduce fever.<br>• Maintain hydration with oral and IV fluids.<br>• Correct electrolyte imbalance.<br>• Arrhythmias should be treated.<br>• Small doses of heparin might decrease possibility of pulmonary emboli.<br>• **Early detection increases client's chance of survival.** |

**Endocrine Effects** By blocking the inhibitory action of dopamine on prolactin release, there is an increase in circulating prolactin levels. This increase can cause breast enlargement (gynecomastia), which can occur in males as well as females, and irregular menses including anovulatory cycles and infertility.

**Sexual Dysfunction** Sexual dysfunction manifests as ejaculatory and erectile disturbances in men, and anorgasmia and decreased lubrication in women. Both experience decreased libido. These drug-related sexual dysfunctions are often responsible for nonadherence to medications.

**Anticholinergic Effects** Anticholinergic effects are more common with low-potency dopamine receptor antagonists such as chlorpromazine. As previously mentioned, these effects include: blurred vision, dry mouth, constipation, and urinary hesitancy, dry eyes, and inhibition of ejaculation or impotence in men (see Table 21-5).

**Skin and Eye Effects** Clients might experience photosensitivity reactions consisting of severe sunburn or rash. It is for this reason that clients should be encouraged to wear sunglasses and use sun block when outside in the sun.

**Adverse Reactions/Toxic Effects** These untoward reactions are serious and can be fatal.
- Agranulocytosis (rare) (see Table 21-5)
- Neuroleptic malignant syndrome (see Table 21-5)

## Drug Interactions

- CNS depressants (alcohol, antihistamines, benzodiazepines, barbiturates): Can increase the CNS respiration depression and hypotensive effects
- Antidepressants (TCAs and MAOIs): May increase sedative anticholinergic effects
- Levodopa (a drug used to treat Parkinson's disease) can counteract the antipsychotic effects of the phenothiazines
- Antithyroid agents: May increase risk of agranulocytosis
- Lithium: May decrease absorption and produce adverse neurologic effects
- Hypotensives: Can increase hypotensive effects of these agents

## Use with Caution

- **Extreme caution in the elderly:** They are extremely susceptible to TD. Always "start low and go slow."
- History of seizures
- Urinary retention
- Glaucoma
- Prostatic hypertrophy
- Hypoglycemia

## Contraindications

- Pregnancy. The weeks 4 to 10 are particularly dangerous. During the remainder of the pregnancy, the lowest possible dosage is desirable. However, it is advised that all antipsychotic medication is discontinued, to avoid neonatal toxicity (Keltner & Folks, 2001).
- Poorly controlled seizure disorders
- Severe CNS depression, comatose states
- Severe cardiovascular disease
- Bone marrow depression
- Liver, renal, or cardiac insufficiency

## Client and Family Teaching

Refer to Box 21-7 for guidelines for client and family teaching with the standard antipsychotic medications. Refer to Table 21-5 for the nursing interventions and teaching points for the various side effects of the standard antipsychotic medications.

# Atypical (Novel) Antipsychotic Agents

These newer atypical agents first emerged in the early 1990s with the advent of clozapine (Clozaril). This was a breakthrough drug in many ways, and a miracle drug for some; however, unfortunately, this drug causes agranulocytosis in approximately 1% of clients. The atypical agents that eventually followed do not share this same disadvantage. These newer agents not only target the positive symptoms (hallucinations, delusions) but also allow improvement in the quality of life for people with schizophrenia by mitigating the negative symptoms as well (lack of motivation, poverty of speech, blunted affect, poor self care, and social withdrawal). Cognitive enhancement, however, might not be evident for several months (personal communication from Dorothy A. Varchol, June 2003).

## Box 21-7 Client and Family Teaching: Standard Antipsychotics

1. Full therapeutic response can take at least 6 weeks.
2. Do not abruptly withdraw from long-term therapy. If client is having sexual difficulty, gaining weight, please contact the physician.
3. Use sun block and wear protective clothing when in the sun. These drugs can potentiate the effects of sunburn.
4. Rise slowly from a sitting or lying position to prevent a sudden drop in blood pressure.
5. Wear sunglasses to minimize the photosensitivity inherent in these medications.
6. Take sips of water and chew sugarless chewing gum. Good oral hygiene can minimize the effects of dry mouth.
7. Do not take alcohol while on these drugs. They potentiate the CNS side effects of each.
8. Smoking might increase the metabolism of some antipsychotics, which might require a dosage adjustment to maintain a therapeutic effect.
9. Do not take any over-the-counter medication without your health care provider's approval.
10. Notify your health care provider if you become pregnant or are planning to become pregnant. These drugs might not be safe during the first trimester.
11. Refer frequently to the written material provided for you by your health care system on the side effects and what might help the side effects of these antipsychotic medications; keep the list in a place where it can be easily referred to.
12. **Report immediately** occurrence of any of the following to your health care provider:
    - Sore throat
    - Fever
    - Malaise
    - Unusual bleeding
    - Difficulty urinating
    - Muscle twitching
    - Severe headache
    - Rapid heart rate
    - Dark-colored urine
    - Pale stools
    - Yellow tinge to skin or eyes

## *Therapeutic Uses*

- Schizophrenia
- Management of manifestations of psychotic disorders
- Treatment of acute mania associated with bipolar disorder: Olanzapine (Zyprexa)

**Unlabeled Uses**
- Anorexia: Olanzapine (Zyprexa)
- Maintenance of treatment response in schizophrenic disorders: Olanzapine (Zyprexa)
- Treatment of resistant mania and for prophylaxis in bipolar mood disorder: Clozapine (Clozaril)

## *Overall Benefits*

The atypical agents are often chosen as first-line treatment because:
1. They have few or no EPS or tardive dyskinesia incidents.
2. They treat the distressing positive symptoms as well as the disabling negative symptoms of schizophrenia.
3. For example, people on these drugs become more animated and behave in more socially acceptable ways; the rate of rehospitalization is lower for such people than for those on the standard antipsychotic agents.
4. They might improve the neurocognitive defects associated with schizophrenia.
5. Clients who have been refractory with conventional agents frequently respond to these drugs.

## *Overall Cautions*

Specific cautions for each individual atypical agent are listed in Table 21-6. However, there are universal precautions that need to be applied to all of the atypicals. These newer antipsychotic medications are used with caution in:
1. People who drink alcohol or take other medications
2. Children, the elderly, and pregnant women: The safety of these drugs has not been studied in these groups of people.

3. Lactating women: The newer antipsychotic medications can pass into breast milk and cause problems in a baby, including behavior changes.

### Adverse Effects and Interactions

The following are common adverse effects for the atypical antipsychotic agents; however, each drug causes these effects to different degrees. Assess for these in your client's who are taking any one of these drugs.

- **Sedation** from blockage of histamine receptors
- **Orthostatic hypotension** from blockage of alpha-adrenergic receptors
- **Weight gain** from blockade of $5HT_2$ receptors (except ziprasidone and aripiprazole). Weight gain is a major factor in noncompliance and predisposes to obesity, diabetes, and/or heart disease.
- Dry mouth, blurred vision, urinary retention, constipation, and tachycardia from blockade of cholinergic receptors.
- Medication interactions. Check with the health care provider as to safety with concurrent medications (e.g., with aripiprazole [Abilify]). Can have serious interactions with alpha blockers, antihypertensives, diuretics, quinidine, fluoxetine, paroxetine, carbamazepine, antifungals, and more.

Because all of the newer novel antipsychotics share different individual properties, they are briefly addressed in Table 21-6. For the usual dosage and highlighted properties of each, please refer to Table 8-3 in the chapter on schizophrenia.

## ANTIMANIC AND MOOD-STABILIZING MEDICATIONS

This section discusses (1) lithium and (2) alternative antimanic and mood-stabilizing agents.

**Lithium** has traditionally been the drug of choice for controlling manic episodes in people with bipolar disorder, and for prophylaxis against recurrent mania and depression. Lithium helps prolong the time before a manic, hypomanic, or mixed episode. It is not as effective in clients with rapid cycling. Because lithium has such a narrow therapeutic index, lithium serum levels should be monitored regularly, and the client and family should be aware of the early signs and symptoms of lithium toxicity (Table 21-7).

*Text continued on p. 626*

Table 21-6 **Highlights of Atypical/Novel Antipsychotics**

| Drug | Therapeutic Use | Adverse Effects | Toxic Reactions | Contraindication/Precautions | Nursing Alerts |
|---|---|---|---|---|---|
| **Clozapine (Clozaril) (NOT A FIRST-LINE DRUG)** | 1. Refractory schizophrenia<br>2. Has mood stabilizing effects that might be effective in delusional major depression and psychosis associated with Parkinson's | 1. Sedation<br>2. Orthostasis<br>3. Anticholinergic symptoms<br>4. Weight gain<br>5. Dizziness<br>6. Tachycardia<br>7. Hypotension<br>8. Hypersalivation in up to 30% | 1. Agranulocytosis in 0.8% to 1%<br>2. Seizures in 5% | **Do not use:**<br>1. Myeloproliferative disorders<br>2. History of clozapine-induced agranulocytosis<br>3. With drugs having potential to suppress bone marrow function<br>4. Severe CNS depression<br>5. Comatose state<br>6. Breastfeeding | 1. Requires weekly WBC count<br>2. Expensive because of weekly monitoring at beginning of treatment<br>3. Obtain baseline WBC count before treatment<br>4. Monitor BP for hypertension/hypotension<br>5. Supervise for suicidal intent<br>6. Weight-gain management |

*Continued*

**Cautions:**
*History of:*
1. Seizures
2. Cardiovascular disease
3. Impaired respiratory function
4. Hepatic or renal function
5. Alcohol withdrawal
6. Urinary retention
7. Glaucoma
8. Prostatic hypertrophy
9. Pregnancy

*BP*, Blood pressure; *CBC*, complete blood count; *CNS*, central nervous system; *ECG*, electrocardiograph; *EPS*, extrapyramidal side effects; *NMS*, neuroleptic malignant syndrome; *TD*, tardive dyskinesia; *WBC*, white blood cell.

Table 21-6 **Highlights of Atypical/Novel Antipsychotics—cont'd**

| Drug | Therapeutic Use | Adverse Effects | Toxic Reactions | Contraindication/Precautions | Nursing Alerts |
|---|---|---|---|---|---|
| **Risperidone (Risperdal)** | 1. Management of symptoms of psychotic disorders | 1. Sedation<br>2. Weight gain<br>3. Insomnia<br>4. Sexual dysfunction<br>5. Headache<br>6. Constipation<br>7. Dyspepsia, rhinitis, drowsiness, and dizziness<br>8. Abdominal pain and dry skin<br>9. Tachycardia<br>10. Visual disturbances, fever, back pain, and angina<br>11. Agitation<br>12. Anxiety | **Rare:**<br>1. NMS (see Table 21-4)<br>2. Tardive dyskinesia | **Do not use:**<br>1. Cardiac disease<br>2. Cerebrovascular disease<br>3. Dehydration<br>4. With antihypertensives<br>5. Lactation<br>**Cautions:**<br>1. History of seizures<br>2. Elderly<br>3. Pregnancy | 1. Baseline renal and liver function test first<br>2. Orthostasis often at beginning of treatment; monitor BP<br>3. Caution client not to drive or use machinery until body adjusts to medication<br>4. Weight-gain management |

| Olanzapine (Zyprexa) | 1. Psychotic disorders<br>2. Short-term treatment for acute manic states<br>3. Unlabeled uses: Treatment of ulcerative colitis and inflammatory bowel disease | **Frequent:**<br>1. Weight gain<br>2. Somnolence<br>3. Agitation<br>4. Insomnia<br>5. Headache<br>6. Nervousness<br>7. Hostility<br>8. Dizziness<br>9. Rhinitis<br>**Occasional:**<br>1. Anxiety<br>2. Constipation<br>3. Nonaggressive objectionable behavior<br>4. Dry mouth<br>5. Weight gain<br>**Rare:**<br>1. Seizures<br>2. NMS<br>3. EPS<br>4. Dysphagia | **No contraindications known at present:**<br>1. **Not a first-line treatment for** people with increased glucose or people with diabetes; safety in children not established<br>**Cautions:**<br>1. Hepatic or cardiovascular disease<br>2. Those who should avoid anticholinergic drugs | 1. Obtain baseline hepatic function<br>2. Supervise suicidal-risk clients closely<br>3. Tell client and family to avoid dehydration<br>4. Notify physician if pregnancy occurs or is being planned<br>5. Avoid driving or tasks that require alertness until response |

*Continued*

Table 21-6 **Highlights of Atypical/Novel Antipsychotics—cont'd**

| Drug | Therapeutic Use | Adverse Effects | Toxic Reactions | Contraindication/ Precautions | Nursing Alerts |
|------|-----------------|-----------------|-----------------|-------------------------------|----------------|
| | | 6. Postural hypotension<br>7. Fever<br>8. Joint pain<br>9. Restlessness<br>10. Cough<br>11. Dimness of vision<br>**Rare:**<br>1. Tachycardia<br>2. Back/chest/abdominal pain<br>3. Tremor<br>4. Extremity pain | | 3. Elderly/debilitated<br>4. Pregnancy<br>5. History of seizures<br>6. Cerebrovascular disease<br>7. Conditions predisposing to hypotension<br>8. Clients at risk for aspiration pneumonia | to drug is established<br>6. **Dietary teaching is essential with medications that alter metabolism, and predispose to obesity, diabetes, and/or heart disease** (personal communication from Dorothy A. Varchol, June 2003) |
| **Quetiapine (Seroquel)** | 1. Management of manifestations in psychotic disorders | **Frequent:**<br>1. Headache<br>2. Sedation/drowsiness<br>3. Dizziness<br>4. Orthostasis | 1. Overdose produces heart block, decreased BP, hypokalemia (weakness), and tachycardia | **No known contraindications:**<br>1. Not advised for breastfeeding mothers; safety in pregnancy | 1. Obtain baseline CBC and hepatic function tests before initiation of treatment and periodically |

**Occasional:**
1. Constipation
2. Postural hypotension
3. Tachycardia
4. Dry mouth
5. Dyspepsia
6. Rash
7. Weakness
8. Abdominal pain
9. Rhinitis

**Rare:**
1. Back pain
2. Fever
3. Weight gain

or children not established

**Cautions:**
1. Elderly
2. Alzheimer's dementia
3. History of breast cancer
4. Cardiovascular disease
5. Cerebrovascular disease
6. Dehydration
7. History of drug abuse or drug dependencies
8. Hypothyroidism

2. Tell client and family to avoid exposure to extreme heat
3. Take medication as ordered; do not stop or increase dosage
4. Drowsiness generally subsides during continued therapy
5. Avoid driving or performing tasks that require alertness until response to drug is established

*Continued*

**Table 21-6 Highlights of Atypical/Novel Antipsychotics—cont'd**

| Drug | Therapeutic Use | Adverse Effects | Toxic Reactions | Contraindication/Precautions | Nursing Alerts |
|------|-----------------|-----------------|-----------------|------------------------------|----------------|
| | | | | | 6. Avoid alcohol<br>7. Change positions slowly to reduce hypotensive effects |
| **Ziprasidone (Geodon)** | 1. Treatment of schizophrenia | **Most common:**<br>1. Somnolence<br>2. EPS<br>3. Respiratory disorder | **Cardiac:**<br>1. Prolongation of the $QT_c$ interval; prolonging the $QT_c$ interval can cause cardiac arrthymias and heart attack, leading to death | **Do not use:**<br>*History of:*<br>1. Irregular heartbeats<br>2. Prolonged $QT_c$ interval (ECG)<br>3. Other heartbeat disturbances<br>*Also:*<br>1. With electrolyte disturbance<br>2. When other drugs that prolong the $QT_c$ interval are being taken; this | 1. Baseline ECG should be obtained<br>2. Caution your clients to avoid becoming overheated in hot weather and during exercise; ziprasidone might increase risk of heat stroke<br>**Teach clients:**<br>1. Do not take over-the-counter |

drugs/herbs without checking with a health care provider or pharmacist
2. Give client a list of drugs that can cause heart irregularity so they know what to avoid

is a long list, and these drugs are not to be mixed (e.g., Serentil, Mellaril, Thorazine, Orap, many more); go to *www.health.msn. com* (Drugs and Herbs)

**Cautions:**
1. Elderly
2. Pregnancy
3. Renal problems

3. Alert clients to call health care provider immediately if they experience symptoms that might indicate heart rhythm problems such as dizziness, palpitations, or fainting

*Continued*

Table 21-6 **Highlights of Atypical/Novel Antipsychotics—cont'd**

| Drug | Therapeutic Use | Adverse Effects | Toxic Reactions | Contraindication/ Precautions | Nursing Alerts |
|------|-----------------|-----------------|-----------------|-------------------------------|----------------|
|      |                 |                 |                 |                               | 4. Use caution when driving, operating machinery, or performing other hazardous activities; ziprasidone might cause dizziness or drowsiness |
|      |                 |                 |                 |                               | 5. Avoid alcohol or use with caution |
|      |                 |                 |                 |                               | 6. Rise slowly to prevent dizziness or falls from dizziness |

| Aripiprazole (Abilify) | 1. Treatment of schizophrenia | **Frequent:**<br>1. Anxiety<br>2. Constipation<br>3. Headache<br>4. Insomnia<br>5. Nausea<br>6. Vomiting<br>**Less frequent:**<br>1. Lightheadedness/dizziness<br>2. Orthostatic hypotension<br>3. Rhinitis<br>4. Drowsiness<br>5. Tremors<br>**Rare:**<br>1. Blurred vision | 1. Akathisia<br>2. Fever<br>3. Skin rash<br>4. TD<br>**Rare:**<br>1. Dysphasia<br>2. Heat stroke<br>3. NMS<br>4. Seizures | **Do not use:**<br>1. Breastfeeding<br>**Cautions:**<br>*History of:*<br>1. Heart disease<br>2. Stroke<br>3. Dehydration<br>4. Seizures<br>5. Alzheimer's disease<br>6. Swallowing<br>7. Allergies<br>*Also:*<br>1. Elderly<br>2. Pregnant women | 1. Rise slowly to prevent dizziness or falls from dizziness<br>2. Drink plenty of fluids to prevent dehydration<br>3. Refrain from driving or using machinery if dizziness or drowsiness occurs |

Lithium is not effective in 30% to 50% of people with bipolar disease, and, as mentioned earlier, it is less effective in bipolar subtypes (e.g., rapid cycling).

Regarding **alternative antimanic and mood-stabilizing drugs**, traditionally two anticonvulsants have been used in clients who do not respond to lithium, or could not tolerate the side effects. These are carbamazepine (Tegretol) and valproic acid, and both are effective with rapid cycling bipolar disorder. Clonazepam (Klonopin), a benzodiazepine, has also been used with some success as treatment, or adjunct treatment, of acute mania. Currently there are a number of other anticonvulsant medications that seem to be effective in treating bipolar disorder, such as gabapentin (Neurontin) and lamotrigine (Lamictal). The latest of the anticonvulsant agents at this writing is topiramate (Topamax). These and the calcium channel blocker Verapamil are identified in Table 21-8.

## Lithium

### Therapeutic Uses

- Acute manic phase of bipolar disorder
- Prophylaxis treatment for mania
- Depression
- Bulimia
- Schizophrenia
- Premenstrual syndrome
- Prophylaxis of vascular headache
- Neutropenia

### Mechanism of Action

Lithium affects storage, release, and reuptake of neurotransmitters. Antimanic effects result from increase in norepinephrine reuptake, and increase in serotonin receptors producing antimanic and antidepressant effects (Hodgson & Kizior, 2003). Besides the serotonergic properties, and the effects on norepinephrine, lithium stabilizes calcium channels and decreases neuronal activity via effects on second messenger systems, all of which might add to its therapeutic profile (Keltner & Folks, 2001).

**Table 21-7 Side Effects of Lithium and Signs of Toxicity**

| Level | Sign* | Interventions |
|---|---|---|
| **Expected Side Effects** 0.4-1 mEq/L (therapeutic levels) | Fine hand tremors, polyuria, and mild thirst. Mild nausea and general discomfort. Weight gain | Symptoms might persist throughout therapy. Symptoms often subside during treatment. Weight gain might be helped with diet, exercise, and nutritional management. |
| **Early Signs of Toxicity** <1.5 mEq/L | Nausea, vomiting, diarrhea, thirst, polyuria, slurred speech, muscle weakness | Medication should be withheld, blood lithium levels drawn, and the dose reevaluated. |
| **Advanced Signs of Toxicity** 1.5-2.0 mEq/L | Coarse hand tremor, persistent gastrointestinal upset, mental confusion, muscle hyperirritability, electroencephalographic changes, incoordination | Use interventions outlined earlier or later, depending on severity of circumstances. |
| **Severe Toxicity** 2.0-2.5 mEq/L | Ataxia, serious electroencephalographic changes, blurred vision, clonic movements, large output of dilute urine, seizures, stupor, severe hypotension, coma. Death is usually secondary to pulmonary complications. | There is no known antidote for lithium poisoning. The drug is stopped and excretion is hastened. Gastric lavage and treatment with urea, mannitol, and aminophylline all hasten lithium excretion. |
| >2.5 mEq/L | Confusion, incontinence of urine or feces, coma, cardiac arrhythmia, peripheral circulatory collapse, abdominal pain, proteinuria, oliguria, and death | Hemodialysis might also be used in severe cases. |

Data from Hodgson & Kizior. (2003). pp. 670-672; Lehne (2001), p 334.
*Careful monitoring is needed because the toxic levels of lithium are close to the therapeutic levels.

Table 21-8 **Alternative Antimanic and Mood-Stabilizing Drugs**

| Drug | Dose | Type | Major Concern/Side Effect |
|---|---|---|---|
| Divalproex | 750-1500 mg/day | Anticonvulsant | • **Baseline liver function tests should be done and monitored at regular intervals** (6-12 months). Hepatotoxicity, although rare, has been reported with fatalities in children.<br>• Thrombocytopenia and platelet dysfunction can occur. Check for bruises and monitor platelet count. Signs and symptoms to watch for: Fever, chills, right upper quadrant pain, dark-colored urine, malaise, and jaundice.<br>• Common side effects: Sedation, gastrointestinal upset, tremors, weight gain, and (rarely) alopecia.<br>• Can be used as initial treatment. |
| Lamotrigine (Lamictal) | 50-40 mg/day | Anticonvulsant | • Tolerated well. Low-dose titration to reduce risk of rashes. **Rarely, the rash can progress to a potentially life-threatening condition** (one person per 1000) |
| Carbamazepine (Tegretol) | 600-1600 mg/day | Anticonvulsant | • **Agranulocytosis** and **aplastic anemia** are most serious side effects. |

- Blood levels should be monitored through first 8 weeks because drug induces liver enzymes that speed its own metabolism. (Check complete blood count [CBC] when checking blood levels.) Dose should be adjusted to maintain serum level of 6-8 mg/L.
- Sedation, fatigue, nausea, and dizziness are the most common problems.
- Diplopia, incoordination, and sedation can signal excessive levels.
- Because the action decreases sodium and calcium ions, hyponatremia might occur.

**Other Agents Used To Treat Acute Mania in Bipolar Disorder**

| | | |
|---|---|---|
| Gabapentin (Neurontin) | 300-1800 mg/day | Anticonvulsant |

- No evidence to support; use as a first- or second-line agent (Preston et al, 2005).
- Tolerated well. Associated with somnolence, dizziness, gastrointestinal upset, headache, blurred or double vision, clumsiness, and tremor.

| | | |
|---|---|---|
| Topiramate (Topamax) | 50-300 mg/day | Anticonvulsant |

- Lack of research to support efficacy for bipolar disorder.
- If weight gain desirable, it may be desirable for selected clients (Preston et al, 2005).

*Continued*

Table 21-8 **Alternative Antimanic and Mood-Stabilizing Drugs—cont'd**

| Drug | Dose | Type | Major Concern/Side Effect |
|------|------|------|---------------------------|
| Topiramate (Topamax)—cont'd | | | • Adverse effects include weight loss, cognitive side effects, fatigue, dizziness, and paresthesias. |
| Clonazepam (Klonopin) | 1-6 mg/day | Benzodiazepine | • Used in the treatment or as an adjunct; can facilitate the effects of other antimanics.<br>• Same as those of all benzodiazepines (e.g., sedation, ataxia, incoordination). |
| Verapamil | 160-480 mg/day | Calcium channel blocker | • As an adjunct in combination with lithium or in combination with a neuroleptic.<br>• Might help prevent antidepressant switches into mania.<br>• Might be more responsive in lithium responders.<br>• Taper off gradually to prevent rebound psychiatric and physical symptoms. |

The major disadvantage of lithium is that improvement is gradual. Antimanic effects begin 5 to 7 days after the onset of treatment. However, it can take up to 3 weeks to adequately control the symptoms of mania. Therefore, other agents are given in conjunction with lithium to help control the mania until the lithium reaches a therapeutic level (0.8 to 1.4 mEq/L). Effective medications include antipsychotic agents, such as olanzapine or haloperidol, or potent benzodiazepines such as lorazepam or clonazepam. Lithium levels are best obtained approximately 12 hours after the administration of the last dose.

## Clinical Dosage

As mentioned in Chapter 7, blood levels are initially drawn weekly or biweekly until therapeutic levels are reached. For acute mania, a blood level of 0.8 to 1.4 mEq/L would be within the initial range. For maintenance therapy, lithium levels should range from 0.4 to 1.0 mEq/L; however, levels of 0.6 to 0.8 mEq/L are effective for most. Levels higher than 1.5 mEq can result in significant toxicity. A typical maintenance dose is 300 mg of lithium carbonate tid or qid. The therapeutic window between therapeutic levels and toxic levels is very small with lithium. Therefore, plasma levels should be monitored routinely. In the beginning, levels should be monitored every 2 to 3 days to keep the levels within the therapeutic range. During maintenance therapy, drug levels should be monitored every 1 to 3 months.

## Metabolism

Lithium has a short half-life, necessitating the drug to be administered in divided daily doses. Lithium is secreted in the kidneys. It must be used with extreme caution in people with renal impairment.

Low sodium levels or sodium depletion will decrease renal excretion of lithium. When this happens, the drug can accumulate in the body, and toxicity results. Therefore, maintaining normal sodium levels is vital, and diuretics, diarrhea, and dehydration can all cause lithium retention by the kidneys, which potentiates the occurrence of lithium toxicity.

## Adverse Effects

There are essentially two categories of adverse effects: (1) adverse effects when lithium levels are excessive; and (2) adverse effects when lithium levels are at therapeutic levels.

**Adverse Effects When Lithium Levels Are Excessive** Refer to Table 21-7 for the expected side effects, and the early, advanced and severe signs of toxicity. Interventions for the different levels of toxicity are included.

**Adverse Effects When Lithium Levels Are within Therapeutic Levels** Several responses occur early in treatment and then usually subside. Refer to Table 21-7 under Expected Side Effects for a list of these. Approximately 30% of people experience transient fatigue, muscle weakness, headache, confusion, and memory impairment. Polyuria and thirst occur in up to 50% of clients and can persist throughout treatment.

Rare reports of weight gain, acne, muscle twitching, eye pain, and headache and vision problems have been made. Other concerns are:

**Renal Toxicity** For some people who have been on lithium for long periods, degenerative changes in the kidney are noted. Therefore, kidney function should be assessed before treatment is started, and every 6 to 12 months thereafter (Schatzberg, Cole, & DeBattista, 1997).

**Goiter** Reports of goiter with chronic administration of lithium have also been identified. This is usually benign. However, measurement of thyroid hormones should be obtained prior to treatment, and annually thereafter as well.

## Drug Interactions

- Drugs that might increase effects of lithium
  - Alcohol
  - Diuretics (promote sodium loss)
  - Hypotensive agents
- Drugs that can cause hyperkalemia, such as potassium-sparing diuretics and potassium supplements

- Anticholinergic drugs, which can cause urinary hesitancy, although the administration of these drugs with anticholinergic effects cannot always be avoided (e.g., antipsychotics, antidepressants)
- Concurrent use of lithium with carbamazepine, fluoxetine, fluvoxamine, haloperidol, phemothiagines, TCAs, and verapamil might increase the risk for neurotoxicity (Fuller & Sajatovic, 2000)
- Phenytoin, which can enhance lithium toxicity

### Use with Caution

- Renal impairment
- Elderly clients
- Those with sodium depletion or on diuretic therapy
- Thyroid disorders
- Dialysis
- Hypovolemia
- Coronary or cerebrovascular insufficiency

### Contraindications

- Pregnancy and lactation
- Myocardial infarction
- Coronary insufficiency
- Angina
- Evidence of coronary artery disease

**Client and Family Teaching** A useful guideline for client and family teaching is found in Box 21-8.

## Alternative Antimanic and Mood-Stabilizing Drugs

Three anticonvulsants have demonstrated efficacy in the treatment of bipolar disease. These agents are divalproex (Depakote), carbamazepine (Tegretol), and lamo- trigine (Lamictal) (Preston et al, 2005). Lamotrigine is generally well tolerated. However, there is one rare and potentially fatal toxic effect and clients are urged to seek immediate medical advice upon the appearance of a rash. Most rashes that appear with the administration of lamotrigine are benign.

## Box 21-8 Client and Family Teaching: Lithium

The client and the client's family should be instructed about the following, encouraged to ask questions, and given the material in written form as well.

1. Lithium can treat your current emotional problem and will also help prevent relapse. So, it is important to continue with the drug after the current episode is resolved.
2. Because therapeutic and toxic dosage ranges are so close, your lithium blood levels must be monitored very closely, more frequently at first, then once every several months after that.
3. Lithium is not addictive.
4. Maintain a normal diet and normal salt and fluid intake (2500 to 3000 ml/day, or six 12-oz glasses). Lithium decreases sodium reabsorption by the renal tubules, which could cause sodium depletion. A low sodium intake causes a relative increase in lithium retention, which could lead to toxicity.
5. Withhold drug if excessive diarrhea, vomiting, or diaphoresis occurs. Dehydration can raise lithium levels in the blood to toxic levels. Inform your health care provider if you have any of these problems.
6. Diuretics (water pills) are contraindicated with lithium.
7. Lithium is irritating to the gastric mucosa. Therefore, take your lithium with meals.
8. Periodic monitoring of renal functioning and thyroid function is indicated with long-term use. Discuss your follow-up with your health care provider.
9. Avoid taking any over-the-counter medications without checking first with your health care provider.
10. If weight gain is significant, you might need to see a health care provider or nutritionist.
11. Many self-help groups have been developed to provide support for bipolar patients and their families. The local self-help group is (give name and phone number).
12. You can find out more information by calling (give name, phone number, and/or website).

Data from Maxmen, J.S., & Ward, N.G. (2002). *Psychotropic drugs fast facts* (3rd ed.). New York: WW Norton; Schatzberg, A.F., Cole, J.O., & DeBattista, C. (1991). *Manual of clinical psychopharmacology*. Washington, DC: American Psychiatric Press; Preston, J., & Johnson, J. (1995). *Clinical psychopharmacology made ridiculously simple*. Miami: MedMaster.

1. **Divalproex sodium (Depakote)** has long been approved for the primary treatment of mania. Divalproex is effective in treating cases of mixed mania and rapid cycling. Divalproex and carbamazepine are both effective in treating mania secondary to general medical conditions. The use of these drugs requires initial evaluation and ongoing monitoring (see Table 21-8). Because of rare reports of elevated liver enzymes, baseline liver function tests should be done and monitored at frequent intervals.

2. **Carbamazepine (Tegretol)** is a good choice for manic episodes when lithium or divalproex are ineffective, contraindicated, or not tolerated. It is especially effective in clients with rapid-cycling or secondary mania (Keltner & Folks, 2001). The most serious side effect of carbamazepine is agranulocytosis; mild-to-moderate leukopenia and thrombocytopenia might also occur. A baseline evaluation needs to be done before treatment is started. Complete blood cell count and examination of a blood smear should be performed weekly during the first month of therapy and can be done at progressively longer intervals as treatment continues (Keltner & Folks, 2001).

3. **Clonazepam (Klonopin)**, a BZ, has been effectively used in treatment or as an adjunct for the treatment of acute mania.

4. A number of **other agents,** many of them newer (e.g., gabapentin (Neurontin), topiramate (Topomax), as well as calcium channel blockers, are being used with some effectiveness in the treatment of bipolar disorder. Refer to Table 21-8 for an overview of these drugs.

# APPENDIX A

# References

About Campral (acamprosate calcium) http:www.campral.
com/about campral/index.aspx. Retrieved July, 27, 2005.

Aguilera, D. (1998). *Crisis intervention: Theory and methodology* (8th ed.). St. Louis: Mosby.

Alvarez, C. (2002). Communication with angry and aggressive clients. In E.M. Varcarolis (Ed.): *Foundations of psychiatric nursing* (4th ed.). Philadelphia: W.B. Saunders.

American Academy of Pediatrics. (2001). Clinical practice guidelines: Treatment of the school-aged child with attention-deficit/hyperactivity disorder, *Pediatrics, 108*(4), 1033-1044.

American Nurses Association. (2000). *Scopes and standards of psychiatric–mental health clinical nursing practice*. Washington, DC: American Nurses Association.

American Psychiatric Association. (2000a). *Diagnostic and statistical manual of mental disorders* (4th ed., text revision). Washington, DC: American Psychiatric Press.

American Psychiatric Association. (2000b). *Practice guidelines for the treatment of psychiatric disorders (compendium 2000)*. Washington, DC: American Psychiatric Press.

Association of Women's Health Obstetric and Neonatal Nurses (AWHONN). (June 2004). Dietary supplements and women. Paper given at AWHONN convention, June, 26-30, Tampa, FL.

Basco, M.R., & Rush, A.J. (1996). *Cognitive behavioral therapy for bipolar disorder*. New York: Guilford Press.

Beeder, A.B., & Mellman, R.B. (1992). Treatment of patients with psychopathology and substance abuse.

In J. Lowinson, P. Ruiz, R. Millman, & J. Langrod (Eds.), *Substance abuse: A comprehensive textbook* (2nd ed.). Baltimore: Williams & Wilkins.

Borson, S. (1997). Delirium and confusional states. In D.L. Dunner (Ed.), *Current psychiatric therapy* (vol. 2). Philadelphia: W.B. Saunders.

Burnside, I. (1988). *Nursing and the aged* (3rd ed.). New York: McGraw-Hill.

Chiles, J.A., & Strosahl, K. (1997). Assessment, crisis management, and treatment of the suicidal patient. In D.L. Dunner (Ed.), *Current psychiatric therapy* (2nd ed., pp. 547-551). Philadelphia: W.B. Saunders.

Chitty, K.K., & Maynard, C.K. (1986). Managing manipulation. *Journal of Psychosocial and Mental Health Nursing Services, 34*(2), 9.

Dee, V. (1991). How can we become more aware of culturally specific body language and use this awareness therapeutically? *Journal of Psychosocial Nursing and Mental Health Services, 29*(11), 39-40.

Delaney, C. (1999). Reducing recidivism: Medication versus psychosocial rehabilitation. *Journal of Psychosocial Nursing and Mental Health Services, 36*(11), 28-34.

DiMatteo, M.R., & DiNicola, D.D. (1982). *Achieving patient compliance: The psychology of the medical practitioner's role.* Elmsford, NY: Pergamon Press.

Dochterman, J.M. and Bulechek, G.M. (Eds.) (2004). *Nursing interventions classification,* (4th ed.) St. Louis, MO:Mosby.

Dubin, W.R., & Weiss, K.J. (1991). *Handbook of psychiatric emergencies.* Springhouse, PA: Springhouse.

Dunner, D.L. (1997). *Current psychiatric theory* (2nd ed.). Philadelphia: W.B. Saunders.

Dunner, D.L., & Rosenbaum, J.F. (1999). *The Psychiatric Clinics of North America annual of drug therapy.* Philadelphia: W.B. Saunders.

Eells, T. (1995). Relational therapy of grief disorders. In J.J.P. Barber & P. Crits-Christoph (Eds.), *Dynamic therapies for psychiatric disorders (axis 1)* (pp. 86-419). New York: Basic Books.

Egan, G. (2004). *The skilled helper: A problem-management and opportunity-development approach to helping* (7th ed.). Pacific Grove, CA: Brooks/Cole.

Ekman, P. (1972). *Darwin and facial expression: A century of research in review.* New York: Academic Press.

Feldhaus, K.L., Koziol-McLain, J., Amsbury, H.L., et al. (1997). Accuracy of three brief screening questions for detecting partner violence in the emergency department. *JAMA*, 227, 1357-1361.

Ferreira, L., Figueira, M.L., Bessa-Peixoto, A., et al. (2003). Psychomotor and anxiolytic effects of mexazolam in patients with GAD. *Clinical Drug Investigation, 23*(4), 235-243.

Finfgeld, D.L. (1999). Use of brief interventions to treat individuals with drinking problems. *Journal of Psychosocial Nursing, 37*(4), 23-30.

Fuller, M.A., & Sajatovic, M. (2000). *Drug information handbook* (2nd ed.). Cleveland, OH: Levi-Comp.

Gahlinger, P.M. (2004). Club drugs: MDMA, gamma-hydroxybutyrate (GHB), rohypnol, and ketamine. *American Family Physcisian, 69*(11) June 1, 2004. *http://www.aafp.org/afp/20040601/2619.html*. Retrieved 2/25/05.

Gamble, C., & Brennan, G. (2000). *Working with serious mental illness: A manual for clinical practice*. London, England: Baillére Tindall/Harcourt Health Sciences.

Goldberg, R.J. (1998). *Practical guide to the care of the psychiatric patient* (2nd ed.). St. Louis: Mosby.

Goodwin, J. (1985). *The talk book: The intimate science of communicating in close relationships*. New York: Ballantine.

Gorman, L.M., Sultan D.F., & Raines, M.L. (1996). *Davis's manual of psychosocial nursing for general patient care*. Philadelphia: F.A. Davis.

Greden, J. (November 17, 1995). *Better outcomes with difficult cases*. Presented at the U.S. Psychiatric and Mental Health Congress, New York.

Green, A.I., Mooney, J.J., Posner, J.A., & Schildkraut, J.J. (1995). Mood disorders: Biological aspects. In H.I. Kaplan & B.J. Sadock (Eds.), *Comprehensive textbook of psychiatry* (4th ed.). Baltimore: Williams & Wilkins.

Gregory, R.J. (1994). Grief and loss among Eskimos attempting suicide in western Alaska. *American Journal of Psychiatry, 15*(12), 1815.

Hagerty, B.K. (1984). *Psychiatric mental health assessment*. St. Louis: Mosby.

Hall, E.T. (1983). Excerpts from an interview conducted by Carol Travis. *GEO, 25*(3), 12.

Hall, E.T. (1997). *Beyond culture*. Garden City, NJ: Anchor Press.

Harvard Mental Health Letter. (August 1996). *Alcohol dependence: Treatment of alcoholism.* Boston: Harvard Medical School Publication Group.

Hill, S.S. (1998). Practice guidelines for major disorders. In G.P. Koocher, J.C. Norcross, & S.S. Hill (Eds.), *Psychologists' desk reference.* New York: Oxford University Press.

Hodgson, B.B., & Kizior, R.J. (1999). *Nurse's drug handbook 1999.* Philadelphia: W.B. Saunders.

Hodgson, B.B., & Kizior, R.J. (2003). *Saunders nursing handbook 2003.* Philadelphia: W.B. Saunders.

Hoff, L.A. (1995). *People in crisis: Understanding and helping* (4th ed.). San Francisco: Jossey-Bass.

Hoffman, L., & Halmi, K.A. (1997). Treatment of anorexia nervosa. In D.L. Dunner (Ed.), *Current psychiatric therapy* (vol. 2). Philadelphia: W.B. Saunders.

Hogarty, G.E. (1999). *Schizophrenia and modern mental health services.* National Alliance for the Mentally III. Available online at *http://www/nami.org/research.*

Hollander, E. (1999). Anxiety disturbances. In R.E. Hales, S.C. Yudofsky, & J.A. Talbott (Eds.), *The American Psychiatric Press textbook of psychiatry* (3rd ed., pp. 567-634). Washington, DC: American Psychiatric Press.

Hurt, R.D., Offord, K.P., Croghan, I.T., et al. (1996). Mortality following inpatient addictions treatment: Role of tobacco use in community-based cohort. *JAMA, 275,* 1097-1103.

Ibrahim, K. (2005). People with eating disorders. In E.M. Varcarolis, Carson, V.B., & Shoemaker, N.C. (Eds.), *Foundations of psychiatric nursing* (5th ed.). Philadelphia: W.B. Saunders.

Ingram, C.A. (1991). How can we become more aware of culturally specific body language and use this awareness therapeutically? *Journal of Psychosocial Nursing, 29*(11), 39-40.

Jin, C.Y., & McCance-Katz, E.F. (2003). *Substance abuse: Cocaine use disorders.* In A. Tasman, J. Kay, and J.A. Lieberman (Eds.), *Psychiatry* (2nd ed., A. pp. 1010-1036). Chichester, West Sussex, England: John Wiley & Sons, Ltd.

Johnson, M., Maas, M., & Moorehead, S. (2000). *Nursing outcomes classification* (2nd, ed.). St. Louis: Mosby.

Kanas, N. (1996). *Group therapy for schizophrenic patients.* Washington, DC: American Psychiatric Press.

Kaplan, H.I., & Sadock, B.J. (2002). *Pocket handbook of clinical psychiatry* (9th ed.). Baltimore: Lippincott-Williams & Wilkins.

Keller, M. (November 18, 1995). Depression in adults. Presented at the U.S. Psychiatric and Mental Health Congress, New York.

Keltner, N.L. & Folks, D.G. (2001). *Psychotropic drugs* (3rd ed.). St. Louis: Mosby.

Kobayashi, M., Smith, T.P., & Norcross, J.C. (1998). Enhancing adherence. In G.P. Koocher, J.C. Norcross, & S.S. Hill (Eds.), *Psychologists' desk reference*. New York: Oxford University Press.

Korn, M.L., & Weiss, M. (May 17-22, 2003). *ADHD in adults: New perspective and treatments*. Presented at the American Psychiatric Association 156th annual meeting, San Francisco.

Kramer-Howe, K. (2002). Care for the dying and those who grieve. In E. Varcarolis (Ed.), *Foundations of psychiatric mental health nursing* (4th ed.). Philadelphia: W.B. Saunders.

Krupnick, S.L.W., & Wade, A.J. (1993). *Psychiatric care planning*. Springhouse, PA: Springhouse.

Kübler-Ross, E. (1969). *On death and dying*. New York: Macmillan.

Lazarus, R.S. (1993). Why we should think of stress as a subset of emotion. In L. Goldberger & S. Breznitz (Eds.), *Handbook of stress: Theoretical and clinical aspects* (2nd ed.). New York: The Free Press.

Lehne, R.A. (2004). *Pharmacology for nursing care* (4th ed.). Philadelphia: W.B. Saunders.

Lerner, B.H. (1997). From careless consumptives to recalcitrant patients: The historical construction of noncompliance. *Social Science and Medicine, 45*(9), 1423-1431.

Limon, L. (2000, March 10-14). *Use of alternative medicine in women's health*. Presented at the annual meeting of the American Pharmaceutical Association, Washington DC.

Lin, K., Anderson, D., & Poland, R.E. (1997). Ethnic and cultural considerations in psychopharmacotherapy. In D.L. Dunner (Ed.), *Current psychiatric therapy* (2nd ed.). Philadelphia: W.B. Saunders.

Linehan, M.M. (1993). *Cognitive behavioral treatment of borderline personality disorder*. New York: Guilford Press.

Lloyd-Williams, M. (1995). Bereavement referrals to a psychiatric service: An audit. *European Journal of Cancer Care, 4*(1), 17.

Lyons, M.A. (1998). The phenomenon of compulsive overeating in a select group of professional women. *Journal of Advanced Nursing, 27*(9), 1158-1164.

Mairo, R.D. (1997). Anger and aggression. In D.L. Dunner (Ed.), *Current psychiatric therapy* (2nd ed.). Philadelphia: W.B. Saunders.

Marris, P. (1975). *Loss and change.* Garden City, NY: Anchor Books.

Maxmen, J.S., & Ward, N.G. (1995). *Psychotropic drugs fast facts* (2nd ed.). New York: W.W. Norton.

Maxmen, J.S., & Ward, N.G. (2003). *Psychotropic drugs fast facts* (3rd ed.). New York: W.W. Norton.

McGee, D.E., & Linehan, M.M. (1997). Cluster B personality disorders. In D.L. Dunner (Ed.), *Current psychiatric therapy* (2nd ed., pp. 433-438). Philadelphia: W.B. Saunders.

Meichenbaum, D., & Turk, D.C. (1987). *Facilitating treatment adherence: A practitioner's guidebook.* New York: Plenum Press.

Meier, S.T., & Davis, S.R. (1989). *The elements of counseling* (2nd ed.). Pacific Grove, CA: Brooks/Cole.

Moore, J.M., & Hartman, C.R. (1988). Developing a therapeutic relationship. In C.K. Beck, R.P. Rawlins, & S.R. Williams (Eds.), *Mental health psychiatric nursing.* St. Louis: Mosby.

Moorhead, S., Johnson, M., Mass, M. (2004). *Nursing outcome classification* (NOC) (3rd ed.). St. Louis: Mosby.

Moscato, B. (1988). The one-to-one relationship. In H.S. Wilson & C.S. Kneisel (Eds.), *Psychiatric nursing* (3rd ed.). Menlo Park, CA: Addison-Wesley.

NANDA International. (2005-2006). *Nursing diagnoses: Definitions and classification 2005-2006.* Philadelphia: NANDA International.

National Alliance for the Mentally Ill. (April 16, 1999). Senators Domenici and Wellstone Introduced Mental Health Equitable Treatment Act of 1999. *NAMI E-News,* 99(116). Available online at *http://www.nami.org.*

National Institute of Mental Health. (1995). *Suicide.* NIMH.

O'Malley, S.S., Jaffe, A.J., Chang, G., et al. (1992). Naltrexone and coping skills therapy for alcohol dependence. *Archives of General Psychiatry, 49,* 881-887.

O'Malley, S.S., Jaffe, A.J., Rode, S., et al. (1996). Experience of a "slip" among alcoholics treated with naltrexone or placebo. *American Journal of Psychiatry, 153,* 281-283.

Pages, K.P. (1997). Bulimia nervosa. In D.L. Dunner (Ed.), *Current psychiatric therapy* (vol. 2). Philadelphia: W.B. Saunders.

Palmer-Erbs, V.K., & Manos, E. (1998). Are we there yet? When will we be there? Designing collaboration plans for future psychiatric nursing practice. *Journal of Psychosocial Nursing and Mental Health Services, 36*(4), 10-12.

Paquette, M., & Rodemich, C. (1997). *Psychiatric nursing diagnosis care plans for DSM-IV.* Sudbury, MA: Jones and Bartlett.

Parsons, R.D., & Wicks, R.J. (1994). *Counseling strategies and intervention techniques for human services* (4th ed.). Needham Heights, MA: Allyn & Bacon.

Pascualy, M., & Raskind, M.A. (1997). Alzheimer's disease. In D.L. Dunner (Ed.), *Current psychiatric therapy* (vol. 2). Philadelphia: W.B. Saunders.

Patterson, W., et al. (1983). Evaluation of suicidal patients. The SAD PERSONS Scale. *Psychosomatics, 24*(4), 343.

Peplau, H.E. (1952). *Interpersonal relations in nursing.* New York: G.P. Putnam & Sons.

Post, R.M. (1992). Anticonvulsants and novel drugs. In E.S. Paykel (Ed.), Handbook of affective disorders (2nd ed., pp. 387-418). New York: Guilford Press.

Postrado, L.T., & Lehman, A.F. (1995). Quality of life and clinical predictors of rehospitalization of persons with severe mental illness. *Psychiatric Services, 46*(11), 1161-1165.

Preston, J., & Johnson, J. (2004). *Clinical psychopharmacology made ridiculously simple.* Miami, FL: MedMaster, Inc.

Preston, J.D., O'Neal, J.H., & Talaga, M.C. (2005). *Handbook of clinical psychopharmacology for therapists* (4th ed.). Oakland, CA: New Harbinger Publications, Inc.

Prigerson, H.G., Franke, E., Kasl, S.V., et al. (1995). Complicated grief and bereavement-related depression as distinct disorders: Preliminary empirical validation in elderly bereaved spouses. *American Journal of Psychiatry 152,* 22-30.

Profiri, F. (1998). Personality disorders. In E.M. Varcarolis (Ed.), *Foundations of psychiatric mental health nursing* (3rd ed., pp. 507-537). Philadelphia: W.B. Saunders.

Public Policy Committee of the Board of Directors and the NAMI Department of Public Policy and Research. (1999). Public Policy Platform of the National Alliance for the Mentally III (NAMI) (3rd ed.). Section 4: Services and Supports for Adults. Available online at *http://www.nami.org/update/platform/services.htm*.

Raynor, J. (2002). Biological basis for understanding psychotropic drugs. In E. Varcarolis (Ed.), *Foundations of psychiatric mental health nursing* (4th ed.). Philadelphia: W.B. Saunders.

Ries, R.K., Sloan, K.L., & Miller, N.S. (1997). Concept, diagnosis, and treatment of dual diagnosis. In D.L. Dunner (Ed.), *Current psychiatric therapy* (vol. 2). Philadelphia: W.B. Saunders.

Roberts, J.K.A. (1984). *Differential diagnosis in neuropsychiatry* (p. 26). New York: John Wiley.

Robers, L.J., & Marlatt, G.A. (1998). Guidelines for relapse prevention. In G.P. Koocher, J.C. Norcross, & S.S. Hill (Eds.), *Psychologists' desk reference*. New York: Oxford University Press.

Robertson, R.G., & Paradiso, S. (1997). Treatment of psychiatric disorders, including dementia, associated with cerebrovascular disease. In D.L. Dunner (Ed.), *Current psychiatric therapy* (vol. 2). Philadelphia: W.B. Saunders.

Robinson, D. (1997). *Good intentions: The nine unconscious mistakes of nice people.* New York: Warner Books.

Rogers, S. (1998). To work or not to work: That is not the question. *Journal of Psychosocial Nursing and Mental Health Services, 36*(4), 42-46.

Sadock, B.J., & Sadock, V.A. (Eds.). (1999). *Kaplan and Sadock's comprehensive textbook of psychiatry* (7th ed.). Philadelphia: Lippincott, Williams and Wilkins.

St. John, D. (2003). *Aripiprazole/abilify.* University of Jowa Department of Psychiatry. Available online at the Virtual Hospital at *www.vh.org/adult/patient/psychiatry/medications/aripiprazole.html*.

Salzman, C. (1997). Overview of the treatment of geriatric disorders. In D.L. Dunner (Ed.), *Current psychiatric therapy* (vol. 2). Philadelphia: W.B. Saunders.

Saxon, A.J. (1997). Treatment of opioid dependence. In D.L. Dunner (Ed.), *Current psychiatric therapy* (vol. 2). Philadelphia: W.B. Saunders.

Schatzberg, A.F., Cole, J.O., & DeBattista, C. (1997). *Manual of clinical psychopharmacology* (3rd ed.). Washington, DC: American Psychiatric Press.

Schofield, R. (1999). Empowerment education for individuals with serious mental illness. *Journal of Psychosocial Nursing, 36*(11), 35-42.

Schultz, J.M., & Videbeck, S.D. (2005). *Lippincott's manual of psychiatric nursing care plans* (7th ed.). Philadelphia: Lippincott Williams and Wilkins.

Shea, S.C. (1998). *Psychiatric interviewing: The art of understanding* (2nd ed.). Philadelphia: W.B. Saunders.

Sieh, A., & Brentin, L.K. (1997). *The nurse communicates.* Philadelphia: W.B. Saunders.

Skidmore-Roth, L. (Ed.) (2005). Mosby's nursing drug reference 2005. St. Louis, MO:Elsevier Mosby.

Slaby, A.E. (1994). *Handbook of psychiatric emergencies* (4th ed.). Norwalk, CT: Appleton & Lange.

Smith, L.S. (1994). Coping with the "problem" resident. *Nursing Care, 43*(1), 40-41.

Smith, S. (1992). *Communications in nursing.* St. Louis: Mosby.

Smith-DiJulio, K. (2002). Families in crisis: Family violence. In E.M. Varcarolis (Ed.), *Psychiatric mental health nursing* (4th ed.). Philadelphia: W.B. Saunders.

Steinhauer, E. (2003). Current topic review: Psychosocial treatment of bipolar disorder. *Medscape Psychiatry and Mental Health, 8*(1). Available online at *www.medscape.com/viewarticle/457054.*

Stern, T.A., Herman, J.B., & Slavin, P.L. (2004). Massachusetts General Hospital Guide to primary care psychiatry, 2nd ed. New York: McGraw-Hill Medical Publishing Division.

Stone, M.H. (1997). Cluster C personality disorders. In D.L. Dunner (Ed.), *Current psychiatric therapy* (2nd ed., pp. 439-445). Philadelphia: W.B. Saunders.

Stone, S. (1999). Refractory schizophrenia. *Journal of Psychosocial Nursing, 37*(2), 19-23.

Stuart, G.W., & Laraia, M.T. (1998). *Pocket guide to psychiatric nursing* (4th ed.). St. Louis: Mosby.

UC Berkeley Wellness Letter. (Jan 2004). SAM-e. *www.berkeleywellness.com/html/ds/dsSAM.e.php.* Retrieved 2/15/05.

U.S. Department of Health and Human Services (2002). Buprenorphine: about buprenorphine therapy. http://buprenorphine.samha.gov/about.html. Retrieved 8/30/2005.

Vaillant, G.E. (1988). What can long-term follow-up teach us about relapse and prevention of relapse in addictions? *British Journal of Addictions, 83*:1147-1157.

Varcarolis, E.M. (Ed.). (2002). *Psychiatric mental health nursing* (4th ed.). Philadelphia: W.B. Saunders.

Varcarolis, E.M., Carson, V.B., & Shoemaker, N.C. (Eds.). (2005). *Psychiatric mental health nursing* (5th ed.). Philadelphia: W.B. Saunders.

Volpicelli, J.R., Alterman, A.I., Hayashida, M., et al. (1992). Naltrexone in the treatment of alcohol dependence. *Archives of General Psychiatry, 49,* 876-880.

Weeks, S.M. (1999). Disaster mental health services: A personal perspective. *Journal of Psychosocial Nursing, 37*(2), 14-18.

Weissman, M.M., et al. (1989). Suicidal ideation and suicide attempts in panic disorder and attacks. *New England Journal of Medicine, 321,* 1209.

Woody, G.E., McNicholas, L.F., & Fudala, P.J. (2003). Substance abuse: Opioid use disorders. In A. Tasman, J. Kay & J.A. Lieberman (Eds.) *Psychiatry* (2nd ed., pp. 1102-1118). Chichester, West Sussex, England: John Wiley & Sons, Ltd.

World Federation of Societies of Biological Psychiatry. (2002). Guidelines for the pharmacological treatment of anxiety, obsessive-compulsive, and posttraumatic stress disorders.

World Health Organization. (1992). *International statistical classification of diseases and related health problems* (10th revision). Geneva: World Health Organization.

*World Journal of Biological Psychiatry, 3*(4), 171-199.

Zajecka, J. (November 16, 1995). *Treatment strategies for depression complicated by anxiety disorder.* Presented at the U.S. Psychiatric and Mental Health Congress, New York.

Zale, C.F., O'Brian, M.M., Trestman, R.L., & Siever, L.J. (1997). Cluster A personality disorders. In D.L. Dunner (Ed.), *Current psychiatric therapy* (2nd ed., pp. 427-432). Philadelphia: W.B. Saunders.

Zerbe, K.J. (1999). *Women's mental health in primary care.* Philadelphia: W.B. Saunders.

Zuckerman, E.L. (1995). *Clinician's thesaurus* (4th ed.). New York: Guilford Press.

# APPENDIX B

# NANDA Nursing Diagnoses 2005-2006 Taxonomy II

**Domain 1   Health Promotion**
*Class 1   Health Awareness*

*Class 2   Health Management*
Effective therapeutic regimen management
Ineffective therapeutic regimen management
Ineffective family therapeutic regimen management
Ineffective community therapeutic regimen management
Health-seeking behaviors (specify)
Ineffective health maintenance
Impaired home maintenance
Readiness for enhanced management of therapeutic regimen
Readiness for enhanced nutrition

**Domain 2   Nutrition**
*Class 1   Ingestion*
Ineffective infant feeding pattern
Impaired swallowing
Imbalanced nutrition: Less than body requirements
Imbalanced nutrition: More than body requirements
Risk for imbalanced nutrition: More than body requirements

*Class 2   Digestion*

*Class 3   Absorption*

*Class 4   Metabolism*

*Class 5   Hydration*
Deficient fluid volume
Risk for deficient fluid volume
Excess fluid volume
Risk for imbalanced fluid volume
Readiness for enhanced fluid balance

**Domain 3   Elimination**
*Class 1   Urinary Function*
Impaired urinary elimination
Urinary retention
Total urinary incontinence
Functional urinary incontinence
Stress urinary incontinence
Urge urinary incontinence
Reflex urinary incontinence
Risk for urge urinary incontinence
Readiness for enhanced urinary elimination

*Class 2   Gastrointestinal Function*
Bowel incontinence
Diarrhea
Constipation
Risk for constipation
Perceived constipation

*Class 3   Integumentary System*

*Class 4   Respiratory Function*
Impaired gas exchange

**Domain 4   Activity/Rest**
*Class 1   Sleep/Rest*
Disturbed sleep pattern
Sleep deprivation
Readiness for enhanced sleep

*Class 2   Activity/Exercise*
Risk for disuse syndrome
Impaired physical mobility
Impaired bed mobility
Impaired wheelchair mobility

Impaired transfer ability
Impaired walking
Deficient diversional activity
Delayed surgical recovery
Sedentary lifestyle

*Class 3    Energy Balance*
Energy field disturbance
Fatigue

*Class 4    Cardiovascular/Pulmonary Responses*
Decreased cardiac output
Impaired spontaneous ventilation
Ineffective breathing pattern
Activity intolerance
Risk for activity intolerance
Dysfunctional ventilatory weaning response
Ineffective tissue perfusion (specify: renal, cerebral, car-
    diopulmonary, gastrointestinal, peripheral)

*Class 5    Self Care*
Dressing/grooming self-care deficit
Bathing/hygiene self-care deficit
Feeding self-care deficit
Toileting self-care deficit

**Domain 5    Perception/Cognition**
*Class 1    Attention*
Unilateral neglect

*Class 2    Orientation*
Impaired environmental interpretation syndrome
Wandering

*Class 3    Sensation/Perception*
Disturbed sensory perception (specify: visual, auditory,
    kinesthetic, gustatory, tactile, olfactory)

*Class 4    Cognition*
Deficient knowledge (specify)
Readiness for enhanced knowledge (specify)
Acute confusion
Chronic confusion

Impaired memory
Disturbed thought processes

*Class 5 Communication*
Impaired verbal communication
Readiness for enhanced communication

**Domain 6 Self-Perception**
*Class 1 Self-Concept*
Disturbed personal identity
Powerlessness
Risk for powerlessness
Hopelessness
Risk for loneliness
Readiness for enhanced self-concept

*Class 2 Self-Esteem*
Chronic low self-esteem
Situational low self-esteem
Risk for situational low self-esteem

*Class 3 Body Image*
Disturbed body image

**Domain 7 Role Relationships**
*Class 1 Caregiving Roles*
Caregiver role strain
Risk for caregiver role strain
Impaired parenting
Risk for impaired parenting
Readiness for enhanced parenting

*Class 2 Family Relationships*
Interrupted family processes
Readiness for enhanced family processes
Dysfunctional family processes: Alcoholism
Risk for impaired parent/infant/child attachment

*Class 3 Role Performance*
Effective breastfeeding
Ineffective breastfeeding
Interrupted breastfeeding
Ineffective role performance
Parental role conflict
Impaired social interaction

**Domain 8    Sexuality**
*Class 1    Sexual Identity*

*Class 2    Sexual Function*
Sexual dysfunction
Ineffective sexuality patterns

*Class 3    Reproduction*

**Domain 9    Coping/Stress Tolerance**
*Class 1    Post-trauma Responses*
Relocation stress syndrome
Risk for relocation stress syndrome
Rape-trauma syndrome
Rape-trauma syndrome: Silent reaction
Rape-trauma syndrome: Compound reaction
Post-trauma syndrome
Risk for post-trauma syndrome

*Class 2    Coping Responses*
Fear
Anxiety
Death anxiety
Chronic sorrow
Ineffective denial
Anticipatory grieving
Dysfunctional grieving
Impaired adjustment
Ineffective coping
Disabled family coping
Compromised family coping
Defensive coping
Ineffective community coping
Readiness for enhanced coping (individual)
Readiness for enhanced family coping
Readiness for enhanced community coping
Risk for dysfunctional grieving

*Class 3    Neurobehavioral Stress*
Autonomic dysreflexia
Risk for autonomic dysreflexia
Disorganized infant behavior
Risk for disorganized infant behavior
Readiness for enhanced organized infant behavior
Decreased intracranial adaptive capacity

**Domain 10    Life Principles**
*Class 1    Values*

*Class 2    Beliefs*
Readiness for enhanced spiritual well-being

*Class 3    Value/Belief/Action Congruence*
Spiritual distress
Risk for spiritual distress
Decisional conflict (specify)
Noncompliance (specify)
Risk for impaired religiosity
Impaired religiosity
Readiness for enhanced religiosity

**Domain 11    Safety/Protection**
*Class 1    Infection*
Risk for infection

*Class 2    Physical Injury*
Impaired oral mucous membrane
Risk for injury
Risk for perioperative positioning injury
Risk for falls
Risk for trauma
Impaired skin integrity
Risk for impaired skin integrity
Impaired tissue integrity
Impaired dentition
Risk for suffocation
Risk for aspiration
Ineffective airway clearance
Risk for peripheral neurovascular dysfunction
Ineffective protection
Risk for sudden infant death syndrome

*Class 3    Violence*
Risk for self-mutilation
Self-mutilation
Risk for other-directed violence
Risk for self-directed violence
Risk for suicide

## Class 4   Environmental Hazards
Risk for poisoning

## Class 5   Defensive Processes
Latex allergy response
Risk for latex allergy response

## Class 6   Thermoregulation
Risk for imbalanced body temperature
Ineffective thermoregulation
Hypothermia
Hyperthermia

# Domain 12   Comfort
## Class 1   Physical Comfort
Acute pain
Chronic pain
Nausea

## Class 2   Environmental Comfort

## Class 3   Social Comfort
Social isolation

# Domain 13   Growth/Development
## Class 1   Growth
Delayed growth and development
Risk for disproportionate growth
Adult failure to thrive

## Class 2   Development
Delayed growth and development
Risk for delayed development

# APPENDIX C

# DSM-IV-TR Classification

## MULTIAXIAL SYSTEM

| | |
|---|---|
| Axis I | Clinical Disorders<br>Other Conditions That May Be a Focus<br>of Clinical Attention |
| Axis II | Personality Disorders<br>Mental Retardation |
| Axis III | General Medical Conditions |
| Axis IV | Psychosocial and Environmental Problems |
| Axis V | Global Assessment of Functioning |

NOS = Not Otherwise Specified.

An *x* appearing in a diagnostic code indicates that a specific code number is required.

An ellipsis (. . .) is used in the names of certain disorders to indicate that the name of a specific mental disorder or general medical condition should be inserted when recording the name (e.g., 293.0 Delirium Due to Hypothyroidism).

If criteria are currently met, one of the following severity specifiers may be noted after the diagnosis:

Mild

Moderate

Severe

From American Psychiatric Association. (2000). *Diagnostic and statistical manual of mental disorders* (4th ed., text revision). Washington, DC: American Psychiatric Association.

If criteria are no longer met, one of the following specifiers may be noted:
In Partial Remission
In Full Remission
Prior History

# DISORDERS USUALLY FIRST DIAGNOSED IN INFANCY, CHILDHOOD, OR ADOLESCENCE

## Mental Retardation

*Note:* These are coded on Axis II.

| | |
|---|---|
| 317 | Mild Mental Retardation |
| 318.0 | Moderate Mental Retardation |
| 318.1 | Severe Mental Retardation |
| 318.2 | Profound Mental Retardation |
| 319 | Mental Retardation, Severity Unspecified |

## Learning Disorders

| | |
|---|---|
| 315.00 | Reading Disorder |
| 315.1 | Mathematics Disorder |
| 315.2 | Disorder of Written Expression |
| 315.9 | Learning Disorder NOS |

## Motor Skills Disorder

| | |
|---|---|
| 315.4 | Developmental Coordination Disorder |

## Communication Disorders

| | |
|---|---|
| 315.31 | Expressive Language Disorder |
| 315.32 | Mixed Receptive-Expressive Language Disorder |
| 315.39 | Phonologic Disorder |
| 307.0 | Stuttering |
| 307.9 | Communication Disorder NOS |

## Pervasive Developmental Disorders

| | |
|---|---|
| 299.00 | Autistic Disorder |
| 299.80 | Rett's Disorder |
| 299.10 | Childhood Disintegrative Disorder |

| | |
|---|---|
| 299.80 | Asperger's Disorder |
| 299.80 | Pervasive Developmental Disorder NOS |

## Attention-Deficit and Disruptive Behavior Disorders

| | |
|---|---|
| 314.xx | Attention-Deficit/Hyperactivity Disorder |
| .01 | Combined Type |
| .00 | Predominantly Inattentive Type |
| .01 | Predominantly Hyperactive-Impulsive Type |
| 314.9 | Attention-Deficit/Hyperactivity Disorder NOS |
| 312.xx | Conduct Disorder |
| .81 | Childhood-Onset Type |
| .82 | Adolescent-Onset Type |
| .89 | Unspecified Onset |
| 313.81 | Oppositional Defiant Disorder |
| 312.9 | Disruptive Behavior Disorder NOS |

## Feeding and Eating Disorders of Infancy or Early Childhood

| | |
|---|---|
| 307.52 | Pica |
| 307.53 | Rumination Disorder |
| 307.59 | Feeding Disorder of Infancy or Early Childhood |

## Tic Disorders

| | |
|---|---|
| 307.23 | Tourette's Disorder |
| 307.22 | Chronic Motor or Vocal Tic Disorder |
| 307.21 | Transient Tic Disorder |
| | *Specify if:* Single Episode/Recurrent |
| 307.20 | Tic Disorder NOS |

## Elimination Disorders

| | |
|---|---|
| ——.— | Encopresis |
| 787.6 | With Constipation and Overflow Incontinence |
| 307.7 | Without Constipation and Overflow Incontinence |
| 307.6 | Enuresis (Not Due to a General Medical Condition) |
| | *Specify type:* Nocturnal Only/Diurnal Only/Nocturnal and Diurnal |

**Other Disorders of Infancy, Childhood, or Adolescence**

| | |
|---|---|
| 309.21 | Separation Anxiety Disorder |
| | *Specify if:* Early Onset |
| 313.23 | Selective Mutism |
| 313.89 | Reactive Attachment Disorder of Infancy or Early Childhood |
| | *Specify type:* Inhibited Type/Disinhibited Type |
| 307.3 | Stereotypic Movement Disorder |
| | *Specify if:* With Self-Injurious Behavior |
| 313.9 | Disorder of Infancy, Childhood, or Adolescence NOS |

# DELIRIUM, DEMENTIA, AND AMNESTIC AND OTHER COGNITIVE DISORDERS

## Delirium

| | |
|---|---|
| 293.0 | Delirium Due to . . . *[indicate the general medical condition]* |
| \_\_\_.\_\_ | Substance Intoxication Delirium *(refer to Substance-Related Disorders for substance-specific codes)* |
| \_\_\_.\_\_ | Substance Withdrawal Delirium *(refer to Substance-Related Disorders for substance-specific codes)* |
| \_\_\_.\_\_ | Delirium Due to Multiple Etiologies *(code each of the specific etiologies)* |
| 780.09 | Delirium NOS |

## Dementia

| | |
|---|---|
| 294.xx | Dementia of the Alzheimer's Type, With Early Onset *(also code 331.0 Alzheimer's disease on Axis III)* |
| .10 | Without Behavioral Disturbance |
| .11 | With Behavioral Disturbance |
| 294.xx | Dementia of the Alzheimer's Type, with Late Onset *(also code 331.0 Alzheimer's disease on Axis III)* |
| .10 | Without Behavioral Disturbance |
| .11 | With Behavioral Disturbance |

| | |
|---|---|
| 290.xx | Vascular Dementia |
| .40 | Uncomplicated |
| .41 | With Delirium |
| .42 | With Delusions |
| .43 | With Depressed Mood |

*Specify if:* With Behavioral Disturbance *Code presence or absence of a behavioral disturbance in the fifth digit for* Dementia Due to a General Medical Condition:
  0 = Without Behavioral Disturbance
  1 = With Behavioral Disturbance

| | |
|---|---|
| 294.1x | Dementia Due to HIV Disease<br>*(also code 042 HIV on Axis III)* |
| 294.1x | Dementia Due to Head Trauma<br>*(also code 854.00 head injury on Axis III)* |
| 294.1x | Dementia Due to Parkinson's Disease<br>*(also code 332.0 Parkinson's disease on Axis III)* |
| 294.1x | Dementia Due to Huntington's Disease<br>*(also code 333.4 Huntington's disease on Axis III)* |
| 294.1x | Dementia Due to Pick's Disease<br>*(also code 331.1 Pick's disease on Axis III)* |
| 294.1x | Dementia Due to Creutzfeldt-Jakob Disease<br>*(also code 046.1 Creutzfeldt-Jakob disease on Axis III)* |
| 294.1x | Dementia Due to . . . *[indicate the general medical condition not listed above]* *(also code the general medical condition on Axis III)* |
| \_\_\_.\_\_ | Substance-Induced Persisting Dementia *(refer to Substance-Related Disorders for substance-specific codes)* |
| \_\_\_.\_\_ | Dementia Due to Multiple Etiologies *(code each of the specific etiologies)* |
| 294.8 | Dementia NOS |

## Amnestic Disorders

| | |
|---|---|
| 294.0 | Amnestic Disorder Due to . . . *[indicate the general medical condition]*<br>*Specify if:* Transient/Chronic |
| \_\_\_.\_\_ | Substance-Induced Persisting Amnestic Disorder *(refer to Substance-Related Disorders for substance-specific codes)* |
| 294.8 | Amnestic Disorder NOS |

**Other Cognitive Disorders**

 294.9  Cognitive Disorder NOS

# MENTAL DISORDERS DUE TO A GENERAL MEDICAL CONDITION NOT ELSEWHERE CLASSIFIED

 293.89  Catatonic Disorder Due to . . . *[indicate the general medical condition]*

 310.1  Personality Change Due to . . . *[indicate the general medical condition]*
     *Specify type:* Labile Type/Disinhibited Type/Aggressive Type/Apathetic Type/Paranoid Type/Other Type/Combined Type/Unspecified Type

 293.9  Mental Disorder NOS Due to . . . *[indicate the general medical condition]*

# SUBSTANCE-RELATED DISORDERS

*The following specifiers may be applied to Substance Dependence as noted:*
[a]With Physiologic Dependence/without Physiologic Dependence
[b]Early Full Remission/Early Partial Remission/Sustained Full Remission/Sustained Partial Remission
[c]In a Controlled Environment
[d]On Agonist Therapy
*The following specifiers apply to Substance-Induced Disorders as noted:*
[I]With Onset during Intoxication
[W]With Onset during Withdrawal

**Alcohol-Related Disorders**

*Alcohol Use Disorders*

 303.90  Alcohol Dependence[a,b,c]
 305.00  Alcohol Abuse

*Alcohol-Induced Disorders*

 303.00  Alcohol Intoxication
 291.81  Alcohol Withdrawal
     *Specify if:* With Perceptual Disturbances

| 291.0 | Alcohol Intoxication Delirium |
|---|---|
| 291.0 | Alcohol Withdrawal Delirium |
| 291.2 | Alcohol-Induced Persisting Dementia |
| 291.1 | Alcohol-Induced Persisting Amnestic Disorder |
| 291.x | Alcohol-Induced Psychotic Disorder |
| .5 | With Delusions[I,W] |
| .3 | With Hallucinations[I,W] |
| 291.89 | Alcohol-Induced Mood Disorder[I,W] |
| 291.89 | Alcohol-Induced Anxiety Disorder[I,W] |
| 291.89 | Alcohol-Induced Sexual Dysfunction[I] |
| 291.89 | Alcohol-Induced Sleep Disorder[I,W] |
| 291.9 | Alcohol-Related Disorder NOS |

## Amphetamine (or Amphetamine-Like)–Related Disorders

### Amphetamine Use Disorders

| 304.40 | Amphetamine Dependence[a,b,c] |
|---|---|
| 305.70 | Amphetamine Abuse |

### Amphetamine-Induced Disorders

| 292.89 | Amphetamine Intoxication |
|---|---|
| | *Specify if:* With Perceptual Disturbances |
| 292.0 | Amphetamine Withdrawal |
| 292.81 | Amphetamine Intoxication Delirium |
| 292.xx | Amphetamine-Induced Psychotic Disorder |
| .11 | With Delusions[I] |
| .12 | With Hallucinations[I] |
| 292.84 | Amphetamine-Induced Mood Disorder[I,W] |
| 292.89 | Amphetamine-Induced Anxiety Disorder[I] |
| 292.89 | Amphetamine-Induced Sexual Dysfunction[I] |
| 292.89 | Amphetamine-Induced Sleep Disorder[I,W] |
| 292.9 | Amphetamine-Related Disorder NOS |

## Caffeine-Related Disorders

### Caffeine-Induced Disorders

| 305.90 | Caffeine Intoxication |
|---|---|
| 292.89 | Caffeine-Induced Anxiety Disorder[I] |
| 292.89 | Caffeine-Induced Sleep Disorder[I] |
| 292.9 | Caffeine-Related Disorder NOS |

## Cannabis-Related Disorders

### Cannabis Use Disorders

304.30 Cannabis Dependence[a,b,c]
305.20 Cannabis Abuse

### Cannabis-Induced Disorders

292.89 Cannabis Intoxication
*Specify if:* With Perceptual Disturbances
292.81 Cannabis Intoxication Delirium
292.xx Cannabis-Induced Psychotic Disorder
.11 With Delusions[I]
.12 With Hallucinations[I]
292.89 Cannabis-Induced Anxiety Disorder[I]
292.9 Cannabis-Related Disorder NOS

## Cocaine-Related Disorders

### Cocaine Use Disorders

304.20 Cocaine Dependence[a,b,c]
305.60 Cocaine Abuse

### Cocaine-Induced Disorders

292.89 Cocaine Intoxication
*Specify if:* With Perceptual Disturbances
292.0 Cocaine Withdrawal
292.81 Cocaine Intoxication Delirium
292.xx Cocaine-Induced Psychotic Disorder
.11 With Delusions[I]
.12 With Hallucinations[I]
292.84 Cocaine-Induced Mood Disorder[I,W]
292.89 Cocaine-Induced Anxiety Disorder[I,W]
292.89 Cocaine-Induced Sexual Dysfunction[I]
292.89 Cocaine-Induced Sleep Disorder[I,W]
292.9 Cocaine-Related Disorder NOS

## Hallucinogen-Related Disorders

### Hallucinogen Use Disorders

304.50 Hallucinogen Dependence[b,c]
305.30 Hallucinogen Abuse

## Hallucinogen-Induced Disorders

| | |
|---|---|
| 292.89 | Hallucinogen Intoxication |
| 292.89 | Hallucinogen Persisting Perception Disorder (Flashbacks) |
| 292.81 | Hallucinogen Intoxication Delirium |
| 292.xx | Hallucinogen-Induced Psychotic Disorder |
| .11 | With Delusions[I] |
| .12 | With Hallucinations[I] |
| 292.84 | Hallucinogen-Induced Mood Disorder[I] |
| 292.89 | Hallucinogen-Induced Anxiety Disorder[I] |
| 292.9 | Hallucinogen-Related Disorder NOS |

# Inhalant-Related Disorders

## Inhalant Use Disorders

| | |
|---|---|
| 304.60 | Inhalant Dependence[b,c] |
| 305.90 | Inhalant Abuse |

## Inhalant-Induced Disorders

| | |
|---|---|
| 292.89 | Inhalant Intoxication |
| 292.81 | Inhalant Intoxication Delirium |
| 292.82 | Inhalant-Induced Persisting Dementia |
| 292.xx | Inhalant-Induced Psychotic Disorder |
| .11 | With Delusions[I] |
| .12 | With Hallucinations[I] |
| 292.84 | Inhalant-Induced Mood Disorder[I] |
| 292.89 | Inhalant-Induced Anxiety Disorder[I] |
| 292.9 | Inhalant-Related Disorder NOS |

# Nicotine-Related Disorders

## Nicotine Use Disorder

| | |
|---|---|
| 305.1 | Nicotine Dependence[a,b] |

## Nicotine-Induced Disorder

| | |
|---|---|
| 292.0 | Nicotine Withdrawal |
| 292.9 | Nicotine-Related Disorder NOS |

# Opioid-Related Disorders

## Opioid Use Disorders

| | |
|---|---|
| 304.00 | Opioid Dependence[a,b,c,d] |
| 305.50 | Opioid Abuse |

## Opioid-Induced Disorders

| | |
|---|---|
| 292.89 | Opioid Intoxication |
| | *Specify if:* With Perceptual Disturbances |
| 292.0 | Opioid Withdrawal |
| 292.81 | Opioid Intoxication Delirium |
| 292.xx | Opioid-Induced Psychotic Disorder |
| .11 | With Delusions[I] |
| .12 | With Hallucinations[I] |
| 292.84 | Opioid-Induced Mood Disorder[I] |
| 292.89 | Opioid-Induced Sexual Dysfunction[I] |
| 292.89 | Opioid-Induced Sleep Disorder[I,W] |
| 292.9 | Opioid-Related Disorder NOS |

## Phencyclidine (or Phencyclidine-Like)–Related Disorders

### Phencyclidine Use Disorders

| | |
|---|---|
| 304.60 | Phencyclidine Dependence[b,c] |
| 305.90 | Phencyclidine Abuse |

### Phencyclidine-Induced Disorders

| | |
|---|---|
| 292.89 | Phencyclidine Intoxication |
| | *Specify if:* With Perceptual Disturbances |
| 292.81 | Phencyclidine Intoxication Delirium |
| 292.xx | Phencyclidine-Induced Psychotic Disorder |
| .11 | With Delusions[I] |
| .12 | With Hallucinations[I] |
| 292.84 | Phencyclidine-Induced Mood Disorder[I] |
| 292.89 | Phencyclidine-Induced Anxiety Disorder[I] |
| 292.9 | Phencyclidine-Related Disorder NOS |

## Sedative-, Hypnotic-, or Anxiolytic-Related Disorders

### Sedative, Hypnotic, or Anxiolytic Use Disorders

| | |
|---|---|
| 304.10 | Sedative, Hypnotic, or Anxiolytic Dependence[a,b,c] |
| 305.40 | Sedative, Hypnotic, or Anxiolytic Abuse |

### Sedative-, Hypnotic-, or Anxiolytic-Induced Disorders

| | |
|---|---|
| 292.89 | Sedative, Hypnotic, or Anxiolytic Intoxication |
| 292.0 | Sedative, Hypnotic, or Anxiolytic Withdrawal |

|        | *Specify if:* With Perceptual Disturbances |
|--------|---------------------------------------------|
| 292.81 | Sedative, Hypnotic, or Anxiolytic Intoxication Delirium |
| 292.81 | Sedative, Hypnotic, or Anxiolytic Withdrawal Delirium |
| 292.82 | Sedative-, Hypnotic-, or Anxiolytic-Induced Persisting Dementia |
| 292.83 | Sedative-, Hypnotic-, or Anxiolytic-Induced Persisting Amnestic Disorder |
| 292.xx | Sedative-, Hypnotic-, or Anxiolytic-Induced Psychotic Disorder |
| .11    | With Delusions[I,W] |
| .12    | With Hallucinations[I,W] |
| 292.84 | Sedative-, Hypnotic-, or Anxiolytic-Induced Mood Disorder[I,W] |
| 292.89 | Sedative-, Hypnotic-, or Anxiolytic-Induced Anxiety Disorder[W] |
| 292.89 | Sedative-, Hypnotic-, or Anxiolytic-Induced Sexual Dysfunction[I] |
| 292.89 | Sedative-, Hypnotic-, or Anxiolytic-Induced Sleep Disorder[I,W] |
| 292.9  | Sedative-, Hypnotic-, or Anxiolytic-Related Disorder NOS |

## Polysubstance–Related Disorder

| 304.80 | Polysubstance Dependence[a,b,c,d] |
|--------|-----------------------------------|

## Other (or Unknown) Substance–Related Disorders

### *Other (or Unknown) Substance Use Disorders*

| 304.90 | Other (or Unknown) Substance Dependence[a,b,c,d] |
|--------|--------------------------------------------------|
| 305.90 | Other (or Unknown) Substance Abuse |

### *Other (or Unknown) Substance–Induced Disorders*

| 292.89 | Other (or Unknown) Substance Intoxication |
|--------|-------------------------------------------|
|        | *Specify if:* With Perceptual Disturbances |
| 292.0  | Other (or Unknown) Substance Withdrawal |
|        | *Specify if:* With Perceptual Disturbances |
| 292.81 | Other (or Unknown) Substance-Induced Delirium |

292.82    Other (or Unknown) Substance–Induced
          Persisting Dementia
292.83    Other (or Unknown) Substance–Induced
          Persisting Amnestic Disorder
292.xx    Other (or Unknown) Substance–Induced
          Psychotic Disorder
   .11     With Delusions[I,W]
   .12     With Hallucinations[I,W]
292.84    Other (or Unknown) Substance–Induced
          Mood Disorder[I,W]
292.89    Other (or Unknown) Substance–Induced
          Anxiety Disorder[I,W]
292.89    Other (or Unknown) Substance–Induced
          Sexual Dysfunction[I]
292.89    Other (or Unknown) Substance–Induced
          Sleep Disorder[I,W]
292.9     Other (or Unknown) Substance–Induced
          Disorder NOS

## SCHIZOPHRENIA AND OTHER PSYCHOTIC DISORDERS

295.xx    Schizophrenia

*The following Classification of Longitudinal Course applies to all subtypes of Schizophrenia:*

Episodic with Interepisode Residual Symptoms (*specify if:* With Prominent Negative Symptoms)/Episodic with No Interepisode Residual Symptoms

Continuous (*specify if:* With Prominent Negative Symptoms)

Single Episode in Partial Remission (*specify if:* With Prominent Negative Symptoms)/Single Episode in Full Remission

Other or Unspecified Pattern

   .30     Paranoid Type
   .10     Disorganized Type
   .20     Catatonic Type
   .90     Undifferentiated Type
   .60     Residual Type
295.40    Schizophreniform Disorder
          *Specify if:* Without Good Prognostic Features/
          with Good Prognostic Features
295.70    Schizoaffective Disorder
          *Specify type:* Bipolar Type/Depressive Type

297.1      Delusional Disorder
*Specify type:* Erotomanic Type/Grandiose Type/Jealous Type/Persecutory Type/Somatic Type/Mixed Type/Unspecified Type

298.8      Brief Psychotic Disorder
*Specify if:* With Marked Stressor(s)/without Marked Stressor(s)/with Postpartum Onset

297.3      Shared Psychotic Disorder

293.xx    Psychotic Disorder Due to . . . *[indicate the general medical condition]*

  .81      With Delusions

  .82      With Hallucinations

___.___   Substance-Induced Psychotic Disorder *(refer to Substance-Related Disorders for substance-specific codes)*
*Specify if:* With Onset During Intoxication/with Onset During Withdrawal

298.9      Psychotic Disorder NOS

## MOOD DISORDERS

*Code current state of Major Depressive Disorder or Bipolar I Disorder in fifth digit:*

1 = Mild

2 = Moderate

3 = Severe without Psychotic Features

4 = Severe with Psychotic Features

*Specify:* Mood-Congruent Psychotic Features/Mood-Incongruent Psychotic Features

5 = In Partial Remission

6 = In Full Remission

0 = Unspecified

*The following specifiers apply (for current or most recent episode) to Mood Disorders as noted:*

[a]Severity/Psychotic/Remission Specifiers/[b]Chronic/[c]with Catatonic Features/[d]with Melancholic Features/[e]with Atypical Features/[f]with Postpartum Onset

*The following specifiers apply to Mood Disorders as noted:*

[g]With or without Full Interepisode Recovery/[h]with Seasonal Pattern/[i]with Rapid Cycling

## Depressive Disorders

| | |
|---|---|
| 296.xx | Major Depressive Disorder |
| .2x | Single Episode[a,b,c,d,e,f] |
| .3x | Recurrent[a,b,c,d,e,f,g,h] |
| 300.4 | Dysthymic Disorder |
| | *Specify if:* Early Onset/Late Onset |
| | *Specify:* With Atypical Features |
| 311 | Depressive Disorder NOS |

## Bipolar Disorders

| | |
|---|---|
| 296.xx | Bipolar I Disorder |
| .0x | Single Manic Episode[a,c,f] |
| | *Specify if:* Mixed |
| .40 | Most Recent Episode Hypomanic[g,h,i] |
| .4x | Most Recent Episode Manic[a,c,f,g,h,i] |
| .6x | Most Recent Episode Mixed[a,c,f,g,h,i] |
| .5x | Most Recent Episode Depressed[a,b,c,d,e,f,g,h,i] |
| .7 | Most Recent Episode Unspecified[g,h,i] |
| 296.89 | Bipolar II Disorder[a,b,c,d,e,f,g,h,i] |
| | *Specify (current or most recent episode):* Hypomanic/Depressed |
| 301.13 | Cyclothymic Disorder |
| 296.80 | Bipolar Disorder NOS |
| 293.83 | Mood Disorder Due to . . . *[indicate the general medical condition]* |
| | *Specify type:* With Depressive Features/with Major Depressive-Like Episode/with Manic Features/with Mixed Features |
| —·— | Substance-Induced Mood Disorder *(refer to Substance-Related Disorders for substance-specific codes)* |
| | *Specify type:* With Depressive Features/with Manic Features/with Mixed Features |
| | *Specify if:* With Onset During Intoxication/ with Onset during Withdrawal |
| 296.90 | Mood Disorder NOS |

# ANXIETY DISORDERS

| | |
|---|---|
| 300.01 | Panic Disorder without Agoraphobia |
| 300.21 | Panic Disorder with Agoraphobia |
| 300.22 | Agoraphobia without History of Panic Disorder |
| 300.29 | Specific Phobia |

*Specify type:* Animal Type/Natural
　　Environment Type/Blood-Injection-Injury
　　Type/Situational Type/Other Type

300.23　Social Phobia
*Specify if:* Generalized

300.3　Obsessive-Compulsive Disorder
*Specify if:* With Poor Insight

309.81　Posttraumatic Stress Disorder
*Specify if:* Acute/Chronic
*Specify if:* With Delayed Onset

308.3　Acute Stress Disorder

300.02　Generalized Anxiety Disorder

293.84　Anxiety Disorder Due to ... *[indicate the
　　general medical condition]*
*Specify if:* With Generalized Anxiety/with
　　Panic Attacks/with Obsessive-Compulsive
　　Symptoms

___.___　Substance-Induced Anxiety Disorder
　　*(refer to Substance-Related Disorders for
　　substance-specific codes)*
*Specify if:* With Generalized Anxiety/with
　　Panic Attacks/with Obsessive-Compulsive
　　Symptoms/with Phobic Symptoms
*Specify if:* With Onset during Intoxication/
　　with Onset During Withdrawal

300.00　Anxiety Disorder NOS

## SOMATOFORM DISORDERS

300.81　Somatization Disorder

300.82　Undifferentiated Somatoform Disorder

300.11　Conversion Disorder
*Specify type:* With Motor Symptom or Deficit/
　　with Sensory Symptom or Deficit/with
　　Seizures or Convulsions/with Mixed
　　Presentation

307.xx　Pain Disorder
　.80　　Associated with Psychologic Factors
　.89　　Associated with Both Psychologic Factors
　　　　and a General Medical Condition
*Specify if:* Acute/Chronic

300.7　Hypochondriasis
*Specify if:* With Poor Insight

300.7　Body Dysmorphic Disorder

300.82　Somatoform Disorder NOS

# FACTITIOUS DISORDERS

| | |
|---|---|
| 300.xx | Factitious Disorder |
| .16 | With Predominantly Psychologic Signs and Symptoms |
| .19 | With Predominantly Physical Signs and Symptoms |
| .19 | With Combined Psychologic and Physical Signs and Symptoms |
| 300.19 | Factitious Disorder NOS |

# DISSOCIATIVE DISORDERS

| | |
|---|---|
| 300.12 | Dissociative Amnesia |
| 300.13 | Dissociative Fugue |
| 300.14 | Dissociative Identity Disorder |
| 300.6 | Depersonalization Disorder |
| 300.15 | Dissociative Disorder NOS |

# SEXUAL AND GENDER IDENTITY DISORDERS

## Sexual Dysfunctions

*The following specifiers apply to all primary Sexual Dysfunctions:*
Lifelong Type/Acquired Type
Generalized Type/Situational Type
Due to Psychologic Factors/Due to Combined Factors

### *Sexual Desire Disorders*

| | |
|---|---|
| 302.71 | Hypoactive Sexual Desire Disorder |
| 302.79 | Sexual Aversion Disorder |

### *Sexual Arousal Disorders*

| | |
|---|---|
| 302.72 | Female Sexual Arousal Disorder |
| 302.72 | Male Erectile Disorder |

### *Orgasmic Disorders*

| | |
|---|---|
| 302.73 | Female Orgasmic Disorder |
| 302.74 | Male Orgasmic Disorder |
| 302.75 | Premature Ejaculation |

## Sexual Pain Disorders

| | |
|---|---|
| 302.76 | Dyspareunia (Not Due to a General Medical Condition) |
| 306.51 | Vaginismus (Not Due to a General Medical Condition) |

## Sexual Dysfunction Due to a General Medical Condition

| | |
|---|---|
| 625.8 | Female Hypoactive Sexual Desire Disorder Due to . . . *[indicate the general medical condition]* |
| 608.89 | Male Hypoactive Sexual Desire Disorder Due to . . . *[indicate the general medical condition]* |
| 607.84 | Male Erectile Disorder Due to . . . *[indicate the general medical condition]* |
| 625.0 | Female Dyspareunia Due to . . . *[indicate the general medical condition]* |
| 608.89 | Male Dyspareunia Due to . . . *[indicate the general medical condition]* |
| 625.8 | Other Female Sexual Dysfunction Due to . . . *[indicate the general medical condition]* |
| 608.89 | Other Male Sexual Dysfunction Due to . . . *[indicate the general medical condition]* |
| \_\_\_.\_\_ | Substance-Induced Sexual Dysfunction *(refer to Substance-Related Disorders for substance-specific codes)* |
| | *Specify if:* With Impaired Desire/with Impaired Arousal/with Impaired Orgasm/ with Sexual Pain |
| | *Specify if:* With Onset during Intoxication |
| 302.70 | Sexual Dysfunction NOS |

## Paraphilias

| | |
|---|---|
| 302.4 | Exhibitionism |
| 302.81 | Fetishism |
| 302.89 | Frotteurism |
| 302.2 | Pedophilia |
| | *Specify if:* Sexually Attracted to Males/ Sexually Attracted to Females/Sexually Attracted to Both |
| | *Specify if:* Limited to Incest |

# IMPULSE-CONTROL DISORDERS NOT ELSEWHERE CLASSIFIED

312.39    Trichotillomania
312.30    Impulse-Control Disorder NOS

# ADJUSTMENT DISORDERS

309.xx    Adjustment Disorder
.0        With Depressed Mood
.24       With Anxiety
.28       With Mixed Anxiety and Depressed Mood
.3        With Disturbance of Conduct
.4        With Mixed Disturbance of Emotions and
          Conduct
.9        Unspecified
          *Specify if:* Acute/Chronic

# PERSONALITY DISORDERS

*Note:* These are coded on Axis II.
301.0     Paranoid Personality Disorder
301.20    Schizoid Personality Disorder
301.22    Schizotypal Personality Disorder
301.7     Antisocial Personality Disorder
301.83    Borderline Personality Disorder
301.50    Histrionic Personality Disorder
301.81    Narcissistic Personality Disorder
301.82    Avoidant Personality Disorder
301.6     Dependent Personality Disorder
301.4     Obsessive-Compulsive Personality Disorder
301.9     Personality Disorder NOS

# OTHER CONDITIONS THAT MAY BE A FOCUS OF CLINICAL ATTENTION

## Psychologic Factors Affecting Medical Condition

316       . . . *[Specified psychologic factor] Affecting . . .*
          *[indicate the general medical condition]*
          *Choose name based on nature of factors:*
          Mental Disorder Affecting Medical Condition
          Psychologic Symptoms Affecting Medical
          Condition
          Personality Traits or Coping Style Affecting
          Medical Condition
          Maladaptive Health Behaviors Affecting
          Medical Condition

Stress-Related Physiologic Response
Affecting Medical Condition
Other or Unspecified Psychologic Factors
Affecting Medical Condition

## Medication-Induced Movement Disorders

| | |
|---|---|
| 332.1 | Neuroleptic-Induced Parkinsonism |
| 333.92 | Neuroleptic Malignant Syndrome |
| 333.7 | Neuroleptic-Induced Acute Dystonia |
| 333.99 | Neuroleptic-Induced Acute Akathisia |
| 333.82 | Neuroleptic-Induced Tardive Dyskinesia |
| 333.1 | Medication-Induced Postural Tremor |
| 333.90 | Medication-Induced Movement Disorder NOS |

## Other Medication-Induced Disorder

| | |
|---|---|
| 995.2 | Adverse Effects of Medication NOS |

## Relational Problems

| | |
|---|---|
| V61.9 | Relational Problem Related to a Mental Disorder or General Medical Condition |
| V61.20 | Parent-Child Relational Problem |
| V61.10 | Partner Relational Problem |
| V61.8 | Sibling Relational Problem |
| V62.81 | Relational Problem NOS |

## Problems Related to Abuse or Neglect

| | |
|---|---|
| V61.21 | Physical Abuse of Child *(code 995.54 if focus of attention is on victim)* |
| V61.21 | Sexual Abuse of Child *(code 995.53 if focus of attention is on victim)* |
| V61.21 | Neglect of Child *(code 995.52 if focus of attention is on victim)* |
| \_\_\_.\_\_ | Physical Abuse of Adult |
| V61.12 | (if by partner) |
| V62.83 | (if by person other than partner) *(code 995.81 if focus of attention is on victim)* |
| \_\_\_.\_\_ | Sexual Abuse of Adult |
| V61.12 | (if by partner) |
| V62.83 | (if by person other than partner) *(code 995.83 if focus of attention is on victim)* |

## Additional Conditions That May Be a Focus of Clinical Attention

| | |
|---|---|
| V15.81 | Noncompliance With Treatment |
| V65.2 | Malingering |
| V71.01 | Adult Antisocial Behavior |
| V71.02 | Child or Adolescent Antisocial Behavior |
| V62.89 | Borderline Intellectual Functioning |
| | *Note:* This is coded on Axis II. |
| 780.9 | Age-Related Cognitive Decline |
| V62.82 | Bereavement |
| V62.3 | Academic Problem |
| V62.2 | Occupational Problem |
| 313.82 | Identity Problem |
| V62.89 | Religious or Spiritual Problem |
| V62.4 | Acculturation Problem |
| V62.89 | Phase of Life Problem |

# ADDITIONAL CODES

| | |
|---|---|
| 300.9 | Unspecified Mental Disorder (nonpsychotic) |
| V71.09 | No Diagnosis or Condition on Axis I |
| 799.9 | Diagnosis or Condition Deferred on Axis I |
| V71.09 | No Diagnosis on Axis II |
| 799.9 | Diagnosis Deferred on Axis II |

# APPENDIX D

# Assessment Tools

## Appendix D-1A Types of Assessment Data

**History of Present Illness**
- Chief complaint
- Development and duration of problems
- Help sought and tried
- Effect of problem on child's life at home and school
- Effect of problem on family and sibling's life

**Developmental History**
- Pregnancy, birth, neonatal data
- Developmental milestones
- Description of eating, sleeping, elimination habits, and routines
- Attachment behaviors
- Types of play
- Social skills and friendships
- Sexual activity

**Development Assessment**
- Psychomotor
- Language
- Cognitive
- Interpersonal-social
- Academic achievement
- Behavior (response to stress, changes in the environment)
- Problem solving and coping skills (impulse control, delay of gratification)
- Energy level and motivation

## Appendix D-1A **Types of Assessment Data—cont'd**

**Neurologic Assessment**
- Cerebral functions
- Cerebellar functions
- Sensory functions
- Reflexes
- Cranial nerves
- Functions can be observed in developmental assessment and while playing games involving a specific ability (e.g., "Simon Says, touch your nose.")

**Medical History**
- Review of body systems
- Trauma, hospitalization, operations, and child's response
- Illnesses or injuries affecting the central nervous system
- Medications (past and current)
- Allergies

**Family History**
- Illnesses in related family members (e.g., seizures, mental disorders, mental retardation, hyperactivity, drug and alcohol abuse, diabetes, cancer)
- Background of family members (occupation, education, social, activities, religion)
- Family relationships (separation, divorce, deaths, contact with extended family, support system)

**Mental Status Assessment**
- General appearance
- Activity level
- Coordination/motor function
- Affect
- Speech
- Manner of relating
- Intellectual functions
- Thought processes and content
- Characteristics of child's play

## Appendix D-1B Child/Adolescent Mental Status Assessment

### General Appearance
- Size—height and weight
- General health and nutrition
- Dress and grooming
- Distinguishing characteristics
- Gestures and mannerisms
- Looks/acts younger or older than chronological age

### Speech
- Rate, rhythm, intonation
- Pitch and modulation
- Vocabulary and grammar appropriate to age
- Mute, hesitant, talkative
- Articulation problems
- Other expressive problems
- Unusual characteristics (pronoun reversal, echolalia, gender confusion, neologisms)

### Intellectual Functions
- Fund of general information
- Ability to communicate (follow directions, answer questions)
- Memory
- Creativity
- Sense of humor
- Social awareness
- Learning and problem solving
- Conscience (sense of right and wrong, accepts guilt and limits)

### Characteristics of Child's Play
- Age appropriate use of toys
- Themes of play
- Imagination and pretend play
- Role and gender play
- Age-appropriate play with peers
- Relationship with peers (empathy, sharing, waiting for turns, best friends)

### Activity Level
- Hyperactivity/hypoactivity
- Tics, other body movements

## Appendix D-1B Child/Adolescent Mental Status Assessment—cont'd

- Autoerotic and self-comforting movements (thumb sucking, ear/hair pulling, masturbation)

### Coordination/Motor Function
- Posture
- Gait
- Balance
- Gross motor movement
- Fine motor movement
- Writing and drawing skills
- Unusual characteristics (bizarre postures, tiptoe walking, hand flapping, head banging, hand biting)

### Manner of Relating
- Eye contact
- Ability to separate from caregiver, be independent
- Attitude toward interviewer
- Behavior during interview (ability to have fun/play, low frustration tolerance, impulsive, aggressive)

### Thought Processes and Content
- Orientation
- Attention span
- Self-concept and body image
- Sex role, gender identity
- Ego-defense mechanisms
- Perceptual distortions (hallucinations, illusions)
- Preoccupations, concerns, and unusual ideas
- Fantasies and dreams

Adapted from Goodman, J.D., & Sours, J. (1987). *The child mental status examination* (2nd ed.). New York: Basic Books; reprinted with permission.

## Appendix D-1C **Stages of Development**

| FREUD | ERIKSON | SULLIVAN |
| --- | --- | --- |
| **ORAL-BIRTH—½-2 yrs.** Pleasure—Pain Principle Goal: Immediate release of tension and immediate gratification. *ID*—Major agency of mind present. Source of all psychic energy. Seat of instincts. Behavior—*Demanding,* impulsive irrational, asocial, selfish, trustful, *omnipotent, dependent.* Primary thought processes. Unconscious Instincts—source-energy-aim-object Mouth—primary source of pleasure. | **INFANCY TRUST vs. MISTRUST** First task is to develop a basic sense of trust. Trust requires a feeling of 1) Physical comfort 2) Minimal experience of fear or uncertainty If this occurs, the child will extend trust to new experience. Egocentric. *Danger* second half of first year. Discontinue care may increase the natural sense of loss, as the child gradually recognizes his separateness from his mother, to a basic sense of mistrust that may last through life. | **INFANCY-BIRTH—1½ yrs.** Mothering object relieves tension through empathic intervention and tenderness. Relief to tension yields satisfaction and security and symbol of good mother. Goal—Pursuit of satisfaction (Biol) Pursuit of security (Psych) Denial of relief yields anxiety and symbol of Bad Mother. Anxiety in mother yields anxiety and fear in child via empathy. These states are experienced by the child in diffuse-undifferentiated manner. *Task of Infancy*—To learn to count on others for satisfaction and security "to trust." |

## ANAL 2–3½ or 4 yrs.

Begin to develop *Ego*

Reality principle—postpone immediate discharge of energy and seek actual object to satisfy needs.

Learning to defer pleasure. Gaining satisfaction from tolerating some tension mastering impulses.

Toilet training

Reality testing—ambivalence

Retaining/letting go

Power struggle

*Ego*—functions on conscious, preconscious and unconscious levels. Ego is in touch with reality functions primarily on *Reality Principle.*

Ego—problem solves, perceives, thinks, mediates ID impulses.

An unconscious level (except for suppression).

## EARLY CHILDHOOD
### Autonomy vs. Shame/Doubt

With muscular maturation the child experiments holding on and letting go. Begins to attach enormous value to his autonomous will.

Danger—Development of a deep sense of shame/doubt, if he is deprived of the opportunity to rebel and therefore learns to expect defeat in any battle of wills with those who are bigger and stronger.

## CHILDHOOD 1½–6 yrs.

Muscular maturation and learning to communicate verbally. Learning social skills through consensual validation. Beginning to develop self system via reflected appraisals

    Self System—Good me
                  Bad me
                  Not me

Levels of awareness
    Aware
    Selective inattention
    Dissociation

*TASK*—To learn to delay satisfaction of wishes with relative comfort.

*Continued*

Appendix D-1C **Stages of Development—cont'd**

| FREUD | ERIKSON | SULLIVAN |
|---|---|---|
| **PHALLIC 3½-7 yrs.** | **PLAY AGE INITIATIVE vs. GUILT** | **JUVENILE 6-9 yrs.** |
| Superego develops via incorporating moral values, ideals and judgments of right and wrong that are held by parents superego is primarily unconscious and functions on reward and punishment principle (Pride and Guilt). Sexual identity attained via resolving oedipal conflict by identifying with parent of same sex. | During this stage child's imagination is greatly expanded because of: | Oedipal conflict occur *only* with IPR with individual parents (same as well as opposite) is distorted and child's satisfaction and security needs are not met. *Task*—To develop satisfying interpersonal relationships with his peers |
| | 1. increased ability to move around freely | |
| | 2. increased ability to communicate It is an age on intrusive, activity, and curiosity and consuming fantasies which lead to feelings of guilt and anxiety. Also the stage of the establishment of conscience. If this tendency to feel guilty is "overburdened by all too eager adults," the child may develop a deep-seated conviction that he is essentially bad, with a resultant stifling of initiative or a conversion of his moralism to vindictiveness. | Involves competition and compromise. Absorbed in learning to deal with ever-widening outside world peers and other adults. Reflections and revisions of self-image and parental images. |
| Conflict differs for boy and girl mastubatory activity. | | |

**LATENCY 7-12 yrs.**
De-sexualization. Libido diffused. Involved in learning social skills, exploring, building, collecting, accomplishing, hero worship. Peer group loyalty begins. Gang and scout behavior. Growing independence from family.

**SCHOOL AGE—INDUSTRY vs. INFERIORITY**
A long period of sexual latency before puberty is the age when the child wants to learn how to do and make things with others. In learning to accept instruction and to win recognition by producing "things," he opens the way for the capacity of work enjoyment. The danger in this period is the development of a sense of inadequacy and inferiority in a child who does not receive recognition.

**PRE-ADOLENCE 9-12 yrs.**
*Task*—Is to develop intimate IPR with chum of same sex. Pal perceived to be much like one-self in interest, feelings and mutual collaboration. Normal homosexuality.

**ADOLESCENCE**
(Developed by Anna Freud)
Fluctuation regarding emotional stability physical maturation. Very ambivalent and labile, seeking life-goals and emancipation from parents. Independence re-appraisal of parents and self; intense peer loyalty.

**ADOLESCENCE: IDENTITY vs IDENTITY DIFFUSION**
The physiological revolution that comes with puberty (rapid body growth and sexual maturity) forces the young person to question "all sameness and continuities relied on earlier" and to refight many of the earlier battles.

**ADOLESCENCE**
Physical maturation, swift all in emotional stability.
**Early Adolescence 12-14 yrs**
Establishing satisfying relationships with opposite sex.
**Late Adolescence 14-21 yrs**
Interdependent and establishing durable sexual relations with a select member of the opposite sex.

*Continued*

Appendix D-1C **Stages of Development—cont'd**

| FREUD | ERIKSON | SULLIVAN |
|-------|---------|----------|
| **ADOLESENCE—cont'd** | *Development Task*—Is to integrate childhood identification "with the basic biological driven, native endowment and the opportunities offered in social roles. The danger is that identity diffusion, temporarily unavoidable in this period of physical and psychological upheaval, may result in a permanent inability to integrate a personal identity. | |
| | **YOUNG ADULTHOOD INTIMACY vs. ISOLATION** Only as a young person begins to feel more secure in his identity is he able to establish intimacy with himself (with his inner-life) and with others, both in friendships and eventually | |
| **ADULTHOOD** Increasing objectivity regarding self, realistic in regard to one's level of aspiration, code of values, and ability to achieve. Establishment of effective hetero- | | **ADULTHOOD** Has successfully negotiated the previous tasks. **Late Adulthood** To learn to accept and seek needed. |

sexual LPR both in love union and in non-sexual IPR with opposite sex. Freud's definition of a healthy person is one who has the ability "to love and to work."

in a love-based mutually satisfying sexual relationship with a member of the opposite sex. A person who cannot enter wholly into an intimate relationship because of the fear of losing his identity may develop a deep sense of isolation.

### ADULTHOOD GENERATIVITY vs. SELF-ABSORPTION

Out of the intimacies of adulthood grows generativity the mature person's interest in establishing and guiding the next generation. The lack of this results in self-absorption and frequently in a "prevading sense of stagnation and interpersonal improvement."

*Continued*

Appendix D-1C **Stages of Development—cont'd**

| FREUD | ERIKSON | SULLIVAN |
|-------|---------|----------|
| Adulthood—cont'd | **SENESCENCE—INTEGRITY/DISGUST** The person who has achieved a satisfying intimacy with other human beings and who has adapted to the triumphs and disappointments of his generative activities as parent and coworker, reaches the end of his life with a certain ego integrity. The person would also have a sense of what his life is and was and of its place in the flow of history. Without this "accured ego integration," there is despair, usually marked by a display of displeasure and distrust. | |

Adapted from original sources by Erikson, Freud, and Sullivan. Data compiled by the faculty of the Nursing Department and the Borough of Manhattan Community College, New York.

## Appendix D-2 Hamilton Rating Scale for Anxiety

Max Hamilton designed this scale to help clinicians gather information about anxiety states. The symptom inventory provides scaled information that classifies anxiety behaviors and assists the clinician in targeting behaviors and achieving outcome measures. Provide a rating for each indicator based on the following scale:

0 = None
1 = Mild
2 = Moderate
3 = Disabling
4 = Severe, Grossly Disabling

| Item | Symptoms | Rating |
|------|----------|--------|
| Anxious mood | Worries, anticipation of the worst, fearful anticipation, irritability | _____ |
| Tension | Feelings of tension, fatigability, startle response, moved to tears easily, trembling, feelings of restlessness, inability to relax | _____ |
| Fear | Of dark, of strangers, of being left alone, of animals, of traffic, of crowds | _____ |
| Insomnia | Difficulty in falling asleep, broken sleep, unsatisfying sleep and fatigue on waking, dreams, nightmares, night terrors | _____ |
| Intellectual (cognitive) | Difficulty in concentration, poor memory | _____ |
| Depressed mood | Loss of interest, lack of pleasure in hobbies, depression, early waking, diurnal swings | _____ |
| Somatic (sensory) | Tinnitus, blurring of vision, hot and cold flushes, feelings of weakness, prickling sensation | _____ |
| Somatic (muscular) | Pains and aches, twitchings, stiffness, myoclonic jerks, grinding of teeth, unsteady voice, increased muscular tone | _____ |

*Continued*

## Appendix D-2 Hamilton Rating Scale for Anxiety—cont'd

| Item | Symptoms | Rating |
|------|----------|--------|
| Cardiovascular symptoms | Tachycardia, palpitations, pain in chest, throbbing of vessels, fainting feelings, missing beat | _____ |
| Respiratory symptoms | Pressure of constriction in chest, choking feelings, sighing, dyspnea | _____ |
| Gastrointestinal symptoms | Difficulty in swallowing, wind, abdominal pain, burning sensations, abdominal fullness, nausea, vomiting, borborygmi, looseness of bowels, loss of weight, constipation | _____ |
| Genitourinary symptoms | Frequency of micturition, urgency of micturition, amenorrhea, menorrhagia, development of frigidity, premature ejaculation, loss of libido, impotence | _____ |
| Autonomic symptoms | Dry mouth, flushing, pallor, tendency to sweat, giddiness, tension headache, raising of hair | _____ |
| Behavior at interview | Fidgeting, restlessness or pacing, tremor of hands, furrowed brow, strained face, sighing or rapid respiration, facial pallor, swallowing, belching, brisk tendon jerks, dilated pupils, exophthalmos | _____ |

Adapted from Hamilton, M. (1959). The assessment of anxiety states by rating. *British Journal of Medical Psychology, 32*, 50-55; reprinted with permission.

## Appendix D-3 Sample Items from the Beck Depression Inventory

Name _____ Date _____

The questionnaire provides groups of statements. Clients are asked to read all statements in the group and to circle the number that best describes their feelings. The following are two samples.

1. 0 I get as much satisfaction out of things as I used to.
   1 I don't enjoy things the way I used to.
   2 I don't get real satisfaction out of anything anymore.
   3 I am dissatisfied or bored with everything.
2. 0 I have not lost interest in other people.
   1 I am less interested in other people than I used to be.
   2 I have lost most of my interest in other people.
   3 I have lost all of my interest in other people.

## Appendix D-4 Mania Questionnaire

*Use this questionnaire to help determine if you need to see a mental health professional for diagnosis and treatment of mania or manic-depression or bipolar disorder.*

*Instructions:* You might reproduce this scale and use it on a weekly basis to track your moods. It also might be used to show your doctor how your symptoms have changed from one visit to the next. Changes of 5 or more points are significant. This scale is not designed to make a diagnosis of mania or take the place of a professional diagnosis. If you suspect you are manic, please consult with a mental health professional as soon as possible.

The 18 items below refer to how you have felt and behaved DURING THE PAST WEEK. For each item, indicate the extent to which it is true by circling the appropriate number next to the item.

**Key:**

| | |
|---|---|
| 0 = **Not at all** | 3 = **Moderately** |
| 1 = **A little** | 4 = **Quite a lot** |
| 2 = **Somewhat** | 5 = **Very much** |

*Continued*

## Appendix D-4 Manla Questionnaire—cont'd

| | |
|---|---|
| 1. My mind has never been sharper. | 0 1 2 3 4 5 |
| 2. I need less sleep than usual. | 0 1 2 3 4 5 |
| 3. I have so many plans and new ideas that it is hard for me to work. | 0 1 2 3 4 5 |
| 4. I feel a pressure to talk and talk. | 0 1 2 3 4 5 |
| 5. I have been particularly happy. | 0 1 2 3 4 5 |
| 6. I have been more active than usual. | 0 1 2 3 4 5 |
| 7. I talk so fast that people have a hard time keeping up with me. | 0 1 2 3 4 5 |
| 8. I have more new ideas than I can handle. | 0 1 2 3 4 5 |
| 9. I have been irritable. | 0 1 2 3 4 5 |
| 10. It's easy for me to think of jokes and funny stories. | 0 1 2 3 4 5 |
| 11. I have been feeling like "the life of the party." | 0 1 2 3 4 5 |
| 12. I have been full of energy. | 0 1 2 3 4 5 |
| 13. I have been thinking about sex. | 0 1 2 3 4 5 |
| 14. I have been feeling particularly playful. | 0 1 2 3 4 5 |
| 15. I have special plans for the world. | 0 1 2 3 4 5 |
| 16. I have been spending too much money. | 0 1 2 3 4 5 |
| 17. My attention keeps jumping from one idea to another. | 0 1 2 3 4 5 |
| 18. I find it hard to slow down and stay in one place. | 0 1 2 3 4 5 |

## Appendix D-5 Brief Psychiatric Rating Scale

DIRECTIONS: Place an X in the appropriate box to represent level of severity of each symptom.

Patient Name _____ Physician _____
Patient SS# _____ UT# _____ HH# _____ Date _____

| | Not Present | Very Mild | Mild | Moderate | Mod. Severe | Severe | Extremely Severe |
|---|---|---|---|---|---|---|---|
| SOMATIC CONCERN—preoccupation with physical health, fear of physical illness, hypochondriasis | ❑ | ❑ | ❑ | ❑ | ❑ | ❑ | ❑ |
| ANXIETY—worry, fear, over-concern for present or future, uneasiness | ❑ | ❑ | ❑ | ❑ | ❑ | ❑ | ❑ |
| EMOTIONAL WITHDRAWAL—lack of spontaneous interaction, isolation deficiency in relating to others | ❑ | ❑ | ❑ | ❑ | ❑ | ❑ | ❑ |
| CONCEPTUAL DISORGANIZATION—thought processes confused, disconnected, disorganized, disrupted | ❑ | ❑ | ❑ | ❑ | ❑ | ❑ | ❑ |
| GUILT FEELINGS—self-blame, shame, remorse for past behavior | ❑ | ❑ | ❑ | ❑ | ❑ | ❑ | ❑ |
| TENSION—physical and motor manifestations of nervousness, over-activation | ❑ | ❑ | ❑ | ❑ | ❑ | ❑ | ❑ |
| MANNERISMS AND POSTURING—peculiar, bizarre, unnatural motor behavior (not including tic) | ❑ | ❑ | ❑ | ❑ | ❑ | ❑ | ❑ |
| GRANDIOSITY—exaggerated self-opinion, arrogance, conviction of unusual power or abilities | ❑ | ❑ | ❑ | ❑ | ❑ | ❑ | ❑ |
| DEPRESSIVE MOOD—sorrow, sadness, despondency, pessimism | ❑ | ❑ | ❑ | ❑ | ❑ | ❑ | ❑ |

*Continued*

| Appendix D-5 Brief Psychiatric Rating Scale—cont'd | Not Present | Very Mild | Mild | Moderate | Mod. Severe | Severe | Extremely Severe |
|---|---|---|---|---|---|---|---|
| HOSTILITY—animosity, contempt, belligerence, disdain for others | ❑ | ❑ | ❑ | ❑ | ❑ | ❑ | ❑ |
| SUSPICIOUSNESS—mistrust, belief others harbor malicious or discriminatory intent | ❑ | ❑ | ❑ | ❑ | ❑ | ❑ | ❑ |
| HALLUCINATORY BEHAVIOR—perceptions without normal stimulus correspondence | ❑ | ❑ | ❑ | ❑ | ❑ | ❑ | ❑ |
| MOTOR RETARDATION—slowed, weakened movements or speech, reduced body tone | ❑ | ❑ | ❑ | ❑ | ❑ | ❑ | ❑ |
| UNCOOPERATIVENESS—resistance, guardedness, rejection of authority | ❑ | ❑ | ❑ | ❑ | ❑ | ❑ | ❑ |
| UNUSUAL THOUGHT CONTENT—unusual, odd, strange, bizarre thought content | ❑ | ❑ | ❑ | ❑ | ❑ | ❑ | ❑ |
| BLUNTED AFFECT—reduced emotional tone, reduction in formal intensity of feelings, flatness | ❑ | ❑ | ❑ | ❑ | ❑ | ❑ | ❑ |
| EXCITEMENT—emotional tone, agitation, increased reactivity | ❑ | ❑ | ❑ | ❑ | ❑ | ❑ | ❑ |
| DISORIENTATION—confusion or lack of proper association for person, place, or time | ❑ | ❑ | ❑ | ❑ | ❑ | ❑ | ❑ |

Global Assessment Scale (Range 0-100) _____

From Overall, J.E., & Gorham, D.R. (1962). The Brief Psychiatric Rating Scale. *Psychological Reports, 10,* 799-812; reprinted by permission. Copyright Southern Universities Press, 1962.

## Appendix D-6 Sample Questions to Identify Personality Traits

*The nurse uses a variety of therapeutic techniques to obtain the answers to the following questions. Use your discretion and decide which questions are appropriate to complete your assessment.*

**The following questions are NOT meant to be used in a checklist fashion. They should be woven into the assessment, with only a few of the questions used for each diagnosis. Often the answer to one can eliminate certain diagnoses.**

### Obsessive-Compulsive Personality
1. Do you tend to drive yourself pretty hard, frequently feeling like you need to do just a little more? (yes)
2. Do you think that most people would view you as witty and light-hearted? (no)
3. Do you tend toward being a perfectionist? (yes)
4. Do you tend to keep lists or sometimes feel a need to keep checking things, like is the door locked? (yes)

### Dependent Personality
1. Is it sort of hard for you to argue with your spouse, because you're worried that he or she will really get mad at you and start to dislike you? (yes)
2. When you wake up in the morning, do you need to plan your day around the activities of your husband or wife? (yes)
3. Do you enjoy making most decisions in your house or would you prefer that others make most important decisions? (prefers others to make decision)
4. When you were younger, did you often dream of finding someone who would take care of you and guide you? (yes)

### Avoidant Personality
1. Throughout most of your life, have you found yourself being worried that people won't like you? (yes)
2. Do you often find yourself sort of feeling inadequate and not up to new challenges and tasks? (yes)
3. Do you tend to be very careful about selecting friends, perhaps only having one or two close friends in your whole life? (yes)
4. Have you often felt hurt by others, so that you are pretty wary of opening yourself to other people? (yes)

*Continued*

**Schizoid Personality**
1. Do you tend to really enjoy being around people, or do you much prefer being alone? (much prefers being alone)
2. Do you care a lot about what people think about you as a person? (tends not to care)
3. Are you a real emotional person? (no, feels strongly that he or she is not emotional)
4. During the course of your life, have you had only about one or two friends? (yes)

**Antisocial Personality**
1. If you felt like the situation really warranted it, do you think that you would find it pretty easy to lie? (yes)
2. Have you ever been arrested or pulled over by the police? (yes)
3. Over the years have you found yourself able to take care of yourself in a physical fight? (yes)
4. Do you sometimes find yourself resenting people who give you orders? (yes)

**Histrionic Personality**
1. Do people of the opposite sex frequently find you attractive? (answered with an unabashed "yes")
2. Do you frequently find yourself being the center of attention, even if you don't want to be? (yes)
3. Do you view yourself as being a powerfully emotional person? (yes)
4. Do you think that you'd make a reasonably good actor or actress? (yes)

**Narcissistic Personality**
1. Do you find that, when you get really down to it, most people aren't quite up to your standards? (yes)
2. If people give you a hard time, do you tend to put them in their place quickly? (yes)
3. If someone criticizes you, do you find yourself getting angry pretty quickly? (yes)
4. Do you think that, compared with other people, you are a very special person? (answered with a self-assured "yes")

## Appendix D-6  Sample Questions to Identify Personality Traits—cont'd

### Borderline Personality

1. Do you frequently feel let down by people? (yes)
2. If a friend or family member hurts you, do you sometimes feel like hurting yourself, perhaps by cutting at yourself and burning yourself? (yes)
3. Do you find that other people cause you to feel angry a couple of times per week? (yes)
4. Do you think that your friends would view you as sort of moody? (yes)
5. Does anxiety make you want to self-mutilate? (yes)

### Schizotypal Personality

1. Do you tend to stay by yourself, even though you would like to be with others? (yes)
2. Do you sometimes feel like other people are watching you or have some sort of special interest in you? (yes)
3. Have you ever felt like you had some special powers like ESP or some sort of magical influence over others? (yes)
4. Do you feel that people often want to reject you or that they find you odd? (yes)

### Paranoid Personality

1. Do you find that people often have a tendency to be disloyal or dishonest? (yes)
2. Is it fairly easy for you to get jealous, especially if someone is making eyes at your spouse? (yes)
3. Do you tend to keep things to yourself just to make sure the wrong people don't get the right information? (yes)
4. Do you feel that other people take advantage of you? (yes)

Adapted from Roberts, J.K.A. (1984). *Differential diagnoses in neuropsychiatry*. Chichester: John Wiley & Sons Limited, p. 26; and Shea, S.C. (1998). *Psychiatric interviewing: The art of understanding*. Philadelphia: W.B. Saunders, pp. 420-422; with permission.

## Appendix D-7A Michigan Alcohol Screening Test (MAST): Brief Version

### Scoring Yes to 3 or more indicates alcoholism.

1. Do you feel you are a normal drinker?
2. Do friends or relatives think you are a normal drinker?
3. Have you ever attended a meeting of Alcoholics Anonymous?
4. Have you ever gotten in trouble at work because of drinking?
5. Have you ever lost friends or girlfriends/boyfriends because of drinking?
6. Have you ever neglected your obligations, your family, or your work for 2 or more days in a row because of your drinking?
7. Have you ever had delirium tremens (DTs), severe shaking, or heard voices or seen things that were not there after heavy drinking?
8. Have you ever gone to anyone for help about your drinking?
9. Have you ever been in a hospital because of your drinking?
10. Have you ever been arrested for drunken driving or other drunken behavior?

From Pokorny, A.D., Miller, B.A., & Kaplan, H.B. (1972). The brief MAST: A shortened version of the Michigan Alcohol Screening Test. *American Journal of Psychiatry*, *129*, 342-345; reprinted by permission. Copyright © by 1972 American Psychiatric Association; *http://ajp.psychiatryonline.org*.

## Appendix D-7B Drug Abuse Screening Test (DAST)

The following questions concern information about your involvement with drugs *not including alcoholic beverages* during the past 12 months.

In the statements, "drug abuse" refers (1) to the use of prescribed or OTC drugs in excess of the directions and (2) any nonmedical use of drugs. The various classes of drugs may include cannabis, solvents, antianxiety drugs, sedative-hypnotics, cocaine, stimulants, hallucinogens, and narcotics. Remember that the questions *do not include alcoholic beverages*.

These questions refer to the past 12 months.

## Appendix D-7B Drug Abuse Screening Test (DAST)—cont'd

| | |
|---|---|
| Have you used drugs other than those required for medical purposes? | Yes _____ No _____ |
| Do you abuse more than one drug at a time? | Yes _____ No _____ |
| Are you always able to stop using drugs when you want to? | Yes _____ No _____ |
| Have you had "blackouts" or "flashbacks" as a result of drug use? | Yes _____ No _____ |
| Do you ever feel bad about your drug abuse? | Yes _____ No _____ |
| Does your spouse (or parents) ever complain about your involvement with drugs? | Yes _____ No _____ |
| Have you neglected your family because of your use of drugs? | Yes _____ No _____ |
| Have you engaged in illegal activities in order to obtain drugs? | Yes _____ No _____ |
| Have you ever experienced withdrawal symptoms (felt sick) when you stopped taking drugs? | Yes _____ No _____ |
| Have you had medical problems as a result of your drug use (e.g., memory loss, hepatitis, convulsions, bleeding, etc.)? | Yes _____ No _____ |
| **Scoring:** 1 positive response warrants further evaluation. | Yes _____ No _____ |

From Skinner, H.A. (1982). Drug Abuse Screening Test (DAST). Langford Lance, England: Elsevier Science, p. 363; reprinted with permission.

## Appendix D-7C Brief Nursing Assessment— Emergency Department

*The nurse uses a variety of therapeutic techniques to obtain the answers to the following questions. Use your discretion and decide which questions are appropriate to complete your assessment.*

**If the client is impaired or unable to focus, friends and family members may be able to answer for the client.**
1. What drug(s) did you take before coming to the emergency department/hospital/clinic/session?
2. How did you take the drug(s) (e.g., intravenously, intramuscularly, orally, subcutaneously, smoking, intranasally)?

*Continued*

## Appendix D-7C Brief Nursing Assessment— Emergency Department—cont'd

3. How much did you take (e.g., glasses of beer/wine/ whisky)?
4. When was the last dose taken?
5. How long have you been using the substance? When did you start this last episode of use?
6. How often and how much do you usually use?
7. What kinds of problems have substance use caused for you? With your family/friends? Job? Health? Finances? The law?

## Appendix D-8 Criteria for Hospital Admission for Clients with an Eating Disorder

### Physical Criteria

1. Weight loss over 30% over 6 months
2. Rapid decline in weight
3. Severe hypothermia as a result of loss of subcutaneous tissue or dehydration (temperature less than 36° C or 96.8° F)
4. Inability to gain weight repeatedly with outpatient treatment
5. Heart rate less than 40 beats/minute
6. Systolic blood pressure less than 70 mmHg
7. Hypokalemia (potassium under 3 mEq/L) or other electrolyte disturbances not corrected by oral supplementation
8. Electrocardiograph changes (especially arrhythmias)

### Psychiatric Criteria

1. Suicidal or severely out-of-control self-mutilating behaviors
2. Out-of-control use of laxatives, emetics, diuretics, or street drugs
3. Failure to comply with treatment contract
4. Severe depression
5. Psychosis
6. Family crisis/dysfunction

## Appendix D-9 Functional Dementia Scale

Circle one rating for each item:
1. None or little of the time
2. Some of the time
3. Good part of the time
4. Most or all of the time

Client_____
Observer_____
Position or relation to
  patient_____
Facility_____
Date_____

1 2 3 4  (1)  Has difficulty in completing simple tasks on own (e.g., dressing, bathing, doing arithmetic).

1 2 3 4  (2)  Spends time either sitting or in apparently purposeless activity.

1 2 3 4  (3)  Wanders at night or needs to be restrained to prevent wandering.

1 2 3 4  (4)  Hears things that are not there.

1 2 3 4  (5)  Requires supervision or assistance in eating.

1 2 3 4  (6)  Loses things.

1 2 3 4  (7)  Appearance is disorderly if left to own devices.

1 2 3 4  (8)  Moans.

1 2 3 4  (9)  Cannot control bowel function.

1 2 3 4  (10)  Threatens to harm others.

1 2 3 4  (11)  Cannot control bladder function.

1 2 3 4  (12)  Needs to be watched so doesn't injure self (e.g., by careless smoking, leaving the stove on, falling).

1 2 3 4  (13)  Destructive of materials around him/her (e.g., breaks furniture, throws food trays, tears up magazines).

1 2 3 4  (14)  Shouts or yells.

1 2 3 4  (15)  Accuses others of doing him bodily harm or stealing his/her possessions—when you are sure the accusations are not true.

1 2 3 4  (16)  Is unaware of limitations imposed by illness.

1 2 3 4  (17)  Becomes confused and does not know where he/she is.

1 2 3 4  (18)  Has trouble remembering.

1 2 3 4  (19)  Has sudden changes of mood (e.g., gets upset, angered, or cries easily).

1 2 3 4  (20)  If left alone, wanders aimlessly during the day or needs to be restrained to prevent wandering

## Appendix D-10 Life-Changing Events Questionnaire

| Life-Changing Event | Life Change Unit (LCU) |
| --- | --- |
| **Health** | |
| An injury or illness that: | |
| Kept you in bed a week or more, or sent you to the hospital | 74 |
| Was less serious than above | 44 |
| Major dental work | 26 |
| Major change in eating habits | 27 |
| Major change in sleep habits | 26 |
| Major change in your usual type and/or amount of recreation | 28 |
| **Work** | |
| Change to a new type of work | 51 |
| Change in your work hours or conditions | 35 |
| Change in your responsibilities at work: | |
| More responsibilities | 29 |
| Fewer responsibilities | 21 |
| Promotion | 31 |
| Demotion | 42 |
| Transfer | 32 |
| Troubles at work: | |
| With your boss | 29 |
| With coworkers | 35 |
| With persons under your supervision | 35 |
| Other work troubles | 28 |
| Major business adjustment | 60 |
| Retirement | 52 |
| Loss of job: | |
| Laid off from work | 68 |
| Fired from work | 79 |
| Correspondence course to help you in your work | 18 |

From Miller, M.A., & Rahe, R.H. (1997). Life changes scaling for the 1990s. *Journal of Psychosomatic Research, 43*(3), 279-292.

Six-month totals ≥ 300 LCUs or 1-year totals ≥ 500 LCUs are considered indications of high recent life stress.

## Appendix D-10 **Life-Changing Events Questionnaire—cont'd**

| Life-Changing Event | Life Change Unit (LCU) |
|---|---|
| **Home and Family** | |
| Major change in living conditions | 42 |
| Change in residence: | |
|    Move within the same town or city | 25 |
|    Move to a different town, city, or state | 47 |
| Change in family get-togethers | 25 |
| Major change in health or behavior of family member | 55 |
| Marriage | 50 |
| Pregnancy | 67 |
| Miscarriage or abortion | 65 |
| Gain of a new family member: | |
|    Birth of a child | 66 |
|    Adoption of a child | 65 |
|    A relative moving in with you | 59 |
| Spouse beginning or ending work | 46 |
| Child leaving home: | |
|    To attend college | 41 |
|    Due to marriage | 41 |
|    For other reasons | 45 |
| Change in arguments with spouse | 50 |
| In-law problems | 38 |
| Change in the marital status of your parents: | |
|    Divorce | 59 |
|    Remarriage | 50 |
| Separation from spouse: | |
|    Due to work | 53 |
|    Due to marital problems | 76 |
| Divorce | 96 |
| Birth of a grandchild | 43 |
| Death of spouse | 119 |
| Death of other family member: | |
|    Child | 123 |
|    Brother or sister | 102 |
|    Parent | 100 |

*Continued*

| Appendix D-10 **Life-Changing Events Questionnaire—cont'd** | |
| --- | --- |
| **Life-Changing Event** | **Life Change Unit (LCU)** |
| **Personal and Social** | |
| Change in personal habits | 26 |
| Beginning or ending school or college | 38 |
| Change of school or college | 35 |
| Change in political beliefs | 24 |
| Change in religious beliefs | 29 |
| Change in social activities | 27 |
| Vacation | 24 |
| New close personal relationship | 37 |
| Engagement to marry | 45 |
| Girlfriend or boyfriend problems | 39 |
| Sexual differences | 44 |
| "Falling out" of a close personal relationship | 47 |
| An accident | 48 |
| Minor violation of the law | 20 |
| Being held in jail | 75 |
| Death of a close friend | 70 |
| Major decision regarding your immediate future | 51 |
| Major personal achievement | 36 |
| **Financial** | |
| Major change in finances: | |
|    Increase in income | 38 |
|    Decrease in income | 60 |
|    Investment and/or credit difficulties | 56 |
| Loss or damage of personal property | 43 |
| Moderate purchase | 20 |
| Major purchase | 37 |
| Foreclosure on a mortgage or loan | 58 |

From Miller, M.A., & Rahe, R.H. (1997). Life changes scaling for the 1990s. *Journal of Psychosomatic Research, 43*(3), 279-292.

Six-month totals ≥ 300 LCUs or 1-year totals ≥ 500 LCUs are considered indications of high recent life stress.

## Appendix D-11 Abuse Assessment Screen

1. Have you ever been emotionally or physically abused by your partner or someone important to you?

   Yes _____     No _____

   If yes, by whom? _____

   Number of times _____

2. Within the past year, have you been hit, slapped, kicked, or otherwise physically hurt by someone?

   Yes _____     No _____

   If yes, by whom? _____

   Number of times _____

3. Since you have been pregnant, have you been hit, slapped, kicked, or otherwise physically hurt by someone?

   Yes _____     No _____

   If yes, by whom? _____

   Number of times _____

4. Within the past year, has anyone forced you to have sexual activities?

   Yes _____     No _____

   If yes, by whom? _____

   Number of times _____

5. Are you afraid of your partner or anyone listed above?

   Yes _____     No _____

The Abuse Assessment Screen was developed by the Nursing Research Consortium on Violence and Abuse (1989). Its reproduction and use is encouraged. Used with permission of Peace at Home, Boston, Massachusetts.

## Appendix D-12 SAD PERSONS Scale

| S | Sex | Men kill themselves three times more than women, although women make attempts three times more often than men. |
|---|---|---|
| A | Age | High-risk groups: 19 years or younger; 45 years or older, especially the elderly (65 years or over). |
| D | Depression | Studies report that 35% to 79% of those who attempt suicide manifested a depressive syndrome. |
| P | Previous attempts | Of those who commit suicide, 65% to 70% have made previous attempts. |

*Continued*

## Appendix D-12 SAD PERSONS Scale—cont'd

| | | |
|---|---|---|
| **E** | ETOH | ETOH (alcohol) is associated with up to 65% of successful suicides. Estimates are that 15% of alcoholics commit suicide. Heavy drug use is considered to be in this group and is given the same weight as alcohol. |
| **R** | Rational thinking loss | People with functional or organic psychoses (schizophrenia, dementia) are more apt to commit suicide than those in the general population. |
| **S** | Social supports lacking | A suicidal person often lacks significant others (friends, relatives), meaningful employment, and religious or spiritual supports. All three of these areas need to be assessed. |
| **O** | Organized plan | The presence of a specific plan for suicide (date, place, means) signifies a person at high risk. |
| **N** | No spouse | Repeated studies indicate that people who are widowed, separated, divorced, or single are at greater risk than those who are married. |
| **S** | Sickness | Chronic, debilitating, and severe illness is a risk factor. Suicide risk is two times higher among people with cancer and is high among AIDS clients; clients on hemodialysis or with DTs and respiratory diseases are all at high risk. |
| **Points** | | **Guidelines for Points Intervention** |
| 0-2 | | Treat at home with follow-up care. |
| 3-4 | | Closely follow up and consider possible hospitalization. |
| 5-6 | | Strongly consider hospitalization. |
| 7-10 | | Hospitalize. |

Adapted from Patterson, W., et al. (1983). Evaluation of suicidal patients: The SAD PERSONS Scale. *Psychosomatics, 24*(4), 343; reprinted with permission.

## Appendix D-13 Overt Aggression Scale

**Verbal Aggression**
_____ Makes loud noises, shouts angrily
_____ Yells mild personal insults (e.g., "You're stupid.")
_____ Curses viciously, uses foul language in anger, makes moderate threats to others or self
_____ Makes clear threats of violence towards others or self ("I'm gonna kill you.") or requests help to control self

**Physical Aggression against Objects**
_____ Slams doors, scatters clothing, makes a mess
_____ Throws objects down, kicks furniture without breaking it, marks the wall
_____ Breaks objects, smashes window
_____ Sets fires, throws objects dangerously

**Physical Aggression against Self**
_____ Picks or scratches skin, hits self, pulls hair (with no or minor injury only)
_____ Bangs head, hits fist into objects, throws self onto floor or onto objects (hurts self without serious injury)
_____ Small cuts or bruises, minor burns
_____ Mutilates self; causes deep cuts, bites that bleed, internal injury, fracture, loss of consciousness, loss of teeth

**Physical Aggression against Other People**
_____ Makes threatening gesture, swings at people, grabs at clothes
_____ Strikes, kicks, pushes, pulls hair (without injury to them)
_____ Attacks others, causing mild-moderate physical injury (bruises, sprain, welts)
_____ Attacks others, causing severe physical injury (broken bones, deep lacerations, internal injury)

From Yudofsky, S.C., Silver, J.M., Jackson, W., et al. (1986). The Overt Aggression Scale for the objective rating of verbal and physical aggression. *American Journal of Psychiatry, 143,* 35-39; reprinted with permission. Copyright © by 1986 American Psychiatric Association; *http://ajp.psychiatry online.org.*

## Appendix D-14 Abnormal Involuntary Movement Scale (AIMS)

Public Health Service
Alcohol, Drug Abuse, and
 Mental Health Administration
National Institute of
 Mental Health

NAME:_____
DATE:_____
**Prescribing
 Practitioner:_____**
**CODE:** 0 = None
1 = Minimal,
 may be
 extreme
 normal
2 = Mild
3 = Moderate
4 = Severe

**INSTRUCTIONS:**
**Complete examination
 procedure before
 making ratings**

| **MOVEMENT RATINGS:** | | Rater | Rater |
|---|---|---|---|
| Rate highest severity observed. | | | |
| Rate movements that occur upon activation one *less* than those observed spontaneously. Circle movement as well as code number that applies. | | Date | Date |
| **Facial and Oral Movements** | **1. Muscles of facial expression** (e.g., movements of forehead, eyebrows periorbital area, cheeks, including frowning, blinking, smiling, grimacing) | 0 1 2 3 4 | 0 1 2 3 4 |
| | **2. Lips and perioral area** (e.g., puckering, pouting, smacking) | 0 1 2 3 4 | 0 1 2 3 4 |
| | **3. Jaw** (e.g., biting, clenching, chewing, mouth opening, lateral movement) | 0 1 2 3 4 | 0 1 2 3 4 |
| | 4. **Tongue:** Rate only increases in movement both in and out of mouth, *not* | 0 1 2 3 4 | 0 1 2 3 4 |

| Appendix D-14 **Abnormal Involuntary Movement Scale (AIMS)—cont'd** | | |
|---|---|---|
| | inability to sustain movement. Darting in and out of mouth. | |
| **Extremity Movements** | 5. **Upper (arms, wrists, hands, fingers):** Include choreic movements (i.e., rapid, objectively purposeless, irregular, spontaneous) and athetoid movements (i.e., slow, irregular, complex, serpentine). *Do not include tremor* (i.e., repetitive, regular, rhythmic). | 0 1 2 3 4   0 1 2 3 4 |
| | 6. **Lower (legs, knees, ankles, toes)** (e.g., lateral knee movement, foot tapping, heel dropping, foot squirming, inversion and eversion of foot) | 0 1 2 3 4   0 1 2 3 4 |
| **Trunk Movements** | 7. **Neck, shoulders, hips** (e.g., rocking, twisting, squirming, pelvic gyrations) | 0 1 2 3 4   0 1 2 3 4 |
| **Global Judgments** | 8. **Severity of abnormal movements overall** | 0 1 2 3 4   0 1 2 3 4 |
| | 9. **Incapacitation due to abnormal movements** | 0 1 2 3 4   0 1 2 3 4 |

*Continued*

| Appendix D-14 **Abnormal Involuntary Movement Scale (AIMS)—cont'd** |
|---|

| | | | |
|---|---|---|---|
| | 10. **Patient's awareness of abnormal movements.** Rate only patient's report.<br>No awareness<br>Aware, no distress<br>Aware, mild distress<br>Aware, moderate distress<br>Aware, severe distress | 0 1 2 3 4 | 0 1 2 3 4 |
| **Dental Status** | 11. **Current problems with teeth and/or dentures** | No Yes | No Yes |
| | 12. **Are dentures usually worn?** | No Yes | No Yes |
| | 13. **Edentia?** | No Yes | No Yes |
| | 14. **Do movements disappear in sleep?** | No Yes | No Yes |

**AIMS Examination Procedure**

Either before or after completing the Examination Procedure, observe the patient unobtrusively, at rest (e.g., in waiting room).

The chair to be used in this examination should be a hard, firm one without arms.

1. Ask patient whether there is anything in his/her mouth (i.e., gum, candy) and if there is, to remove it.
2. Ask patient about the *current* condition of his/her teeth. Ask patient if he/she wears dentures. Do teeth or denture bother patient now?
3. Ask patient whether he/she notices any movements in mouth, face, hands, or feet. If yes, ask to describe and to what extent they *currently* bother patient or interfere with his/her activities.
4. Have patient sit in chair with hands on knees, legs slightly apart, and feet flat on floor. (Look at entire body for movements while in this position.)

## Appendix D-14 Abnormal Involuntary Movement Scale (AIMS)—cont'd

5. Ask patient to sit with hands hanging unsupported. If male, between legs; if female and wearing a dress, hanging over knees. (Observe hands and other body areas.)

6. Ask patient to open mouth. (Observe tongue at rest within mouth.) Do this twice.

7. Ask patient to protrude tongue. (Observe abnormalities of tongue movement.) Do this twice.

8. *Ask patient to tap thumb with each finger as rapidly as possible for 10 to 15 seconds; separately with right hand, then with left hand. (Observe facial and leg movement.)

9. Flex and extend patient's left and right arms (one at a time). (Note any rigidity.)

10. Ask patient to stand up. (Observe in profile. Observe all body areas again, hips included.)

11. *Ask patient to extend both arms outstretched in front with palms down. (Observe trunk, legs, and mouth.)

12. *Have patient walk a few paces, turn, and walk back to chair. (Observe hands and gait.) Do this twice.

*Activated movements.

# APPENDIX E

# Defense Mechanisms

| MILD USE | EXTREME EXAMPLE |
|---|---|
| **Repression** | |
| Man forgets wife's birthday after a marital fight. | Woman is unable to enjoy sex after having pushed out of awareness a traumatic sexual incident from childhood. |
| **Sublimation** | |
| Woman who is angry with her boss writes a short story about a heroic woman. By definition, use of sublimation is always constructive. | None. |
| **Regression** | |
| Four-year-old with a new baby brother starts sucking his thumb and wanting a bottle. | Man who loses a promotion starts complaining to others, hands in sloppy work, misses appointments, and comes in late for meetings. |

From Varcarolis, E.M. (2002). *Foundations of psychiatric mental health nursing* (4th ed.). Philadelphia: W.B. Saunders.

| **MILD USE** | **EXTREME EXAMPLE** |
|---|---|

### Displacement

| Patient criticizes a nurse after his family fails to visit. | Child who is unable to acknowledge fear of his father becomes fearful of animals. |
|---|---|

### Projection

| Man who is unconsciously attracted to other women teases his wife about flirting. | Woman who has repressed an attraction toward other women refuses to socialize. She fears another woman will make homosexual advances toward her. |
|---|---|

### Compensation

| Short man becomes assertively verbal and excels in business. | Individual drinks when self-esteem is low to diffuse discomfort temporarily. |
|---|---|

### Reaction-Formation

| Recovering alcoholic constantly preaches about the evils of drink. | Mother who has an unconscious hostility toward her daughter is overprotective and hovers over her to protect her from harm, interfering with her normal growth and development. |
|---|---|

### Denial

| Man reacts to news of the death of a loved one by saying, "No, I don't believe you. The doctor said he was fine." | Woman whose husband died 3 years ago still keeps his clothes in the closet and talks about him in the present tense. |
|---|---|

### Conversion

| Student is unable to take a final examination because of a terrible headache. | Man becomes blind after seeing his wife flirt with other men. |
|---|---|

| MILD USE | EXTREME EXAMPLE |
|---|---|

### Undoing

| | |
|---|---|
| After flirting with her male secretary, a woman brings her husband tickets to a show. | Man with rigid and moralistic beliefs and repressed sexuality is driven to wash his hands when around attractive women to gain composure. |

### Rationalization

| | |
|---|---|
| "I didn't get the raise because the boss doesn't like me." | Father who thinks his son was fathered by another man excuses his malicious treatment of the boy by saying, "He is lazy and disobedient," when that is not the case. |

### Identification

| | |
|---|---|
| Five-year-old girl dresses in her mother's shoes and dress and meets her father at the door. | Young boy thinks a pimp in the neighborhood with money and drugs is someone to look up to. |

### Introjection

| | |
|---|---|
| After his wife's death, husband has transient complaints of chest pains and difficulty breathing—the symptoms his wife had before she died. | Young child whose parents were overcritical and belittling grows up thinking that she is not any good. She has taken on her parent's evaluation of her as part of her self-image. |

### Suppression

| | |
|---|---|
| Businessman who is preparing to make an important speech that day is told by his wife that morning that she wants a divorce. Although visibly upset, he puts the incident aside until after his speech, when he can give the matter his total concentration. | A woman who feels a lump in her breast shortly before leaving for a 3-week vacation puts the information in the back of her mind until after returning from her vacation. |

# APPENDIX F

# Nursing Care in Electroconvulsive Therapy

| | |
|---|---|
| 1. Emotional and educational support to the client and family | 1a. Encourage the client to discuss feelings, including myths regarding ECT. |
| | 1b. Teach the client and the family what to expect with ECT. |
| 2. Pretreatment protocol | 2a. Ascertain if the client and the family have received a full explanation, including the option to withdraw the consent at any time. |
| | 2b. Pretreatment care: |
| | • Withhold food and fluids for 6 to 8 hours before treatment. (Cardiac medication is given with sips of water.) |

Data from Burns, C.M., & Stuart, G.W. (1991). Nursing care in electroconvulsive therapy. *Psychiatric Clinics of North America*, *14(4)*, 971.

*ECG*, Electrocardiographic; *ECT*, electroconvulsive therapy; *EEG*, electroencephalographic.

- Remove dentures, glasses, hearing aids, contact lenses, hairpins, and so on.
- Have client void before treatment.

2c. Preoperative medications (if ordered):
- Give either glycopyrrolate (Robinul) or atropine to prevent potential for aspiration and to help minimize bradyarrhythmias in response to electrical stimulants.

3. Nursing care during the procedure

3a. Place a blood pressure cuff on one of the client's arms.

3b. As the intravenous line is inserted and EEG and ECG electrodes are attached, give a brief explanation to the client.

3c. Clip the pulse oximeter to the client's finger.

3d. Monitor blood pressure throughout treatment.

3e. Medications given:
- Short-acting anesthetic (methohexital sodium [Brevital], thiopental [Pentothal])
- Muscle relaxant (succinylcholine [Anectine])
- 100% oxygen by mask via positive pressure throughout

| | |
|---|---|
| | 3f. Check that the bite block is in place to prevent biting of the tongue. |
| | 3g. Electrical stimulus given (seizure should last 30 to 60 seconds). |
| 4. Posttreatment nursing care | 4a. Have the client go to a properly staffed recovery room (with blood pressure cuff and oximeter in place) where oxygen, suction, and other emergency equipment is available. |
| | 4b. Once the client is awake, talk to the client and check vital signs. |
| | 4c. Often the client is confused, so give frequent orientation reassurance. Orientation statements are brief, distinct, and simple. |
| | 4d. Return the client to the unit after he or she has maintained a 90% oxygen saturation level, vital signs are stable, and mental status is satisfactory. |
| | 4e. Check the gag reflex before giving the client fluids, medicine, or breakfast. |

# APPENDIX G

# Drug Monographs

## aripiprazole
*Category:*
Atypical antipsychotic
*Trade Name:*
Abilify

### Uses

1. Used to treat the symptoms of schizophrenia; targets the positive, negative, and depressive symptoms of schizophrenia
2. Unlabeled use with bipolar disorder and dementia of the Alzheimer's type

### Action

Aripiprazole has unique pharmacologic properties. It acts as a weak stimulator (partial agonist) at dopamine $D_2$ receptors, with the potential for exerting either antagonistic (inhibitory) or agonistic (stimulating) effects to modulate levels of dopamine ($D_2$) activity in the brain.
Aripiprazole:

- Is a partial agonist that uniquely modulates $D_2$ activity in the brain
- Has serotonin antagonists activity at $5\text{-}HT_{2A}$ receptors and partial agonist activity at $5\text{-}HT_{1A}$ receptors
- Has moderate affinity for alpha$_1$-adrenergic and histamine ($H_1$) receptors
- Has no appreciable affinity for cholinergic muscarinic receptors

### Dosages and Routes

*Adults:* 10-15 mg/day is usual therapeutic dose; increments to be made at least after a 2-week interval; dose range 5-30 mg/day; maintain at the lowest therapeutic dose

## Contraindications

Hypersensitivity, seizure disorders, lactation

## Cautions

1. The safety of aripiprazole during pregnancy and breastfeeding is not known.
2. Use with caution in clients with seizure disorders.
3. Because this drug is associated with orthostatic hypotension, use with caution in clients with known:
   - Cardiovascular disease.
   - Cerebrovascular disease.
   - Conditions that would predispose them to hypotension.
4. There are many potential drug interactions with this drug, and the dose of aripiprazole may have to be altered and the client more carefully monitored. Some drugs that can cause potential drug interactions include:
   - Carbamazepine (Tegretol)
   - Ketoconazole (Nisoral)
   - Quinidine
   - Fluoxetine (Prozac)
   - Paroxetine (Paxil)

## Remarks

This medication is usually well tolerated. Positive aspects of this new antipsychotic include no significant weight gain, no changes in plasma glucose levels, and no increase in serum cholesterol or other lipids. The drug does not increase prolactin levels, and so far there have been no reports of heart rhythm abnormalities.

## Adverse Reactions

*More Frequent:* Anxiety, constipation, headache, insomnia, nausea, vomiting

*Less Frequent:* Akathisia, asthenia, cough, fever, lightheadedness, orthostatic hypotension rhinitis, skin rash, somnolence tardive dyskinesia, tremors

*Rare or Very Rare:* Blurred vision, dysphasia, heat stroke, neuroleptic malignant syndrome (NMS), seizures

## Toxic Effects

As with other antipsychotic mediation, NMS has been reported, although it is very rare. The client should be monitored for possible akathisia, fever, skin rash, dysphasia, heat stroke, and seizures throughout maintenance therapy.

### Nursing Measures

1. Monitor blood pressure (BP) lying and standing. Assess for potential orthostatic hypotension. Instruct client to get up slowly from a lying position and dangle the legs before getting out of bed.
2. Although the risk of extrapyramidal symptoms (EPS) is much lower than with older neuroleptic agents, akathisia may have a different basis than other movement disorders. Akathisia is often overlooked. It involves extreme subjective distress with a kind of "anxiety" that involves a physical sense of discomfort partially relieved by moving around. Clients should report these symptoms if they occur.

### Inform Client and Family

1. Although this drug can be taken with or without food, taking the drug in the morning with breakfast may minimize the common side effects of nausea and insomnia.

2. Take the medication on a regular basis and do not miss any doses.
3. Do not stop this medication without first discussing this with the prescriber.
4. Avoid the use of alcohol, which may cause significant drowsiness and disorientation when used with aripiprazole.
5. Avoid driving and other potentially dangerous activities when drowsiness occurs. Drowsiness may diminish over time, but the drowsiness is greater at higher doses.
6. Avoid exposure to excessively warm temperatures. Drink plenty of fluids. Difficulty regulating temperatures has been associated with medications used to treat psychotic symptoms.

## benztropine mesylate

*Category:* Antiparkinsonian
*Trade Name:* Cogentin

### Uses

1. Treatment of Parkinson's disease

2. Treatment of EPS (except tardive dyskinesia) caused by use of neuroleptic/antipsychotic medications

## Action

Cogentin is an anticholinergic agent. This drug increases and prolongs the dopamine activity in the central nervous system (CNS), thereby correcting neurotransmitter imbalances and minimizing involuntary movements.

## Dosages and Routes

- *Adults:* 0.5-1 mg/day PO initially; gradually increase to 4-6 mg/day; *for drug-induced extrapyramidal symptoms:* 1-4 mg IM/PO 1-2 times daily; *for acute dystonic reactions:* 0.5-2 mg IM or IV
- *Elderly:* Use lower doses

## Contraindications

Narrow-angle glaucoma, pyloric or duodenal obstruction, peptic ulcers, prostatic hypertrophy, obstructions of the bladder neck, myasthenia gravis, children under 3 years of age; rarely indicated for children

## Cautions

The elderly and clients with cardiac, liver, or kidney disease or hypertension; also used with caution in clients taking barbiturates or alcohol

## Remarks

The effects of benztropine are cumulative and may not be evident for 2 or 3 days. After 4 to 6 months of long-term maintenance antipsychotic therapy, antiparkinsonian drugs can be used on an as necessary basis or withdrawn. Some clients respond best to the medication being given every day; others do better with divided doses. Long-term use of benztropine with a neuroleptic can predispose a client to tardive dyskinesia.

## Adverse Reactions

*Autonomic:* Dry mouth, blurred vision, nausea, restlessness
*CNS:* Sedation, vertigo, paresthesias
*Cardiovascular:* Palpitations, tachycardia
*Gastrointestinal:* Nausea, vomiting, constipation, paralytic ileus
*Genitourinary:* Dysuria, urinary retention

*Ocular:* Blurred vision, mydriasis, photophobia
*Other:* Anhidrosis (abnormal deficiency of sweat)

## Toxic Effects

*CNS:* Confusion; disorientation; unusual uncontrolled movements, especially around the face

## Nursing Measures

1. Monitor intake and output and observe for urinary retention.
2. Give medication after the client voids to reduce the possibility of urinary retention.
3. Monitor for constipation. Abdominal pain or distention may indicate potential for paralytic ileus.
4. Indications of CNS toxicity (e.g., depression or excitement, hallucinations, psychosis) warrant withholding the drug and informing the physician immediately.

## Inform Client

1. Avoid driving or operating hazardous equipment if drowsiness or dizziness occurs.
2. Tolerance to heat may be reduced owing to a diminished ability to sweat. Plan periods of rest in cool places during the day.
3. Stop taking the medication if CNS toxic effects, difficulty swallowing or speaking, or vomiting occurs. Inform the physician immediately.
4. Monitor urinary output and watch for signs of constipation.
5. Consult with a physician before using any other medication, prescribed or over-the-counter (OTC), once started on benztropine.

## bupropion

*Category:*
Antidepressant, smoking cessation aid
*Trade Names:*
Wellbutrin, Wellbutrin SR (sustained release), Zyban

## Uses

1. Treatment of depression (particularly endogenous)
2. Smoking cessation (Zyban)
3. Unlabeled used in attention deficit hyperactivity disorder in adults and children

## Action

This medication blocks reuptake of neurotransmitters serotonin and norepinephrine at the CNS presynaptic membranes and reduces the firing rate of nonadrenergic neurons, eliminating nicotine withdrawal symptoms.

## Dosages and Routes

- *Adults:* Initially 100 mg 2 times/day; may increase to 100 mg 3 times/day after beginning therapy; gradually increase dose to minimize agitation, motor restlessness, and insomnia; *maximum*: 450 mg/day; maintain on lowest effective dose
- *Sustained-Release (SR):* Initially 150 mg/day as a single dose in the morning; may increase to 300 mg/day at 150 mg 2 times/day as early as day 4; *maximum:* 400 mg/day; maintain on lowest effective dose
- *Smoking Cessation (Zyban):* Initially 150 mg daily for 3 days, then 150 mg 2 times/day
- *Children:* Safety and efficacy not established in those under 18 years old

## Contraindications

Seizure disorder, current or previous diagnosis of bulimia or anorexia, concurrent use of monoamine oxidase inhibitors (MAOIs), head trauma, CNS tumor, recent myocardial infarction (MI), nursing mothers

## Cautions

History of seizures, cranial trauma, concurrent use of antipsychotics or other antidepressants, impaired renal or hepatic function, pregnancy

## Remarks

1. The low overall side effects give this the lowest dropout percentage (9%).
2. No anticholinergic, antihistamine, antiserotonergic, cardiovascular, or sedating side effects.
3. Low mania induction.
4. Low sexual side effects.
5. The seizure risk is significantly higher in "at risk" individuals (e.g., bulimics, those with head injury or a history of seizures).

## Adverse Reactions

*Frequent (18%-32%):*
Constipation, weight gain or loss, nausea, vomiting, anorexia, dry mouth headache, increased sweating, tremor, sedation, insomnia, dizziness, agitation
*Occasional:* Diarrhea, akinesia, blurred vision, tachycardia, confusion, hostility, fatigue

## Toxic Effects

Reactions may include increased seizures with an increase in dosage greater than 150 mg/day in clients with a history of bulimia or seizure disorders.

## Nursing Measures

1. Baseline liver and renal function tests should be periodically performed for those on long-term therapy.
2. Electrocardiograph (ECG) changes may occur with long-term use. Monitor vital signs and assess for changes in cardiac rhythm.
3. Assess for suicidal history and active risk.
4. Assess baseline of depressive level (thoughts, energy level, feelings, appearance, behavior, speech pattern, level of interest and mood).

## Inform Client and Family

1. Full therapeutic effect may take up to 4 weeks.
2. Avoid tasks that require alertness or motor skills until a response to the drug is established.
3. Avoid alcohol, which can increase the risk for seizures.
4. Check with the prescriber before taking OTC drugs.
5. Alert the health care provider if cardiac palpitations or heart beat changes occur.

# buspirone hydrochloride
*Category:* Antianxiety agent
*Trade Name:* BuSpar

## Uses

Management of anxiety disorders

## Action

The exact action of buspirone is not clear.

It may exert a potent presynaptic dopamine antagonist effect in the CNS, resulting in increased dopamine at the synapses. It may also have an effect on serotonin receptors.

## Dosages and Routes

- *Adults and Elderly:* 5 mg PO 2-3 times daily; may increase 5 mg every 3-4 days; *maintenance:* 15-30 mg/day in 2-3 divided doses and not to exceed 60 mg/day

## Contraindications

Severe renal or hepatic impairment, clients on MAOIs

## Cautions

Renal or hepatic impairment, pregnant or lactating women, elderly or debilitated clients

## Remarks

The advantages of buspirone are that it does not cause sedation, tolerance does not develop, and it is not addictive. The drug has a more favorable side effect profile than the benzodiazepines.

## Adverse Reactions

Dizziness, nausea, headache, nervousness, lightheadedness, and excitement, which generally are not major problems; other less common problems may occur (e.g., blurred vision, tachycardia, palpitations, paresthesia, abdominal distention)

## Toxic Effects

Overdose may produce severe nausea, vomiting, dizziness, drowsiness, abdominal distention, and excessive pupil constriction.

## Nursing Measures

1. Offer emotional support to anxious clients.
2. Liver and renal function tests and blood counts should be done regularly for clients on long-term therapy.
3. Assist with ambulation and put other safety features in place if dizziness and lightheadedness occur.

## Inform Client

1. Teach the client to inform the physician:
   - About any medications (prescription or nonprescription),

alcohol, or drugs being taken.
- If she is now or plans to get pregnant.
- If she is breastfeeding an infant.

2. Do not drive a car or operate potentially dangerous machinery until you experience how this medication will affect you.
3. Notify the physician of difficulty breathing, changes in vision, sweating, flushing, or cardiac problems.
4. Improvement may be noted in 7 to 10 days, but it may take 3 to 4 weeks or longer to note therapeutic effects.

## carbamazepine

*Category:* Anticonvulsant, antineuralgic, bipolar disorder
*Trade Names:* Tegretol, Epitol, Mazepine

## Uses

1. Management of generalized tonic-clonic seizures (grand mal) and psychomotor seizures
2. Management of trigeminal neuralgia
3. Potential mood stabilizer, particularly in acute mania; used clinically, but not Food and Drug Administration (FDA) approved at present for this use

## Action

Reduces post-tetanic potentiation at the synapse, preventing repetitive discharge

## Dosages and Routes

- *For Seizures:* PO only (tablets, suspension, and chewable tablets)
- *Adults:* 100-200 mg twice daily, gradually increase until response is attained; *maintenance*: 800-1200 mg/day
- *Children (6-12 Years):* 15-30 mg/kg/day administered in divided doses
  *Note:* Oral suspensions produce higher peak concentrations. Going from tablets to suspension, give in smaller and more frequent doses.

## Contraindications

History of bone marrow depression, history of hypersensitivity to tricyclic antidepressants (TCAs)

## Cautions

Impaired cardiac, hepatic, and renal function; pregnancy or lactation (crosses placenta, appears in breast milk, and accumulates in fetal tissues); administer with meals to reduce gastric irritation

## Remarks

Monitoring drug levels has increased the safety of anticonvulsant therapy.

## Adverse Reactions

*Frequent:* Drowsiness, dizziness, nausea and vomiting
*Infrequent:* Lethargy, visual abnormalities (e.g., spots before the eyes, difficulty focusing), dry mouth, headache, urinary frequency or retention, rash

## Toxic Effects

*Cardiovascular:* Congestive heart failure, edema, aggravation of coronary artery disease, arrhythmias and atrioventricular block, primary thrombophlebitis; some complications have resulted in fatalities
*CNS:* Abrupt withdrawal may precipitate status epilepticus

*Hematologic:* Blood dyscrasias (e.g., aplastic anemia, agranulocytosis, thrombocytopenia, leukopenia, bone marrow depression)
*Hepatic:* Abnormal hepatic function test results, possible jaundice, hepatitis

## Nursing Measures

1. Monitor for therapeutic serum level (3-12 µg/ml).
2. Assess for clinical evidence of early toxic signs (fever, sore throat, mouth ulcerations, easy bruising, unusual bleeding, joint pain).
3. Observe frequently for recurrence of seizure activity.

## Inform Client and Family

1. Blood tests should be repeated frequently during the first 3 months of therapy and at monthly intervals thereafter for 2 to 3 years.
2. Do not abruptly withdraw medications following long-term use; this may precipitate seizures.
3. Avoid tasks that require alertness until

a response to the drug is established.
4. Report visual abnormalities.

## chlorpromazine

*Category:*
Antipsychotic/
neuroleptic,
phenothiazine
*Trade Names:*
Thorazine, Chlorazine

## Uses

1. Management of acute psychotic disorders (schizophrenia, manic phase of a bipolar disorder) and to maintain remission of these psychotic disorders
2. Management of severe behavioral disturbances in children and clients with organic mental disorders
3. Other: Intractable hiccups, acute intermittent porphyria, tetanus, preoperatively, or to control nausea and vomiting

## Action

Chlorpromazine blocks postsynaptic dopamine receptors in the cerebral cortex basal ganglia, hypothalamus, limbic system, brain stem, and medulla. Therefore there is inhibition or alteration of dopamine release, which is thought to be related to the suppression of the clinical manifestations of schizophrenia.

## Dosages and Routes

### Hospitalized: Acute Psychotic Disorders

- *Adults:* PO; gradually increase over several days to maximum of 400 mg q4-6h 25 mg IM; may give an additional 25-50 mg in 1 hour if needed

### Outpatient: Maintenance Dose

- *Adults:* 25 mg tid gradually increased (usual maintenance dose is 400 mg/day); 25-50 mg IM 1-4 times/day; 50-100 mg rectal suppository 3-4 times/day
- *Children:* 0.5 mg/kg PO q4-6h
- *Elderly (Debilitated):* 25 mg PO daily; gradually increased up to 25 mg tid

## Contraindications

Comatose states, alcohol or barbiturate withdrawal states, bone marrow depression, pregnancy, lactation

## Cautions

Seizure disorders, diabetes, hepatic disease, cardiac disease, glaucoma, prostatic hypertrophy, asthma

## Remarks

A "low-potency" neuroleptic, having low neurologic symptoms (EPS) but with a high sedation and autonomic side effects (e.g., hypotension, cardiac, allergic). Food or antacids decrease absorption. A liquid preparation is more rapidly absorbed.

## Adverse Reactions

*Autonomic:* Dry mouth, nasal congestion, constipation or diarrhea, urinary retention or urinary frequency, inhibition of ejaculation and impotence in men
*CNS:* EPS (e.g., pseudoparkinsonism, akathisia, dystonia); possible vertigo or insomnia
*Cardiovascular:* Orthostatic hypotension, hypertension, vertigo, electroencephalogram (EEG) changes
*Endocrine:* Changes in libido, galactorrhea in women, gynecomastia in men

*Ocular:* Photophobia, blurred vision, aggravation of glaucoma
*Other:* Weight gain, allergic reactions (e.g., eczema, skin rashes)

## Toxic Effects

*CNS:* Acute dystonias (e.g., painful neck spasms, torticollis, oculogyric crisis, convulsions); tardive dyskinesia (e.g., choreiform movements of the tongue, face, mouth, jaw, and possibly extremities); the elderly and those on the drug for extended periods of time are more susceptible; often the condition is irreversible
*Hematologic:* Agranulocytosis; stop the drug immediately
*Hepatic:* Jaundice; clinical picture resembles hepatitis
*NMS:* Rare life-threatening syndrome; includes severe rigidity, fever, increased white blood cell (WBC) count, unstable BP, renal failure, tachycardia, and tachypnea; hold all drugs; immediate administration of dantrolene sodium and bromocriptine is the most successful somatic prescription

## Nursing Measures

1. Take BP lying and standing (withhold if systolic is 90 mmHg or below) and notify the physician.
2. Hold the dose with EPS or jaundice.
3. Check frequently for urinary retention.
4. Check for constipation (to avoid impaction).
5. Observe for fever, sore throat, and malaise, and monitor complete blood count (CBC), indicating a blood dyscrasia.

## Inform Client and Family

1. Rise slowly to a sitting position and dangle the legs 5 minutes before standing to minimize orthostatic hypotension.
2. Avoid sun. Use sunscreen when in direct light to avoid skin blotching. Wear long sleeves and hats. The client may experience severe photosensitivity. Advise wearing sunglasses to minimize photophobia.
3. Avoid the use of alcoholic beverages because they enhance CNS depression.
4. Do not operate machinery if drowsiness occurs.

# clozapine

*Category:* Antipsychotic/neuroleptic, tricyclic dibenzodiazepine derivative (atypical)
*Trade Name:* Clozaril

## Uses

Management of severely ill schizophrenic clients who fail to respond to other antipsychotic therapy

## Action

Clozapine may involve antagonism of dopaminergic, serotoninergic, adrenergic, and cholinergic neurotransmitter systems. Its exact action is unknown.

## Dosages and Routes

- *Adults:* PO only: initially, 25 mg 1-2 times/day; may increase by 25-50 mg/day over 2 weeks until 300-450 mg/day achieved; *range;* 200-600 mg/day; *maximum:* 900 mg/day
- *Elderly:* Initially, 25 mg/day; may increase by 25 mg/day; *maximum:* 450 mg/day

## Contraindications

Hypersensitivity to tricyclics, history of severe granulocytopenia, concurrent administration with other drugs having potential to suppress bone marrow function, CNS depression or coma, myeloproliferative disorders

## Cautions

History of seizures; cardiovascular disease; impaired respiratory, hepatic, or rental function; alcohol withdrawal; urinary retention; this drug has potent anticholinergic effects, and extreme caution is advised for clients with prostatic enlargement or narrow-angle glaucoma; also use with caution in pregnant or lactating women

## Remarks

It may take 2 to 4 weeks or as long as 3 to 6 months for therapeutic effects. Because 1% to 2% of people on clozapine develop agranulocytosis, weekly WBC counts must be done.

## Adverse Reactions

*Frequent:* Sedation, salivation, tachycardia, dizziness, constipation (in order of frequency)
*Occasional:* Hypotension or hypertension, gastrointestinal upset, nausea and vomiting, sweating, dry mouth, weight gain
*Rare:* Visual disturbances, diarrhea, rash, urinary abnormalities

## Toxic Effects

*Hematologic:* About 1% to 2% of clients develop agranulocytosis; mild leukopenia may develop
*CNS:* Seizures develop in about 5% of clients on clozapine and up to 15% of clients on dosages over 550 mg/day
*NMS:* Has been reported when clozapine is used concurrently with lithium or other CNS-active agents
*Other:* Dizziness or vertigo, drowsiness, restlessness, akinesia, agitation
*Cardiovascular:* Severe orthostatic hypotension (with or without syncope); marked tachycardia may occur in 25% of clients

## Nursing Measures

1. Check baseline WBC count before initiating treatment.

2. Check weekly WBC count. Hold the drug if the count falls below 3000/mm$^3$ and notify the physician.
3. Check BP lying and standing to assess for potential orthostatic hypotension.
4. Observe for signs of agranulocytosis (e.g., sore throat, fever, malaise).
5. Make baseline assessment of behavior appearance, emotional status, response to environment, speech pattern, and thought content.

## Inform Client and Family

1. Teach about the side effects and toxic effects of the drug and the need for a weekly WBC count.
2. Avoid the use of OTC medications, alcohol, or CNS medications because of potential and severe drug interactions.
3. Immediately report the appearance of lethargy, weakness, fever, sore throat, malaise, mucous membrane ulceration, or other possible signs of infection.
4. Refrain from operating machinery, driving, and performing other tasks that require alertness until a response to the drug is established.
5. Inform the physician if pregnancy occurs.
6. Do not breastfeed an infant if clozapine is being taken.

# diazepam

*Category:* Anxiolytic (antianxiety agent), benzodiazepine
*Trade Name:* Valium

## Uses

1. Management of anxiety disorders and short-term relief of anxiety symptoms
2. Presurgical sedation to allay anxiety and tension
3. Alcohol withdrawal
4. Seizure disorders
5. Anticonvulsant
6. Relief of skeletal muscle spasticity

## Action

One action of the benzodiazepines is to increase the action of gamma-aminobutyric acid (GABA). The benzodiazepines help GABA open a chloride channel in the postsynaptic membrane of many eurons, thereby reducing the neuron's excitability.

## Dosages and Routes

- **Adults:** *Anxiety:* 2-10 mg PO 2-4 times/day or 2-10 mg IM/IV 2-4 times/day; *muscle relaxant:* 2-10 mg PO 2-4 times/day or 5-10 mg IM/IV q3-4h; *convulsions:* 2-10 mg PO 2-4 times/day or 5-10 mg IM/IV at 10-minute intervals; *alcohol withdrawal*: 10 mg PO 3-4 times/day or 10 mg IM/IV initially, followed by 5-10 mg q3-4h
- **Elderly:** 2.5 mg PO bid; *convulsions*: 2-5 mg IM/IV (increase gradually as needed)

## Contraindications

Acute narrow-angle glaucoma, untreated open-angle glaucoma, during or within 14 days of MAOI therapy, depressed or psychotic clients in the absence of anxiety, first-trimester pregnancy, breastfeeding, shock, coma, acute alcohol intoxication

## Cautions

Epilepsy, myasthenia gravis, impaired hepatic or renal function, drug abuse, addiction-prone individuals; injectable diazepam is used with extreme caution in the elderly, the very ill, and people with chronic obstructive pulmonary disease (COPD); may elicit rage reactions in some clients

## Remarks

The benzodiazepines can produce psychologic and physical habituation, dependence, and withdrawal. Therefore they are recommended for short-term therapy (2 to 4 weeks). These drugs need to be used with caution in individuals who have histories of addiction. Withdrawal from these drugs should be gradual in order to minimize withdrawal symptoms.

## Adverse Reactions

**CNS:** Sedation, vertigo, weakness, ataxia, decreased motor performance, confusion
**Ocular:** Double or blurred vision
**Skin:** Urticaria, rash, photosensitivity
**Gastrointestinal:** Change in weight, dry mouth, constipation

## Toxic Effects

*CNS:* Benzodiazepines are
CNS depressants; fairly
safe when used on their
own, but when used in
combination with other
CNS depressants, can
cause death

*Cardiovascular:*
Tachycardia to cardio-
vascular collapse

*Metabolic:* Changes in
liver or renal function
test results

*Injection Sites:* Can cause
venous thrombosis or
phlebitis at injection sites

## Nursing Measures

1. Obtain a drug history
of prescribed and OTC
medications.
2. Periodically monitor
blood cell count and
liver function test
results during pro-
longed therapy.
3. Assess for unexplained
bleeding, petechiae,
fever, and so forth.
4. For IM therapy, aspi-
rate back, administer
deep into large muscle
mass, inject slowly,
and rotate injection
sites.

## Inform Client

1. Avoid alcohol or any
other CNS depressants
(e.g., anticonvulsants,

antidepressants) while
taking a benzodi-
azepine; this could
lead to respiratory
depression.
Check with a
physician before
taking.
2. Avoid driving or
operating hazardous
machinery if drowsi-
ness or confusion
occurs.
3. Avoid abrupt with-
drawal of benzodi-
azepines.

## disulfiram

*Category:*
Alcohol deterrent, alde-
hyde dehydrogenase
inhibitor
*Trade Name:* Antabuse

## Uses

Adjunct treatment for
selected clients with
chronic alcoholism
who want to remain in
a state of enforced
sobriety; a form of
aversion therapy

## Action

Disulfiram inhibits
hepatic enzymes from
normal metabolic break-
down of alcohol,
resulting in high
levels.

## Dosages and Routes

- *Adults:* PO only: initially, a maximum of 250-500 mg daily given as a single dose for 1-2 weeks; *maintenance*: 250 mg daily; not to exceed 500 mg daily

## Contraindications

Severe heart disease, psychosis, and hypersensitivity to disulfiram

## Cautions

Diabetes, hypothyroidism, epilepsy, cerebral damage, nephritis, hepatic disease, pregnancy

## Remarks

Clients must abstain from alcohol intake for at least 12 hours before the initial dose of drug is administered.

## Adverse Reactions

Common side effects experienced during the first 2 weeks of therapy include mild drowsiness, fatigue, headache, metallic or garlic aftertaste, allergic dermatitis, and acne eruptions; symptoms disappear spontaneously with continued therapy or reduced dosage.

## Toxic Effects

*Disulfiram-Alcohol Reaction:* Flushing or throbbing in head and neck, throbbing headache, nausea, copious vomiting, diaphoresis, dyspnea, hyperventilation, tachycardia, hypotension, marked uneasiness, vertigo, blurred vision, confusion; can cause death

## Nursing Measures

1. The client must be able to demonstrate sobriety.
2. The client must be fully aware of the drug's action when taken along with alcohol before treatment commences.
3. In severe disulfiram-alcohol reactions, supportive measures to restore BP and treat for shock in a medical facility are vital.

## Inform Client and Family

1. Avoid any substances that contain alcohol:
   - *Ingestion:* Elixirs, cough syrups, vinegars, vitamin/mineral tonics; be aware that some sauces, soups, ciders, and flavor extracts

(e.g., vanilla, cherry) and some desserts (e.g., flaming desserts, some cakes and pies) are made with alcohol
- *Topical:* Mouthwash, body lotions, liniments, shaving lotion
- *Inhalation:* Avoid inhaling fumes from substances that may contain alcohol (e.g., paints, wood stains, varnishes, "stripping" compounds)
2. Carry a card stating that, if found disoriented or unconscious, the client may be having a disulfiram-alcohol reaction and telling the finder whom to contact for medical care.
3. A disulfiram-alcohol reaction can occur within 5 to 10 minutes after ingestion of alcohol and can last 30 to 60 minutes or longer.
4. Reaction may occur with alcohol up to 14 days after ingesting disulfiram.

## donepezil hydrochloride
*Category:*
Cholinesterase inhibitor
*Trade Name:* Aricept

## Uses

Treatment of mild to moderate dementia of the Alzheimer's type

## Action

The cholinergic system deteriorates in Alzheimer's disease. Donepezil inhibits the breakdown of endogenously released acetylcholine.

## Dosages and Routes

- *Adults and Elderly:* Start with 5 mg PO daily dose. After 6 weeks may increase to 10 mg daily.

## Contraindications

Hypersensitivity to donepezil or piperidine derivatives

## Adverse Reactions

Cholinesterase inhibitors may increase gastric acid secretion; therefore clients should be monitored for gastrointestinal bleeding, especially those at increased risk of developing ulcers (e.g., history of ulcer disease, taking nonsteroidal antiinflammatory medication); use with caution in clients

who have a history of
seizures; prescribe with
care to clients with
asthma or obstructive
pulmonary disease

## Toxic Effects

Common side effects
experienced during the
first 2 weeks of therapy
include mild drowsiness,
fatigue, headache, metal-
lic or garlic aftertaste,
allergic dermatitis, and
acne eruptions; symp-
toms disappear sponta-
neously with continued
therapy or reduced
dosage.

## Adverse Reactions

Syncopal episodes have
been reported in associa-
tion with the use of this
drug.

## Nursing Measures

1. Ascertain what other
   drugs client is taking
   because donepezil has
   the potential to interfere with the activity
   of anticholinergic
   medications.
2. Discuss with family or
   friends who is to
   administer the medica-
   tion to the client to
   prevent dosage
   errors.

## Inform Client and Family

1. Take the drug in
   the evening before
   retiring.
2. The drug may be taken
   with food.
3. In case of accidental
   overdose, call a poison
   control center to
   determine the latest
   recommendations for
   management.

## Duloxetine
*Category:*
Antidepressant
*Trade Name:* Cymbalta

## Uses

1. Diabetic peripheral
   neuropathy
2. Major depression
3. Being studied for
   treatment of stress
   urinary incontinence

## Action

Duloxetine is a duel
reuptake inhibitor of
both serotonin and
norepinephrine.
Besides helping with
depression, the dual
action has the potential
to help with the
physical symptoms
of the disease, such
as vague aches and
pains.

## Dosage and Routes

The recommended daily dose for depression is 60 mg PO.

## Contraindications

*Most significant:* Narrow angle glaucoma
*Significant:* Severe hepatic disease, suicidal ideation
*Possibly Significant:* Bipolar disease

## Cautions

Be especially observant with initial drug use, and monitor use in children and adolescents closely. Always start with low dose in the elderly. Possible increase in suicidal ideation and attempts in children or adolescents. Safety during pregnancy is guarded and neonatal respiratory distress is among adverse effects. Breast-feeding is not advised.

## Remarks

As with all antidepressant therapy, monitor for suicidal ideation.

## Adverse Reactions

*Most Frequent:* Anorexia, constipation, diarrhea, dizziness, drowsiness, fatigue, hyyperhidrosis, insomnia, nausea
*Less Frequent:* Blurred vision, dysuria, alopecia, anxiety, ejaculation difficulty, gastritis, orgasm disorder, skin rash, vomiting, weight loss
*Rare:* Abdominal pain with cramps, acute gingivitis, anemia, back pain, facial edema, irritability, suicidal ideation/behavior, tachycardia, upper respiratory infection.

## Toxic Effects

*Rarely:* Abnormal hepatic function tests, colitis, esophageal compression, gastric ulcer, irritable bowel syndrome, leukocytosis, thrombocytopenia

## Inform Client and Family

1. Desired effect may take up to 3 weeks or more.
2. Should never be taken in conjunction with an SSRI, SSNRI, MAOIs, amphetamines, or thioridazine.
3. Avoid tasks that require alertness or motor skills until a response to the drug is established.
4. Check with the prescriber before taking OTC drugs.

5. Alert health care provider immediately if suicidal ideation occurs.

## fluoxetine hydrochloride

*Category:*
Antidepressant (SSRI)
*Trade Name:* Prozac

## Uses

1. Prozac is an atypical antidepressant medication that is chemically unrelated to TCAs or MAOIs
2. Has been found effective in clients with bulimia and obsessive-compulsive disorder (OCD)

## Action

Fluoxetine is a potent selective serotonin reuptake inhibitor (SSRI) whose use results in an increase in the amount of active serotonin within the synaptic cleft and at the serotonin receptor site. Increased serotonin in these areas appears to modify affective and behavioral disorders.

## Dosages and Routes

- *Adults:* 20 mg/day PO; may reach 40-60 mg in divided doses; do not exceed 80 mg/day
- *Elderly:* Same as for adults
- *Children:* No dosage for children as yet established

## Contraindications

Not to be taken within 14 days of an MAOI; also, client must wait 5 weeks when going from fluoxetine to an MAOI

## Cautions

Use with clients with concomitant systemic illness not studied extensively; caution with pregnant women or women who are breastfeeding, children, and the elderly; caution also with liver disease, renal impairment, or a recent MI

## Remarks

Fluoxetine, like the TCAs and MAOIs, takes from 2 to 5 weeks to produce an elevation of mood. Advantages of this drug are fewer anticholinergic side effects and a low incidence of cardiovascular effects. However, fluoxetine may impair judgment, thinking, and motor skills.

## Adverse Reactions

*General:* Most common side effects reported with fluoxetine are nausea, nervousness and anxiety, insomnia, and vertigo; when these side effects are severe the drug is discontinued; if a rash or urticaria or both develop, the drug should be discontinued; anorexia may appear in some people

## Toxic Effects

See Adverse Reactions

## Nursing Measures

1. Fluoxetine is given in the early morning without consideration to meals.
2. Clients who are potentially suicidal are assessed for suicidal thoughts or actions. Carefully observe taking of medication.
3. If client is underweight and experiences anorexia, the physician should be alerted to reevaluate continuation of medication.

## Inform Client

1. If rash or urticaria appears, notify the physician immediately.
2. Do not drive or operate machinery if drowsiness occurs.
3. Avoid alcoholic beverages.

## fluvoxamine maleate

*Category:*
Antidepressant (SSRI)
*Trade Name:* Luvox

## Uses

Treatment of OCD and depression

## Action

This drug selectively inhibits serotonin neuronal uptake in the CNS, producing an antidepressant effect.

## Dosages and Routes

- *Adults:* 50 mg PO at bedtime; increase by 50 mg every 4-7 days to a maximum of 300 mg/day; give doses over 100 mg in 2 divided doses
- *Children (8-17 Years):* 25 mg PO at bedtime; increase by 25 mg every 4-7 days up to a maximum of 200 mg/day

## Contraindications

Not to be taken within 14 days of MAOI ingestion; concurrent astemizole or terfenadine therapy

## Cautions

History of seizures, heart disease, kidney disease, liver disease, or allergies; this drug should be used during pregnancy only if clearly needed; this medication appears in breast milk

## Remarks

This drug may interact with a variety of other medications, both prescribed and OTC (e.g., lithium, all antidepressants [SSRIs and others], dexfenfluramine, warfarin, phenytoin, benzodiazepines, carbamazepine, clozapine, methadone, propranolol, any MAOI, haloperidol). A careful drug history is warranted for anyone going on this medication.

## Adverse Reactions

*Frequent:* Nausea, vomiting, constipation, upset stomach, delayed ejaculation, decreased libido, urinary frequency, drowsiness, headache, anxiety, tremors, trouble sleeping, dry mouth
*Infrequent:* Dizziness, fatigue, constipation, rash, back pain, visual disturbances

## Toxic Effects

*Cardiac:* Rapid, pounding, or irregular heart beat; chest pain
*CNS:* Confusion; disorientation; unusual uncontrolled movements, especially around the face
*Hematologic:* Bruising or bleeding
*General:* Flu-like symptoms (fever, chills)

## Nursing Measures

1. For clients on long-term therapy, baseline liver/ renal function test and baseline blood counts need to be done and repeated periodically throughout treatment.
2. Perform a suicide assessment and evaluate risk factors. Does the client's history include past suicidal behavior or threats? Identify the client's support system.
3. Obtain a drug history from the client regarding OTC, prescription (especially psychoactive medications, cardiac

medications, and many others), and recreational drugs currently taken. How much and how often does the client use alcohol? Be sure there is good documentation made in the client's chart and that the prescribing health care worker is well informed.

## Inform Client and Family

1. The drug may take up to 4 weeks before improvement is noted.
2. Helpful interventions for common side effects include:
   - Sunglasses for photosensitivity.
   - Sugarless gum and sips of water for dry mouth.
   - Rising and moving slowly to avoid hypotensive effects.
   - Avoiding tasks that require motor skills (e.g., driving a car) until a response to the drug is established.
3. Because of drug interactions, the client should avoid alcohol.

## gabapentin
*Category:*
Anticonvulsant
*Trade Name:* Neurontin

## Uses

1. Adjunctive therapy in the treatment of partial seizures with and without secondary generalization in adults with epilepsy; neuropathic pain
2. Used experimentally with selected refractory bipolar clients

## Action

This drug may be related to increased GABA synthesis rate, increased GABA accumulation, or binding to as-yet-undefined receptor sites in the brain to produce anticonvulsant activity. The exact mechanism is not known.

## Dosages and Routes

- *PO:* 100-, 300-, or 400-mg capsules
- *Adults:* Effective dose is 900-1800 mg given in divided doses (tid); titration to an effective dose can take place rapidly, giving 300 mg on day 1 (hs), 300 mg bid (q12h) on day 2, and 300 mg tid (q8h) on day 3; continue increasing dose up to 1800 mg when indicated
- *Elderly:* In elderly clients with compromised renal function, dose needs to be adjusted

## Contraindications

Clients who have demonstrated hyperactivity to the drug or its ingredients

## Cautions

In clients with renal impairment, dose needs to be modified; use with caution in pregnant women; safety and effectiveness not established in children under 12

## Adverse Reactions

*Frequent:* Fatigue, somnolence, dizziness, ataxia, nystagmus, tremor, diplopia, rhinitis, hypertension

*Infrequent:* Weight gain, dyspepsia, myalgia, nervousness, dysarthria, pharyngitis, nausea and vomiting

## Toxic Effects

Difficulty breathing or tightening of the throat, swelling of lips or tongue, rash, slurred speech, drowsiness, diarrhea

## Nursing Measures

1. Review history of seizure disorder (i.e., type, onset, intensity, frequency, duration, level of consciousness).
2. Assess for seizure activity. Provide safety measures as needed.
3. Obtain baseline assessment, including vital signs.
4. Obtain information on all other medications (e.g., prescription, nonprescription, nutritional supplements, herbal products) that the client is taking.
5. Obtain a history of alcohol frequency and amount. Identify any recreational drugs that the client is taking. These may affect the way the medication will work.

## Inform Client and Family

1. The drug should not be abruptly discontinued because of the possibility of increasing seizure activity.
2. The drug should be taken as prescribed.
3. Gabapentin may cause dizziness, somnolence, and other symptoms of CNS depression; therefore, clients should be advised to refrain from driving a car or operating complex machinery.

4. The client should tell the physician if she:
   - Is about to become pregnant
   - Is breastfeeding

## haloperidol

*Category:*
Antipsychotic/traditional neuroleptic, butyrophenone
*Trade Name:* Haldol

## Uses

1. Management of psychotic disorders
2. Helps control remissions in schizophrenia
3. Controversial use for children with combative, explosive hyperexcitability
4. Control of tics and vocal utterances of Tourette syndrome
5. Useful in acute mania and acute and chronic organic psychosis
6. Management of drug-induced (LSD) psychosis

## Action

This drug blocks the binding of dopamine to the postsynaptic dopamine receptors in the brain.

## Dosages and Routes

- *Adults:* 1-2 mg 2-3 times/day up to 4-6 mg 2-3 times/day (30-40 mg/day may be necessary); *Severe*: 3-5 mg IM q1-8h to control symptoms, then give PO
- *Children:* Note for children under 3 years; for children 3-12 years, 0.05-0.15 mg/kg/day PO in 2-3 divided doses
- *Elderly:* PO; elderly or debilitated clients may require smaller doses than adults

## Contraindications

Hypersensitivity, Parkinson's disease, depression, seizures, coma, alcoholism, during lithium therapy

## Cautions

The elderly; clients on anticoagulant therapy; glaucoma, prostatic hypertrophy, urinary retention, asthma, pregnancy/lactation

## Remarks

This is a "high-potency" neuroleptic with a higher incidence of EPS but a lower incidence of sedation and orthostatic hypotension. Haldol Decanoate E or D given intramuscularly can have effects lasting from 1 to 3 weeks.

## Adverse Reactions

*Autonomic:* Dry mouth, nasal congestion, constipation or diarrhea, urinary retention or urinary frequency, inhibition of ejaculation and impotence in men

*CNS:* EPS (e.g., pseudoparkinsonism, akathisia, dystonia), vertigo, insomnia, headache

*Cardiovascular:* Orthostatic hypotension, hypertension, dizziness, EEG changes

*Endocrine:* Changes in libido, galactorrhea in women, gynecomastia in men

*Ocular:* Photophobia, blurred vision, aggravation of glaucoma

*Other:* Weight gain, allergic reactions such as eczema and skin rashes

## Toxic Effects

*CNS:* Acute dystonias (e.g., painful neck spasms, torticollis, oculogyric crisis, convulsions); tardive dyskinesia (choreiform movements of the tongue, face, mouth, jaw, and possibly extremities); the elderly and those on the drug for extended periods are more susceptible; often irreversible

*Hematologic:* Agranulocytosis (drug immediately stopped)

*Hepatic:* Jaundice; clinical picture resembles hepatitis

*NMS:* Occurs within 24 to 72 hours; fever, rigidity, renal failure, dysrhythmias, and more; hold drug and give dantrolene sodium or bromocriptine immediately

## Nursing Measures

1. Check for signs of tardive dyskinesia (e.g., protrusion of tongue, puffing of cheeks, chewing or puckering of the mouth) and report them to the physician immediately.
2. Observe for other signs of EPS and jaundice.
3. Check for orthostatic hypotension (take blood pressure lying down and standing). Withhold medication if the systolic pressure is 80 mmHg or below.

4. Check frequently for urinary retention.
5. Check for constipation (to avoid impaction).
6. Observe for fever, sore throat, and malaise. Monitor CBC, which may indicate a blood dyscrasia.
7. Monitor renal function during long-term therapy.
8. Monitor blood levels every week.

## Inform Client

1. Rise slowly to a sitting position and dangle the legs 5 minutes before standing to minimize orthostatic hypotension.
2. Use sunscreen when in direct light to avoid skin blotching, and wear sunglasses to prevent photophobia.
3. Avoid the use of alcoholic beverages because they enhance CNS depression.
4. Refrain from operating machinery if drowsiness occurs.

## imipramine hydrochloride
*Category:*
Tricyclic antidepressant
*Trade Name:* Tofranil

## Uses

1. Principal indication for TCAs is the treatment of depression (major, bipolar, or dysthymia)
2. Effective in some organic affective disorders and OCD
3. Used as adjunctive treatment in childhood enuresis and in bulimia
4. Found useful in the treatment of agoraphobia with panic attacks and generalized anxiety disorder

## Action

TCAs block the reuptake of norepinephrine and serotonin into their presynaptic neurons.

## Dosages and Routes

- *Adults:* 50 mg/day PO to start, given in 1-4 divided doses up to 200 mg/day for outpatients; *maintenance*: 50-150 mg/day; *IM*: Do not exceed 100 mg/day in divided doses
- *Children: Childhood enuresis:* 25 mg PO before bedtime; *depression in children over 12 years*: 30-40 mg PO daily initially

- *Elderly:* PO; used with caution, so usually start at lower dose; geriatric clients start on 30-40 mg daily in divided doses initially

## Contraindications

Recent myocardial infarction or cardiac disease, severe renal or hepatic impairment; death may occur if used with an MAOI; however, the two may be cautiously used together in cases of refractory depression; TCAs may also cause fatal cardiac arrhythmias in clients with hyperthyroidism; use with caution in children and adolescents; special cautions for the elderly, especially those with cardiac, respiratory, cardiovascular, hepatic, or gastrointestinal diseases

## Cautions

Renal or hepatic disease, narrow-angle glaucoma; potential for suicide must be assessed; TCAs lower the seizure threshold, so any client with a seizure disorder needs careful monitoring

## Remarks

1. Before receiving TCAs, clients need a thorough physical and cardiac workup.

2. Clients need to know that mood elevation may not occur for 2 to 4 weeks.

## Adverse Reactions

*Anticholinergic:* Dry mouth and nasal passages, constipation, urinary hesitancy, esophageal reflux, blurred vision
*Cardiovascular:* Orthostatic hypotension, hypertension, palpitations
*CNS:* Tachycardia, vertigo, tinnitus, numbness and tingling of extremities, stimulation
*Endocrine:* Galactorrhea, increased or decreased libido, ejaculatory and erectile disturbances, delayed orgasm
*Other:* Weight gain, impotence, cholestatic jaundice, fatigue

## Toxic Effects

*Autonomic:* Intracardiac conduction slowing
*Cardiovascular:* MI, congestive heart failure, arrhythmias, heart block, cardiotoxicity, cerebrovascular accident, shock
*CNS:* Ataxia, neuropathy, EPS, lowered seizure threshold, delirium

*Hematologic:* Bone marrow depression, agranulocytosis

*Psychiatric:* Hallucinations, shift to hypomania, mania, exacerbation of psychosis

## Nursing Measures

1. Monitor BP (both lying and standing) every 2 to 6 hours when initiating therapy.
2. Observe suicidal clients closely during initial therapy.
3. Supervise drug ingestion to prevent hoarding of the drug.
4. Assess for urinary retention.
5. Monitor liver function test results and CBC to assess for signs of cholestatic jaundice and agranulocytosis.
6. Small amount of the drug should be dispensed if the client is to be discharged.
7. Diabetic clients should be closely monitored, especially during early therapy, because hypoglycemia or hyperglycemia may occur in some clients.
8. All clients on TCAs need to be observed for the occurrence of hypomania or manic episodes, urinary retention, orthostatic hypotension, and seizure activity.

## Inform Client

1. Rise slowly to prevent hypotensive effects.
2. Do not drive or use hazardous machinery if drowsiness or vertigo occurs.
3. Do not use OTC drugs in conjunction with a TCA without a physician's approval.
4. The effects of alcohol and imipramine are potentiated when used together, and alcohol use should be discussed with a physician before taking the drug.
5. About 1 to 4 weeks may pass before therapeutic effects are experienced.

## lamotrigine

*Category:* Anticonvulsant, antiepileptic drug [AED]
*Trade Name:* Lamictal

## Uses

1. Adjunctive treatment of partial seizures in adults with epilepsy
2. Bipolar disease

## Action

The precise mechanism by which lamotrigine exerts its anticonvulsant action is unknown. It is thought to be related to the drug's effect on sodium channels.

## Dosages and Routes

- *PO:* 25-, 100-, 150-, or 200-mg tablets
- *Adult, Elderly, and Children Over 16 If Receiving Enzyme-Inducing AEDs but not Valproate; Recommend as Add-on Therapy:* 50 mg qd for 2 weeks, followed by 100 mg/day in 2 divided doses for 2 weeks; *maintenance:* Dose may be increased by 100 mg/day every week up to 300-500 mg in 2 divided doses
- *If Receiving Combination Therapy of Valproic Acid and Enzyme-Inducing AEDs:* 25 mg every other day for 2 weeks, followed by 25 mg qd for 2 weeks; *maintenance:* Dose may be increased by 25-50 mg/day every 1-2 weeks up to 150 mg/day in 2 divided doses
- *Children Age 16 or Under:* Not approved for children under 16 years of age (see Contraindications)

## Contraindications

Incidence of severe, potentially life-threatening rash in pediatric clients (under 16 years of age) is very much higher than that reported in adults using lamotrigine.

## Cautions

Renal impairment, hepatic function impairment, cardiac function impairment; can reduce fetal weight; delayed ossification noted in animals; pregnancy category C; breastfeeding not recommended

## Adverse Reactions

*Frequent:* Dizziness double vision, headache, ataxia (muscular inco-ordination), nausea, blurred vision, somnolence, rhinitis
*Occasional:* Pharyngitis, vomiting, cough, flu-like syndrome, diarrhea, dysmenorrhea, fever, insomnia, dyspepsia
*Infrequent:* Constipation, tremor, anxiety, pruritus, vaginitis

## Toxic Effects

WARNING: Potentially life-threatening rashes have been reported in association with the use of lamotrigine. These rashes occur in approximately 1 in every 1000 adults.

## Nursing Measures

1. Review the history of seizure disorder (i.e., type, onset, intensity, frequency, duration, level of consciousness).
2. Identify what prescription and OTC medications the client is taking.
3. Identify amount and frequency of alcohol intake. Identify any other recreational drugs the client is taking.
4. Identify other medical conditions, particularly renal or hepatic impairment.
5. Obtain baseline vital signs.
6. Report promptly any rash, which may herald a life-threatening medical event.
7. Assess for dizziness or ataxia and provide safety measures.
8. Assess for clinical improvement (e.g., decrease in intensity/ frequency of seizures).

## Inform Client and Family

1. Before initiation of treatment with lamotrigine, the client and family should be instructed that a rash or other signs or symptoms of hypersensitivity (e.g., fever, lymphadenopathy, facial swelling) may herald a serious medical event. The client should report any such occurrence to a physician immediately.
2. Report first signs of a rash to the physician.
3. AEDs should not be abruptly discontinued because of the possibility of increasing seizure frequency, unless safety concerns (e.g., rash) require a rapid withdrawal.
4. Carry an identification card and wear a bracelet to note anticonvulsant therapy.
5. Avoid alcohol, which lowers the seizure threshold.

## lithium carbonate/ citrate

*Category:*
Antimanic
*Trade Names:*
Carbolith, Eskalith, Lithane, Lithizine, Lithonate, Lithobid

## Uses

1. Primarily used to control, prevent, or diminish manic episodes in people with bipolar depression (manic-depressive psychosis)
2. Used experimentally in treatment of alcoholism, premenstrual syndrome, drug abuse, phobias, eating disorders, and rage reactions

## Action

Lithium is an alkali metal salt that behaves in the body much like a sodium ion. Lithium acts to lower concentrations of norepinephrine and serotonin by inhibiting their release and enhancing their reuptake by neurons. The therapeutic effects, as well as the side effects and toxic effects, of lithium are thought to be related to the partial replacement of sodium by lithium in membrane action.

## Dosages and Routes

- *Adults:* *Acute mania:* 600 mg PO 3 times/day; *maintenance:* 300 mg PO 3-4 times/day
- *Children:* Not labeled for pediatric use
- *Elderly:* Starting dose of 300 mg/day; serum levels of 0.4-0.6 mEq/L usually effective in elderly clients

## Contraindications

Pregnancy, nursing mothers, significant cardiovascular or renal disease, schizophrenia, severe debilitation, dehydration, sodium depletion

## Cautions

The elderly, thyroid disease, epilepsy, concomitant use with haloperidol or other antipsychotics, parkinsonism, severe infections, urinary retention, diabetes

## Remarks

Serum lithium levels must be monitored during drug therapy. The therapeutic range is very narrow, and the potential for toxic effects is high if blood levels are not monitored. During the acute stage, blood levels are raised to 1 to 1.4 mEq/L. Maintenance therapy blood levels run from 0.8 to 1.2 mEq/L. Side effects and toxic effects are common at higher doses (1.5 mEq/L or more). Before a client is started on lithium, blood urea nitrogen (BUN), thyroxine, triiodothyronine, and thyroid-stimulating hormone levels should be measured, and an ECG should be done.

## Adverse Reactions

Major long-term risks of lithium therapy are hypothyroidism and impairment of the kidney's ability to concentrate urine; below 1.5 mEq/L, effects may include polyuria, polydipsia, lethargy, fatigue, muscle weakness, headache, mild nausea, fine hand tremor, and inability to concentrate; may experience ankle edema; symptoms disappear during continued therapy

## Toxic Effects

*1.5 to 2 mEq/L:* Vomiting, diarrhea, muscle weakness, ataxia, dizziness, slurred speech, confusion

*2 to 2.5 mEq/L:* Blurred vision, muscle twitching, severe hypotension, persistent nausea and vomiting; thyroid toxicity is common

*2.5 to 3 mEq/L or More:* Urinary and fecal incontinence, seizures, cardiac arrhythmias,

peripheral vascular collapse, death

## Nursing Measures

1. If serum lithium levels are above 1.5 mEq/L or if the client has persistent diarrhea, vomiting, excessive sweating in hot weather, infection, or fever, check with the physician before giving the dose.
2. Check urine specific gravity periodically and teach the client to do so at home (normal is 1.005 to 1.025).
3. Administer lithium with meals.
4. Ensure that the client is well hydrated.

## Inform Client

1. Drink plenty of liquids (2 to 3 L/day) during initial therapy and 1 to 1.5 L/day during the remainder of therapy.
2. Know the side effects and toxic effects of lithium therapy and seek out the physician immediately if problems arise.
3. Have blood lithium levels measured at regular intervals as directed to regulate dosage and prevent toxicity.

4. Maintain a regular diet, thus maintaining the average salt intake (6 to 8 g) required to keep the serum lithium level in the therapeutic range.
5. Avoid alcohol.
6. Be aware that antibiotics (e.g., metronidazole, tetracycline) and nonsteroidal anti-inflammatory agents (e.g., indomethacin) can increase lithium levels.
7. Know that caffeine can lower lithium levels.

## lorazepam
*Category:*
Antianxiety agent, benzodiazipine
*Trade Name:* Ativan

## Uses

1. Treatment of anxiety disorders associated with depression
2. Preoperative sedation
3. Treatment of nausea and vomiting associated with chemotherapy for cancer

## Action

Lorazepam is a CNS depressant, especially in the limbic system and reticular formation. It enhances the action of the inhibitory neurotransmitter GABA, producing a calming effect. It can suppress spread of seizure activity and directly depress motor nerve and muscle function, creating some muscle relaxation.

## Dosages and Routes

- **Adults:** *Anxiety:* 2-3 mg/day PO in 2-3 doses; *insomnia:* 2-4 mg PO at bedtime
- **Elderly:** *Anxiety:* 0.5-1 mg/day PO (may increase gradually); *insomnia:* 0.5-1 mg PO at bedtime

## Contraindications

Acute narrow-angle glaucoma and alcohol intoxication, pregnant clients or lactating mothers, children under 12

## Cautions

Clients with renal or hepatic dysfunction, elderly or debilitated clients, clients with a history of drug abuse or addiction; people taking other CNS depressants (e.g., narcotics, barbiturates, alcohol) may experience a synergistic effect, increasing CNS depression; may reduce digoxin excretion, increasing the potential for toxicity

## Adverse Reactions

*Frequent:* Drowsiness, fatigue, dizziness, incoordination

*Occasional:* Blurred vision, slurred speech, hypotension, headache

*Rare:* Paradoxical CNS restlessness, excitement in the elderly and debilitated

## Toxic Effects

Can have pronounced withdrawal symptoms (e.g., seizures, pronounced restlessness, insomnia, abdominal/muscle cramps) with abrupt withdrawal from the drug

## Nursing Measures

1. Assess for a history of glaucoma, substance abuse, allergies, past reactions to benzodiazepines, and current list of medications.
2. Before long-term therapy, assess CBC and liver function tests in collaboration with the physician.
3. Make sure the client has written information about his or her medications that covers side effects, doses, precautions, and other information.

## Inform Client and Family

1. Avoid tasks that require alertness or motor skills (e.g., driving, operating machinery).
2. Do not take OTC medications or new medications without approval from the physician.
3. Do not drink alcohol or take other CNS depressants while taking this medication.
4. Do not stop this medication abruptly.

## methylphenidate

*Category:* CNS stimulant
*Trade Name:* Ritalin

## Uses

1. Attention deficit disorder (children 6 years and older)
2. Narcolepsy
3. Occasionally for depression in the elderly

## Action

Methylphenidate causes direct release of catecholamines into the synaptic clefts and thus onto postsynaptic receptor sites. It blocks reuptake of catecholamines, thus prolonging their actions, resulting in better impulse control and concentration.

## Dosages and Routes

- *Children 6 Years and Older:* Usual starting dose is 5 mg PO twice daily (breakfast and lunch); most children are maintained on 60 mg/day and should be monitored regularly by the prescribing physician
- *Adults:* Doses may start at 5 mg PO 2-3 times/day; dose range for adults is 10 mg/day to not more than 60 mg/day (20-40 mg/day is usual)
- *Elderly:* Elderly clients using methylphenidate for depression usually maintained on 2.5-20 mg/day PO

## Contraindications

Glaucoma, hypertension, heart problems, or history of Tourette syndrome; people with a history of seizure disorders may experience an increase in number, duration, or severity of seizures

## Cautions

Can cause growth delay in children; can interact with other medications (e.g., alcohol, antidepressants [MAOIs and TCAs], some OTC medications, health food products containing *ma huang*); serious problems can also develop if clients are taking any other amphetamine-type or diet drugs

## Adverse Reactions

*Frequent:* Nervousness and sleeplessness most common; other reactions are loss of appetite, weight loss, nausea, dizziness, heart palpitations, increases in blood pressure, stomach upset, and growth delay in children with prolonged therapy

*Occasional:* Dizziness, dysphoria, joint pain, fever

## Toxic Effects

Potential increased frequency of seizures in people with seizure disorders; chest pain, dysrhythmias; can have serious interactions with other medications and OTC preparations

## Nursing Measures

1. Take a careful inventory of any other medications the client is taking (i.e., prescribed and OTC, health food products). Check with the pharmacy if there might be a problem with compatibility.
2. Medications are best taken shortly before meals and not after 12:00 or 1:00 PM for children or 6:00 PM for adults, because stimulant effect may keep people awake.

## Inform Client and Family

1. Suggest to parents to discuss drug holidays, which can help avoid the side effect of growth delay, with their prescribing health care agent (e.g., physician nurse, therapist).
2. Caution the client and family that the drug may have serious side effects when mixed with other substances. Have the client or family check with the physician before taking any OTC medica-

tions or other drugs or health food products from other sources.
3. If the child must take this medication during school hours, ask the pharmacist to provide an empty labeled container and place no more than 1 week's worth of medication in the bottle. Be sure the medication is secured with a school official.
4. Once the client is stabilized on a dose, methylphenidate can be given in extended-release form. These tablets are to be swallowed whole and never crushed or chewed.
5. Keep tablets dry, tightly capped, and away from direct heat.
6. Keep out of reach of children and pets.

## mirtazapine
*Category:* Antidepressant/alpha-adrenoceptor antagonist
*Trade Name:* Remeron

## Uses

1. Treatment of depression
2. Potential value in treating depressed

clients with sleep or anxiety disturbances

## Action

Mirtazapine is a tetracyclic antidepressant that works by its central presynaptic alpha$_2$-adrenergic antagonist effects, which result in increased release of norepinephrine and serotonin.

## Dosages and Routes

- *Adults:* Initially 15 mg nightly; titrate up to 15-45 mg/day PO, with dose increases made no more frequently than every 1-2 weeks; there is an inverse relationship between dose and sedation
- *Children:* Not available
- *Elderly:* Increase dosage with caution
- *All Ages:* Medication is taken in once daily oral doses

## Contraindications

Hypersensitivity to mirtazapine; do not use MAOIs within 14 days

## Cautions

Alcohol, benzodiazepines, and other CNS depressants should be avoided (they can have an additive CNS effect with this drug); elderly individuals or those with renal or hepatic disease may develop higher serum concentrations than younger individuals; dosages for the elderly should be increased with caution.

## Remarks

The ability to selectively block 5-HT$_2$ and 5-HT$_3$ receptors may account for a low incidence of such symptoms as anxiety, insomnia, nausea, and sexual dysfunction.

## Adverse Reactions

*Frequent:* Dry mouth, constipation, dizziness, tiredness, increased appetite
*Infrequent:* Hypertension, malaise, increased triglycerides, urinary frequency, dyspnea, flu-like symptoms

## Toxic Effects

*Rare:* Seizures, confusion, headache, fever

## Nursing Measures

1. Identify any prescribed or OTC drugs the client may be taking (e.g., MAOIs).

2. Does the client use alcohol or "street drugs"?
3. Assess if the client is pregnant or breast-feeding.

## Inform Client and Family

1. Take this medication at the same time of day. It is generally prescribed once daily.
2. Improvement in energy levels, sleep, and appetite may occur during the first week. Depressive symptoms may take up to 4 to 6 weeks to improve.

## moclobemide (reversible MAO-A)

*Category:*
Antidepressant, reversible inhibitor of monoamine A (RIMA)
*Trade Names:*
Manerix, Aurorix

## Uses

1. Major depression and chronic dysthymia
2. Potential use with attention deficit hyperactivity disorder (ADHD), social phobia, and memory problems related to cognitive disorders

## Action

Moclobemide is a short-acting inhibitor of only the A type of monoamine oxidase, and therefore it does not cause the classic reactions to tyramine-containing foods. The activity of MAO-A enzyme inhibits the metabolism of serotonin, norepinephrine, and dopamine, which seems to account for the antidepressant activity of this drug.

## Dosages and Routes

- *Adults:* Initiated at 300 mg/day (usually in 3 divided doses) and increased gradually if needed; usual therapeutic dose is 300-600 mg/day PO
- *Elderly:* No dosage adjustments are necessary
- *Pediatrics:* Not recommended for children below the age of 18

## Contraindications

Moclobemide should not be given with other antidepressants, (e.g., TCAs, SSRIs, other available MAOIs, buspirone); cimetidine can increase moclobemide serum levels; in depression in which agitation is a predominant clinical symptom, moclobemide should not be used; moclobemide contraindicated in people in acute confusional states

## Cautions

In people with thyrotoxicosis or pheochromocytoma, conventional MAOIs may precipitate hypertensive reactions (caution should be used in these clients if treated with moclobemide); safety in pregnancy has not been established; moclobemide not recommended in nursing mothers; in clients with severe liver dysfunction, moclobemide should be reduced to one third or one half the dose.

## Remarks

Moclobemide results in a minimal BP increase in response to tyramine, is thought to be safer than the traditional MAOIs, and can be used without stringent dietary control. However, it is suggested that moclobemide be given after meals to reduce the likelihood of causing the inhibition of tyramine metabolism.

## Adverse Reactions

*Frequent:* Dry mouth, blurred vision, insomnia, headache, orthostatic hypotension, nausea
*Infrequent:* Constipation, sweating, drowsiness, hypomania, disorientation, tremor, tachycardia, arrhythmias, rash

## Nursing Measures

1. Assess well for suicide potential. Suicide is an inherent possibility in depressed individuals and should be carefully supervised during all phases of treatment.
2. Emphasize to clients that moclobemide should be taken after meals to minimize tyramine potentiation and the possibility of a hypertensive reaction.
3. Identify all other medications, OTC and otherwise, that clients are taking, and identify those that may cause a reaction, especially sympathomimetics and others.

## Inform Client and Family

1. Do not take any OTC or other medications (herbal, natural, or otherwise) without clearing it first with the health care provider.
2. Take this drug after meals for the reasons stated previously

### olanzapine
*Category:* Atypical antipsychotic
*Trade Name:* Zyprexa

## Uses

1. First-line treatment for schizophrenia, targeting both the positive and negative symptoms
2. Other psychotic illness

## Action

Olanzapine blocks various serotonin ($5\text{-}HT_{2A}$) receptors and $D_2$ receptors. It also antagonizes $D_1$ through $D_4$ receptors, $5\text{-}HT_{2C}$ and $5\text{-}HT_3$ receptors, and the $alpha_1$-adrenergic and $H_1$ histamine receptors.

## Dosages and Routes

- *Adults:* Given in 5- to 10-mg doses QD, with a target of 10 mg/day (15 mg/day does not seem to be more effective than 10 mg/day); *range:* 5-20 mg/day
- *PO:* 5-, 7.5-, or 10-mg tablets

## Contraindications

Client pregnant or nursing, hypersensitivity to olanzapine

## Cautions

Olanzapine seems to have a good side effect profile and low potential interactions; carbamazepine may increase olanzapine clearance by 50% at a dose of 200 mg bid, and nicotine may increase olanzapine clearance by 40% in smokers; alcohol may potentiate the CNS effects; olanzapine may potentiate some antihypertensive agents

## Adverse Reactions

*Frequent:* Psychomotor slowing (e.g., somnolence, asthenia), psychomotor activation (e.g., agitation, nervousness, insomnia, hostility), dizziness, weight gain

*Infrequent:* At higher doses, anticholinergic effects (e.g., constipation, dry mouth, increased appetite); mild transient dose-related increases in hepatic transaminase and prolactin levels resolve spontaneously and do not require discontinuation of the drug.

## Nursing Measures

1. Monitor BP.
2. Educate the client on how to minimize postural hypotension.
3. Caution the client that alcohol or benzodiazepines may potentiate hypertension.

## phenelzine sulfate
*Category:*
Antidepressant, MAOI
*Trade Name:* Nardil

## Uses

1. MAOIs used primarily for depression that is refractory to TCA therapy
2. MAOIs particularly effective in atypical depression, agoraphobia, or hypochondriasis
3. Panic disorders

## Action

The antidepressant effect is thought to be due to irreversible inhibition of MAO, thereby increasing the concentration of epinephrine, norepinephrine, serotonin, and dopamine within the presynaptic neurons and at the receptor site.

## Dosages and Routes

- *Adults:* 15 mg PO 3 times daily; increase rapidly to 60 mg daily until therapeutic level is noted
- *Elderly:* Prone to side effects; may be contraindicated in adults older than 60
- *Children:* Not used with children

## Contraindications

MAOIs can cause untoward interactions with certain foodstuffs or cold remedies, which may produce hypertensive crises, cerebrovascular accident, or hyperpyrexia states that can lead to coma or death; therefore, a confused or noncompliant client is at risk with an MAOI; other contraindications include people with congestive heart failure, cardiovascular or cerebrovascular disease, impaired renal function, glaucoma, history of severe headaches, or liver disease; elderly or debilitated clients; and people who are pregnant or who have paranoid schizophrenia.

## Cautions

Depression accompanying alcoholism or drug addiction, manic-depressive states, suicidal tendencies, agitated clients, people with chronic brain syndromes or a history of angina pectoris

## Remarks

Because of the severe interactions of some foodstuffs and medication, clients need comprehensive teaching, teaching aids, and supervision. High-tyramine foods include beer, red wine, aged cheese, dry sausage, fava beans (Italian green beans), brewer's yeast, smoked fish, any kind of liver, avocados, and bologna. Chocolate and coffee should be used in moderation. Those drugs causing severe medication interactions include meperidine (Demerol), epinephrine, local anes-

thetics, decongestants, cough medications, diet pills, and most OTC medications.

## Adverse Reactions

*General:* Constipation, dry mouth, vertigo, orthostatic hypotension, drowsiness or insomnia, weakness, fatigue, weight gain, hypomania, mania, blurred vision, skin rash; muscle twitching is common

## Toxic Effects

*Hypertensive Crisis:* Intense occipital headache, palpitation, stiff neck, fever, chest pain, bradycardia or tachycardia, intracranial bleeding
*Hepatic:* Jaundice, malaise, right upper quadrant pain, change in color or consistency of stools

## Nursing Measures

1. Monitor BP for orthostatic hypotension every 2 to 4 hours during initial therapy.
2. Assess for other potential signs of hypertensive crises.

3. Observe for marked changes in mood (e.g., hypomania, mania).
4. Monitor intake and output and frequency of stools.
5. Have the client dangle legs 5 minutes before standing.
6. Depressed persons are at risk for suicide. Continue to monitor and observe for potential suicidal behaviors.

## Inform Client

1. Inform client and family clearly and carefully about foodstuffs and medications to avoid. Review in detail.
2. Instruct clients taking MAOIs to wear a medical identification tag or bracelet.
3. Caution clients to avoid all OTC drugs unless a physician's approval has been obtained.
4. Caution clients to avoid all alcohol.
5. Encourage clients and their families to go to the emergency room immediately if signs and symptoms of hypertensive crises are suspected. Phentolamine (Regitine) can be given for hypertensive crises.

## quetiapine

*Category:* Atypical antipsychotic (dibenzothiazepine derivative)
*Trade Name:* Seroquel

## Uses

Management of the manifestation of both positive and negative symptoms of schizophrenia

## Action

This drug interacts with multiple neurotransmitter receptors, including serotonin, dopamine, and histamine. The exact mechanism is unknown.

## Dosages and Routes

- *PO:* 25-, 100-, or 200-mg tablets
- *Adults:* Initially, 25 mg bid, then 25-50 mg qd up to a target dose of 300 mg/day given bid within 4-7 days
- *Elderly:* Because plasma clearance is reduced by 30%-50% in elderly individuals, the rate of dose titration may need to be slower and the daily therapeutic target dose lower

## Contraindications

Known hypersensitivity to this medication or any of its ingredients

## Cautions

In clients with preexisting hepatic disorders, in clients who are being treated with potentially hepatotoxic drugs, or if treatment-emergent signs or symptoms of hepatic impairment appear; a liver function test should be done periodically

## Adverse Reactions

*Frequent:* Weight gain, headache, somnolence, postural hypotension, dizziness, tachycardia, agitation, insomnia, dry mouth; may cause sedation and impair motor skills during initial dose titration period
*Infrequent:* Back pain, fever, palpitations, weight gain, hyperthyroidism, rhinitis, leukopenia, ear pain

## Toxic Effects

*Cardiac:* Elevated aspartate transaminase (AST) levels
*Hepatic:* Elevated alanine aminotransaminase (ALT) levels
*Hematologic:* Leukopenia
*Hormonal:* Reduction of thyroxine levels usually during first 2 to 4 weeks of treatment

## Nursing Measures

1. Always monitor clients on antipsychotics for signs of tardive dyskinesia or NMS.
2. Assess for orthostatic hypotension, dizziness, and possible syncope during initial dose titration. Take necessary measures to prevent injury.
3. If the client has a history of seizures or a condition associated with lowered seizure threshold, take necessary precautions.
4. For clients who have known or suspected abnormal hepatic function or clients who develop any signs or symptoms suggestive of new-onset liver disorder during quetiapine therapy, initial assessment and then periodic clinical assessment of transaminase levels are recommended.

## Inform Client and Family

1. The client should inform the physician:
   - If she is about to become pregnant.
   - If she is breastfeeding a baby.
   - About OTC and any prescription drugs he or she is taking (especially antihypertensive drugs).
   - About any and all alcohol and recreational drug consumption.
2. Teach the client to dangle feet before getting out of bed to prevent dizziness.
3. Because this drug may slow cognitive function and motor skills initially, inform the client to refrain from performing activities requiring mental alertness (e.g., driving, using hazardous machinery) until it is certain that the drug does not adversely affect cognitive function.
4. Alcoholic beverages should be avoided while taking quetiapine because both the cognitive and motor effects of alcohol consumption are potentiated with this medication

## risperidone
*Category:* Atypical antipsychotic
*Trade Name:* Risperdal

### Uses

Potent antipsychotic agent; targets negative symptoms (e.g., withdrawal, apathy, negativism) as well as positive symptoms (e.g., hallucinations, delusions, paranoia, hostility) of schizophrenia

### Action

Risperidone is a potent antagonist at $5\text{-}HT_{2A}$ and $D_2$ receptors (serotonin and dopamine)

### Dosages and Routes

- *PO:* Tablets only
- *Adults:* Start with 1 mg bid, increase to 2 mg bid on second day and 3 mg bid on third day
- *Elderly:* Start at 0.5 mg bid; titrate up to a maximum of 3 mg/day

### Contraindications

Hypersensitivity to risperidone

### Cautions

Can cause orthostatic hypotension and tachycardia;

because of these reactions, it should be started at low doses (e.g., 0.5 mg in the elderly and 1 mg for adults); risperidone is associated with dose-related EPS, although often minimal in therapeutic range; use with caution in clients with a history of seizures.

## Adverse Reactions

*Frequent:* Sedation, insomnia, rhinitis, coughing, back or chest pain, erectile problems in men, weight gain, and decreased sexual interest; initial dosing in particular may cause orthostatic hypotension and tachycardia or syncope; some clients report anorexia, polyuria/polydipsia, and/or an increase in dream activity

*Occasional:* Back pain, fever, palpitations, weight gain, hyperthyroidism, rhinitis, leukopenia, ear pain

## Toxic Effects

Number of cases of NMS reported; rare cases of priapism reported

## Nursing Measures

1. The client should know what the medication can do and what it cannot do. This drug can target some of the negative symptoms, and that should be included in client teaching about the drug.
2. The client needs a list of the possible expected side effects and those reactions that would warrant contacting the prescribing nurse, physician, or therapist (e.g., palpitations, erectile problems, sexual disinterest problems that might threaten compliance, dizziness).
3. Teach clients initially to sit on the side of the bed before getting up in the morning (to avoid dizziness when getting up and potential falls).
4. Check to see if the client has had seizures in the past.

## Inform Client and Family

1. When starting medication, be careful driving cars, working around machinery, and crossing

streets. This medication can make people sleepy and perhaps dizzy, especially initially.

2. Do not suddenly stop taking the medication even if there is no immediate return of symptoms. Relapse is a very high risk in the weeks and months after medications have been stopped.

3. The client or family member should notify the doctor if the client is having a sore throat during the first several months of treatment, if NMS appears (the client should have a fact sheet on NMS), or if the client is going to have general or dental surgery or is experiencing chest pain or tachycardia/palpitations.

## sertraline hydrochloride

*Category:*
Antidepressant, SSRI
*Trade Name:* Zoloft

### Uses

1. Major depression
2. OCD

### Action

Sertraline enhances serotoninergic activity in the CNS by blocking reuptake of serotonin in neuronal presynaptic membranes. It has only a very weak effect on dopamine and norepinephrine reuptake.

### Dosages and Routes

- *Adults:* Initially 50 mg PO once daily with morning or evening meal; may be increased no sooner than every week up to a maximum of 200 mg/day
- *Elderly:* Initially 25 mg/day PO once daily, as above; may increase 25 mg every 2-3 days

### Contraindications

Do not use within 2 weeks of an MAOI; safety for children and in pregnancy has not been established; anyone with hypersensitivity to the drug

### Cautions

Severe hepatic or renal insufficiency, elderly and debilitated clients, suicidal clients, and clients with a history of seizures or mania

## Drug Interactions

Cimetidine can increase sertraline concentrations. Other drug interactions with sertraline include an increase in diazepam concentrations, a decrease in tolbutamide, and increased bleeding for clients taking warfarin.

## Adverse Reactions

*Frequent:* Dizziness, headache, tremor, insomnia, somnolence, fatigue, agitation, nausea, dry mouth, loose stools/constipation, sexual dysfunction

*Occasional:* Increased sweating, dyspepsia, anorexia, nervousness, rhinitis, abnormal vision

*Rare:* Rash, vomiting, frequent urination, palpitations, paresthesia, twitching

## Nursing Measures

1. Sertraline is best given in the morning.
2. If the client is hospitalized, watch for signs of cheeking of medications (i.e., instead of swallowing medications, holding them under the tongue or in the cheek for the purpose of saving them and taking an overdose later).

## Inform Client and Family

1. The medication may have to be taken 1 to 3 weeks before improvement is noticed, but often the time is much shorter.
2. If the client is extremely depressed, the client should be given only 1 week's supply at a time.
3. Caution the client about premature discontinuation of therapy, which can result in a relapse. In general, medication should continue for at least 6 months to 1 year after symptoms have subsided.
4. Have the client and family assess for signs of improvement in symptoms, especially in areas such as depressed mood and loss of interest or pleasure in usual activities.
5. Have the client and family watch for signs of suicidal ideation.

## tacrine
*Category:* Reversible cholinesterase inhibitor
*Trade Name:* Cognex

## Uses

Can help mild to moderate dementia in people with Alzheimer's disease; appears to reverse 6 months of dementia progression

## Action

The cholinergic system deteriorates in Alzheimer's dementia. Tacrine inhibits breakdown of endogenously released acetylcholine.

## Dosages and Routes

- *Adults:* 40 mg/day PO (more improvement noticed with 80-160 mg/day); because of 2- to 4-hour half-life, needs qid dosing; start at 10 mg qid (40 mg) and continue 6 weeks if tolerated; every 6 weeks, increase each dose by 10 mg qid; if tolerated, go to 160 mg daily

## Contraindications

Hepatoxic for some clients

## Cautions

Because of elevation in liver enzymes, clients need frequent liver function testing; other drugs can alter (raise or lower) tacrine levels; anticholinergic agents can reverse tacrine's effects; tacrine increases risk of cholinergic agent toxicity; smoking can lower tacrine levels

## Adverse Reactions

*Frequent:* Flu-like symptoms without fever, gastrointestinal symptoms (e.g., nausea, diarrhea, dyspepsia, anorexia, vomiting)

## Toxic Effects

Elevation of ALT; liver function tests must be done and ALT levels monitored weekly for 6 weeks after each dose increase (most common reason for dropouts)

## Nursing Measures

Check for other medications (including smoking) that can alter tacrine levels. Be sure that client has informed the prescribing physician and nurse of all medications he or she is taking.

## Inform Client and Family

1. Clients taking tacrine need to have serum transaminases monitored monthly.
2. Remind the family to let the physician know of any and all medications the client is taking, because tacrine levels are easily altered by some medications.
3. This drug is not a panacea but can be very useful in the early stages of dementia.

## topiramate

*Category:*
Anticonvulsant
*Trade Name:* Topamax

## Uses

1. Adjunct therapy for treatment of partial-onset seizures, tonic-clinic seizures, and seizures associated with Lennox-Gastant syndrome
2. Unlabeled use: May be useful as an adjunctive treatment for clients with rapid cycling bipolar disorder who are nonresponsive to more standard treatments

## Action

Topiramate blocks repetitive, sustained firing of neurons by enhancing the ability of GABA to induce a flux of chloride ions into the neurons, decreasing seizure frequency.

## Dosages and Routes

- *Adults, Elderly, and Children over 17:* Initially 25-50 mg for 1 week; may increase by 25-50 mg/day at weekly intervals; maximum of 1,600 mg/day
- *Children (2-16 Years):* Initially 1-3 mg/kg/day; maximum of 25 mg; may increase by 1-3 mg/kg/day at weekly intervals; *maintenance:* 5-9 mg/kg/day in 2 divided doses

## Contraindications

None known

## Cautions

Sensitivity to topiramate, impaired liver/renal function, predisposition to renal calculi; pregnancy/lactation (unknown if distributed in breast milk; pregnancy category C); age-related renal impairment may require dosage adjustments.

## Remarks

1. Topiramate appears to curb binging and often results in significant weight loss.
2. Topiramate appears to reduce PTSD and possibly borderline personality disorder.
3. People on topiramate show cognitive impairments during acute dosing, particularly regarding attention and word fluency.

## Adverse Reactions

*Frequent (10%-30%):* Somnolence, dizziness, ataxia, nervousness, nystagmus, double vision, paresthesia, nausea, tremors

*Occasional (3%-9%):* Confusion, breast pain, dysmenorrhea, dyspepsia, depression, loss of strength, pharyngitis, weight loss, anorexia, rash, back/abdominal pain, difficulty with coordination, sinusitis, agitation, flu-like symptoms

*Rare (2%-3%):* Increased depression, anger or hostility, dry mouth

## Toxic Effects

Cognitive disturbances (e.g., language problems, like difficulty finding words, difficulty concentrating, and memory disturbances may be severe enough to require withdrawal from drug therapy)

## Nursing Measures

1. Review the history of the seizure disorder and identify safety precautions (e.g., does the client get dizzy and need assistance to ambulate?).
2. Apply routine seizure precautions when hospitalized and assess for needed safety precautions in the home when speaking with the client and family.
3. Assess for renal function, then monitor renal function (e.g., BUN, creatinine).
4. Topiramate decreases the effectiveness of oral contraceptives. Explore other birth control methods with the client if birth control pills are presently being taken.

## Inform Client and Family

1. Since dizziness, drowsiness, and impaired thinking may occur, have the client avoid tasks that require alertness and motor skills (e.g., driving a car) until a response to the drug is established. Drowsiness usually diminishes with continued therapy.
2. Avoid the use of alcohol or other CNS depressants.
3. Do not abruptly discontinue the drug; this may precipitate seizures.
4. Do not break tablets (because of the bitter taste).
5. Maintain adequate fluid intake to decrease the risk of renal stone formation.

## venlafaxine

*Category:*
Antidepressant
*Trade Names:* Effexor, Effexor XR

## Uses

1. Treatment of depression
2. May augment results with psychotherapy
3. Venlaflazine XR used in the treatment of generalized anxiety disorder

## Action

Venlafaxine inhibits reuptake of serotonin and nor-epinephrine and weakly inhibits dopamine reuptake.

## Dosages and Routes

- *Adults and Elderly:* Initially 75 mg/day in 2-3 divided doses with food; may increase by 75 mg/day no sooner than 4-day intervals; maximum 375 mg/day in 3 divided doses; decrease dose by 50% in clients with moderate liver impairment, 25% in mild to moderate renal impairment, and 50% in clients on dialysis
- *Extended Release (XR):* 75 mg/day as a single dose; may increase by 75 mg/day at intervals of at least 4 days; maximum 225 mg/day
- *For Anxiety Disorder:* 37.5-225 mg/day

## Contraindications

Do not use in children under 18 years of age; do not use with MAO inhibitors; wait 14 days after discontinuing MAOIs to start venlafax-

ine; St. John's Wort
may increase sedative-
hypnotic effects

## Cautions

Renal or hepatic impair-
ment, history of mania or
seizures, metabolic or
hemodynamic disease,
hypertension, history of
drug abuse

## Remarks

1. This drug has a
   minimal drug inter-
   action risk.
2. It is effective in
   severe geriatric and
   inpatient melancholic
   depression (first
   choice for this
   indication).
3. It has low sexual side
   effects at dosages
   under 300 mg.
4. It may increase dias-
   tolic blood pressure
   (10-15 mmHg).

## Adverse Reactions

*Frequent (>20%):* Nausea,
   somnolence, headache,
   dry mouth
*Occasional (10%-20%):*
   Dizziness, insomnia,
   constipation, sweating,
   nervousness, loss of
   energy and strength
   (asthenia)

*Rare (<10%):* Anxiety,
   blurred vision, diar-
   rhea, vomiting, tremor,
   abnormal dreams,
   impotence

## Toxic Effects

Sustained increase in dias-
tolic BP (10-15 mmHg)

## Nursing Measures

1. Obtain baseline
   weight and BP,
   and monitor
   periodically.
2. Assess for suicidal
   thoughts or feelings.
3. Assess initial level
   of depressive symp-
   toms (e.g., insomnia,
   energy level, appear-
   ance, behavior,
   speech pattern, level
   of interest, anxiety,
   mood, etc.) and
   reassess during
   treatment.
4. Assess for safety
   concerns (e.g., dizzi-
   ness, somnolence).

## Inform Client and Family

1. Take with food.
2. Do not drive or
   perform tasks that
   require an alert
   response until a
   response to the drug is
   established.

3. Avoid alcohol.
4. Alert the health care provider if planning to become pregnant or breastfeed.
5. Abrupt withdrawal can lead to withdrawal symptoms (e.g., nausea, tachycardia, tinnitus).

## ziprasidone HCl

*Category:*
Antipsychotic (novel/atypical)
*Trade Names:*
Geodon; initially introduced as Zeldox

### Uses

1. First-line treatment for the positive and negative symptoms of schizophrenia (e.g., hallucinations, delusions, lack of motivation and social withdrawal)
2. Because of its pharmacologic effects, has the potential to relieve anxiety and depression often associated with schizophrenia
3. IM preparation useful in the treatment of agitated behavior in people with schizophrenia and schizoaffective disorder
4. Does not cause weight gain; cholesterol and other lipid measures remain essentially unchanged

### Action

Ziprasidone HCl works as a serotonin and dopamine antagonist. It has a high affinity and antagonism for $5HT_{2A}$ and moderate affinity and antagonism for the $D_2$ and $D_3$ receptors. It is also an agonist for the $5HT_{1A}$ receptor and blocks the reuptake of norepinephrine. These neurotransmitter mechanisms suggest a potential for both positive and negative symptoms of schizophrenia and have a potential for relieving anxiety and depression.

### Dosages and Routes

- *Adults:* 40 to 100 mg twice daily (bid) PO; no data available at present for use with the elderly or children and adolescents; IM injection for acute and agitated behaviors

### Contraindications

Presently no data available for the safety of

ziprasidone HCl in pregnant or nursing mothers.

## Cautions

Ziprasidone associated with prolongation of the QTc interval as shown on the ECG; client should receive an ECG before and during treatment with ziprasidone; clinicians need to make their best judgment, based on the overall status of the client, as to whether ziprasidone or another antipsychotic agent is to be used first.

## Adverse Reactions

Most common side effects exhibited during clinical trials include headache, insomnia, somnolence, respiratory disorders, nausea, constipation, dyspepsia, and tachycardia; these effects were generally of mild to moderate severity and rarely led to discontinuation of the drug during drug trials; clients also experienced a reduced incidence of EPS and a low incidence of orthostatic hypotension and anticholinergic effects; transaminase levels increased in some individuals but returned to normal on discontinuance of the drug.

## Nursing Measures

1. The client and family need to be made aware of the ECG changes, and clients should be urged to have their ECG status monitored intermittently.
2. Transaminase levels may be monitored if warranted.
3. The fact that this drug does not cause weight gain and may reduce anxiety and depression associated with schizophrenia may help increase the client's compliance and reduce the potential for relapse. This may well be an excellent first-line treatment once it is determined to be safe for a particular client in terms of his or her cardiac status.

## zolpidem

*Category:*
Nonbenzodiazepine
sedative-hypnotic
*Trade Name:* Ambien

## Uses

Short-term treatment of insomnia

## Action

Zolpidem is thought to bind to the GABA receptors in the CNS, giving the drug sedative, anticonvulsant, and antianxiety properties.

## Dosages and Routes

- *Adults:* 10 mg PO immediately before bedtime
- *Elderly:* 5 mg PO immediately before bedtime

## Contraindications

Safety not established for pregnancy, lactation, and children under age 18.

## Cautions

People with renal or hepatic dysfunction, clients with a history of drug abuse/addictions, depressed and suicidal clients, elderly or debilitated clients

## Side Effects

*Frequent:* Drowsiness, vertigo, double vision, headache, drugged feeling, euphoria, insomnia, nausea
*Occasional:* Palpitations, myalgia, sinusitis, rash

## Adverse Reactions

Rarely; doses over 10 mg associated with psychotic reactions and amnesia

## Nursing Measures

1. Establish a baseline history of sleep patterns.
2. Assess for other medications that the client may be taking that can cause CNS depression, including the level of alcohol consumption.
3. Identify other methods the client has used to induce sleep.
4. Assess for adverse reactions and side effects.

## Inform Client and Family

1. Zolpidem is only for short-term use. Explore other methods of inducing sleep.
2. Do not drive or use machinery once the drug has been taken.
3. Take right before sleep.
4. When taking this drug, do not take other prescribed medications or OTC medications unless they are approved by a physician.
5. Do not consume alcohol while taking this drug

# Index

Page numbers followed by *b* indicate boxed material; page numbers followed by *f* indicate a figure; page numbers followed by *t* indicate a table.